AIDS
PUBLIC POLICY DIMENSIONS

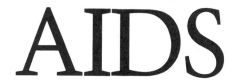

AIDS

PUBLIC POLICY DIMENSIONS

Based on the proceedings of the conference
held January 16 and 17, 1986,
cosponsored by the United Hospital Fund of New York
and the Institute for Health Policy Studies,
School of Medicine, University of California, San Francisco

JOHN GRIGGS
Editor

SALLY J. ROGERS
Vice President for Communications

DAVID A. GOULD
Vice President for Program

GEORGE H. SCHNEIDER
Conference Coordinator

UNITED HOSPITAL FUND OF NEW YORK

362.196
A2882

Copyright © 1987 by the United Hospital Fund of New York

All rights reserved. No part of this publication may be reproduced, stored in a retrieval system, or transmitted in any form or by any means, electronic, mechanical, photocopying, recording, or otherwise (brief quotations used in magazines or newspaper reviews excepted), without the prior permission of the publisher.

Printed in the United States of America.

Library of Congress Cataloging-in-Publication Data

AIDS, public policy dimensions.

    Includes bibliographies and index.
    1. AIDS (Disease)—Government policy—United States—
Congresses. 2. Medical policy—United States—Congresses.
3. Community health services—United States—Congresses.
I. Griggs, John, 1941– . II. United Hospital Fund of
New York. III. University of California, San Francisco.
Institute for Health Policy Studies. [DNLM: 1. Acquired
Immunodeficiency Syndrome—congresses. 2. Public Policy—
United States—congresses. WD 308 A2884 1986]
RA644.A25A37   1987   362.1'969792'00973   86-11388

ISBN 0-934459-35-5

For information, write: Publications Program,
United Hospital Fund of New York,
55 Fifth Avenue, New York, NY 10003.

Cover and interior design: Jeremiah B. Lighter

Table of Contents

University Libraries   v
Carnegie Mellon University
Pittsburgh, Pennsylvania 15213

Preface

For any species that reproduces itself sexually, the appearance of an invariably fatal sexually transmitted disease poses a significant challenge. Since the first few cases of acquired immune deficiency syndrome (AIDS) were described by doctors in New York and California in 1981, the disease has spread and grown to pandemic proportions. According to the World Health Organization, tens of thousands of people in 91 countries around the world have been stricken with AIDS. In the United States alone there have been over 30,000 cases of AIDS, resulting in over 17,000 deaths. Further, as many as two million Americans—and perhaps more—may be infected with the putative AIDS-causing retrovirus. Although AIDS is already causing serious medical, social, and political problems, our society faces the sobering reality that we are still only at the beginning of this tragic episode in human history. Indeed, federal health officials project that by the end of 1991 this country will have seen an estimated 270,000 cases of AIDS, with 179,000 deaths, and no one knows what the ultimate toll may be.

The AIDS epidemic is a complicated one in both medical and sociopolitical terms. While a substantial body of scientific and medical knowledge about AIDS has been accumulated in a relatively short period of time, we still have no cure, no vaccine, nor any proven effective long-term treatment to end the suffering of its victims. The specter of AIDS has stirred up substantial uneasiness, even hysteria, in some communities and has raised a number of important and troublesome public policy issues. We are confronted with the need not only to develop and implement better and more efficient methods of caring for people with AIDS, and more effective measures for treating and preventing the disease, but also to determine the proper roles of the public and the private sectors in responding to this crisis that, according to the National Academy of Sciences, could become a catastrophe.

To respond to some of these public policy issues, the United Hospital Fund of New York and the Institute for Health Policy Studies, of the School of Medicine at the University of California, San Francisco, cosponsored a two-day national conference in New York City in January 1986. Since New York and San Francisco accounted for nearly half of all AIDS cases nationally, the leading health policy organizations in each of these two cities, aware that AIDS was becoming a problem the entire country, not just the major urban centers, would have to face, felt it appropriate that they provide a joint public forum.

AIDS Public Policy Dimensions is based on the proceedings of that conference. Edited and expanded by the conference faculty, a distinguished group of health care administrators, analysts, policymakers, practitioners, scholars, and other experts, the book's 24 chapters confront the most pressing issues in the AIDS epidemic. Drawing upon their own knowledge, research, and personal experience, the authors assess both the most effective approaches to dealing with the problems of AIDS and the implications the epidemic holds for our society.

Mathilde Krim's "Introduction" provides an insightful overview of AIDS and a detailed background for the essays that follow. It is an up-to-date report on what we know about AIDS—and what it betokens—at the beginning of 1987, including the biomedical aspects, current research and prospects for therapies and a vaccine, antibody testing issues, the urgent need for nationwide preventive education, and the continuing failure of much of our national political leadership to face the realities of the growing AIDS crisis.

In Part I, Dr. Philip R. Lee and Professor Peter Arno examine both how our society and its institutions have reacted to the challenge of AIDS and how the current health policy and economic environment, tied in with the concept of "federalism," have affected the responses of federal, state, and local governments to AIDS.

The sociopolitical aspects of AIDS are explored in Part II by Dennis Altman, who also questions the advisability of widespread testing of individuals for antibodies to the AIDS virus; Ronald Bayer, who elaborates on some specific political dimensions of the epidemic; Emily Friedman, who examines the epidemic in the context of the communitarian ethic and warns of the dangers everyone faces when insurers and society begin to discriminate on the basis of disease; and Timothy Westmoreland, who assesses what has and hasn't been done about AIDS at the federal level—and why.

In Part III, the discussion centers around the controversial issue of the placement of AIDS-infected children in public school classrooms. Professor David Rothman examines both public health's historical approaches to risk assessment and the conflict, raised by AIDS, between civil liberties and public health. Attorney Robert Sullivan, who represented the plaintiffs in litigation to keep an AIDS-carrying child out of a New York City schoolroom, describes how bureaucratic bumbling has led understandably to parental alarm—and lawsuits. And on a more philosophical plane, the cultural anxieties that affect society's responses not only to persons with AIDS but also to "otherness" in general are explored by Professor Ralph Johnston, Jr.

The impact of AIDS on the national blood supply and the policies and procedures implemented by blood banks to protect the rights and safety of both blood recipients and donors are examined in Part IV, first by Dr. Johanna Pyndick, who describes the background and development of blood testing programs and their efficacy; then by Nancy Holland, who describes policy formulated by the National Blood Commission with regard to AIDS, and Professor Harvey Sapolsky, who addresses the issue of just whose best interests are being served by current AIDS blood policy.

In Part V, ways of organizing and delivering appropriate levels of acute medical care to different populations of AIDS patients are discussed by Dr. Michael Grieco, of St. Luke's Roosevelt Medical Center in New York City; Dr. Peter Mansell, of M. D. Anderson Hospital and Tumor Institute, Houston; Omar Hendrix, of New York City's municipal hospital system; and Dr. Paul Volberding, of San Francisco General Hospital. Among the topics they cover are resource utilization by AIDS patients in a New York voluntary hospital, the development and effectiveness of both ambulatory clinics and discrete AIDS inpatient units, and the problems of caring for large numbers of intravenous drug-using patients. Such issues as the use of intensive care, the impact of neurological problems on obtaining informed consent, and the availability of experimental drugs are also examined.

Community care and support services for AIDS patients and how—and by whom—these services are being provided in New York City and San Francisco are discussed in Part VI by Richard Dunne, who outlines the pioneering programs of Gay Men's Health Crisis in New York, and Dr. Mervyn Silverman, who describes how a partnership of government and private groups has informed the effectively coordinated response to AIDS in San Francisco. Next, Dr. Lambert King discusses the role hospitals should play in providing these services, and Professor Peter Arno questions to what extent volunteer organizations can be expected to fill the service gap as the epidemic increases. Finally, Dr. Joseph Cimino outlines and comments on New York State's plan for designating selected hospitals as AIDS centers.

AIDS is an expensive disease to treat, and extremely high estimates of annual health care costs for AIDS patients have generated considerable anxiety among providers, policymakers, and insurers. But, in Part VII, a study of AIDS treatment costs at San Francisco General Hospital, reported by Anne Scitovsky, Mary Cline, and Dr. Philip Lee, indicates that average treatment costs need not be as high as some other highly publicized studies have suggested. Their detailed analysis underscores the economic efficacy of the sort of public-private partnership response to AIDS exemplified by programs in San Francisco. AIDS programs and their costs in New York City are discussed by Dr. Jo Ivey Boufford, president of the city's

Health and Hospitals Corporation, and Leslie Strassberg considers the meaning of AIDS from the perspective of one of the nation's major health insurers operating in an area of high AIDS incidence.

In Part VIII, Bruce Vladeck offers a policymaker's assessment and summary of AIDS issues and finds some interesting parallels between AIDS and other contemporary health care issues, as well as some room for optimism—and a long-term need for continuing concern, even beyond AIDS.

Following the main text, three appendices have been added to provide valuable information about some specifics of the AIDS epidemic. Appendix A provides the Centers for Disease Control's clinical definition of AIDS and a list of the medical complications and opportunistic infections that AIDS and AIDS-related complex can entail. Appendix B offers the most up-to-date statistics that the practicalities of book production allow and also provides an international perspective on AIDS, with surveys and statistics on the epidemic in Europe, Africa, the Americas, and elsewhere. Appendix C provides a list of AIDS-related organizations from which additional information and/or assistance may be obtained.

Now to some technical matters: The terminology used in this book reflects what was current and in general use at the time of the conference, and, although consistency has been imposed where it seemed advisable for the sake of clarity or accuracy, individual authors by and large have been allowed their own choice in regard to terminology. Further, it should be noted that statistics in the main text that were current at the time of the conference have been retained, for the most part, as they were and have been updated—and expanded—in Appendix B.

Although hopeful developments in the search for effective treatments for AIDS and for a vaccine are being reported, many of our institutions—both medical and social—are undoubtedly going to be seriously stressed by the effects of AIDS, and the outcome is difficult to predict. We remain in a danger zone. As *AIDS Public Policy Dimensions* makes clear, from a sociological point of view, AIDS has been remarkable in one particular respect that is both awesome and telling; that is, in its apparently catalytic effect on a wide range of society. From many, it has brought forth unusual and hitherto unexpected examples of courage, compassion, generosity, and selflessness; in others it has served merely to elicit expressions of mean-spiritedness, affirming once again the special role of crises in bringing out the best and the worst in all of us.

If human civilization has a moral underpinning, it is surely an at least implied social commitment that calls upon all of us to share, distributively, the burdens of living on this planet. For the reality is that all of our most basic human concerns interlock at some level, regardless of superficial—or even significant—individual differences. And what affects a few of us often will have some eventual impact upon the rest of us in one way or another. Like it or not, we cannot escape to some more or less considerable extent being each other's keepers. That is part and parcel of what it is to be human, and, as several writers here attest, it is a compact that time and again is being honored and renewed in the course of this AIDS epidemic. It is also cause for hope. For, although expressions of communality are not exclusive to the human species, in the long run how we nurture and maintain our sense of common good and individual worth will probably be instrumental in settling the question of whether, as a species, we survive—and avert not only an AIDS catastrophe, but other disasters as well.

JOHN GRIGGS

Introduction

MATHILDE KRIM

As an identified clinical entity, acquired immu ___ syndrome (AIDS) has been among us only a little more than ___ ears. However, the virus that causes it may have been infecting some Americans for as long as ten years when its existence was discovered, in 1983, and its etiological role generally accepted, in 1984. At long last we have now come to realize collectively that AIDS represents a threat to human life that is unparalleled in modern times.

Fortunately, biomedical research has now gained so many profound insights into the workings of cells and viruses that it is not beyond our power to understand the cause, the pathogenesis, and the mechanism of the spread of AIDS, and ultimately to achieve its control. This would surely not have been the case had AIDS appeared even as recently as twenty years ago—a time when mankind, even in the Western world, would have been almost totally defenseless against the AIDS virus. But within two years of its discovery this virus's constitution and its modes of replication and transmission have become known. Promising therapeutic drugs are in clinical trials and some preparations with potential for use as vaccines are ready for testing. The power of contemporary biomedical science and technology is quite certainly equal to the challenge of AIDS.

On the other hand, the threat of AIDS to human societies and institutions, to the economic order, and, potentially, to civil liberties and the very fabric of civilization, in its different forms, may be much more difficult to confront. Not only Western civilization is challenged by AIDS; the worldwide AIDS pandemic now developing is likely to undermine the social order in most countries before medical solutions become widely applicable.

How will different societies respond to AIDS? What value systems will withstand the fear that will sweep through people? Who will know better than to blame the victims? Who will be able to put scientific evidence and rationality above prejudice, and compassion above self-righteousness? No one knows. In most countries, awareness of AIDS itself is still dim, denial common, and a serious dialogue—not to mention, policy development—has hardly begun.

The conference that resulted in this book greatly stimulated the

United States. Even in this country, where outstanding surveillance and communications systems exist, it is taking ng time for people in leadership positions, particularly political piritual leaders, to grasp the enormous future dimensions of the AIDS problem, and to take public positions that promote humane and rational policies. Typically, the convening of a conference entitled "AIDS: Public Policy Dimensions" resulted from an initiative taken by private groups: the United Hospital Fund of New York and the Institute for Health Policy Studies, of the University of California, San Francisco. A few months later, the Institute of Medicine of the National Academy of Sciences undertook its own evaluation of the impact of AIDS in the U.S. It issued a report containing a set of policy recommendations (1986). These recommendations have elicited discussion and comment but, to date, little action. Public officials usually have reacted reluctantly—and continue to do so—to pleas coming from the frontline of the battle against AIDS: the hospitals, the research laboratories, and the self-help community groups.

Dr. C. Everett Koop, the U.S. Surgeon General, recently issued a strong statement regarding the need to warn youth about AIDS and its modes of transmission (1986). Even this courageous stand only echoed the voices of those who, for several years, have witnessed powerlessly how many young people continue to endanger their lives, in the face of AIDS, through engaging in casual sexual encounters and falling prey to the lure of the drug culture.

Why our "leaders" have not led will be the subject of future books. In a dispassionate, scholarly way, this present volume looks at where the U.S. stands now, at the beginning of 1987, in dealing with the public policy dimensions of AIDS.

AIDS Public Policy Dimensions is most important and timely because American society now stands at a crossroads; it can make the effort of' becoming informed and taking appropriate action—including putting to use its lofty moral principles—or it can continue to respond to the danger with "benign neglect." We can summon our collective resources in support of health education, research, and services for those already stricken, or we can abandon the dying and let ignorance, superstition, and misconceptions fuel fear and prejudice. If we choose the latter, we will then see policymakers generate ill-conceived measures that will not protect the public health but will erode everyone's civil liberties. The form that such measures might take has been well illustrated, for example, by Proposition 64, a proposal which was placed on the 1986 California ballot and which would have subjected people seropositive for AIDS virus antibody to job loss and quarantine. Fortunately, it was soundly defeated, but there will be other such challenges. Choices are still possible in dealing with

AIDS, but the time left to make them is running short. This book should help us make wise choices.

AIDS: AN OVERVIEW

As part of this introduction, and because the body of this book does not deal with these topics, it seems useful to review, briefly, how awareness of AIDS has emerged, what we know about its biological and medical aspects, how biomedical research is approaching its control, and what the outcome of the research effort might be.

The term acquired immune deficiency syndrome—AIDS—was coined in 1981 (Gottlieb et al. 1981). The Centers for Disease Control (CDC) gave the condition a narrow clinical definition for the purpose of distinguishing it clearly from other immunodeficiency syndromes (Centers for Disease Control 1982).* This was necessary for the AIDS surveillance program instituted by the CDC in order to follow the spread of the new syndrome in the U.S. population.

The surveillance program soon revealed that cases of AIDS did not occur at random. They were clearly concentrated in certain geographic areas—notably, large urban centers on the East and West coasts—and they seemed to be confined to certain population groups. The groups identified to be at highest risk for AIDS were homosexual men (but not homosexual women), male or female users of illicit drugs taken through intravenous injection, hemophiliacs, some individuals of either sex and of all ages who had received blood transfusions, some individuals of either sex who had had sexual contacts with any of the above, and infants born to mothers with AIDS. Cases diagnosed among non-drug-abusing, non-blood-recipient, exclusively heterosexual adults amounted, until 1985, to only 1 percent of all reported cases of AIDS.

Nevertheless, progressively—and very clearly since 1983—it became obvious that, despite the preponderance of gay men among people with AIDS, AIDS was not a "gay disease": the condition was not necessarily linked to gender, nor to sexual preference, age, or race. AIDS was obviously transmissible through blood or blood products—because it occurred in blood recipients and hemophiliacs—and through sperm—because it was found among male and female sexual partners of men belonging to "high-risk groups." (Evidence that AIDS could also be transmitted by women to men through vaginal secretions emerged later, and the fact of female-to-male transmission is now well-established.)

*For national reporting purposes, the CDC defined AIDS as disease at least moderately predictive of a defect in cell-mediated immunity, e.g., Kaposi's sarcoma, *Pneumocystis carinii* pneumonia, and certain other specified serious opportunistic infections, in previously healthy patients less than 60 years of age. [*See* Appendix A.]

It could be concluded early on, therefore, that AIDS was a condition caused by an infectious agent to which any human being was potentially susceptible. This understanding was supported by reports of the presence of AIDS in certain countries of Central Africa, South America, and the Caribbean, particularly in Haiti, where studies indicated clearly that AIDS was transmitted as a venereal disease, that it affected men and women in virtually equal numbers, and that it was transmissible by both men and women. Moreover, large numbers of infants born to mothers with AIDS also developed the syndrome in these countries (Biggar 1986).

Unfortunately, many people—including some U.S. public health officials—chose to shrug off the Third World's epidemiological pattern as being due mainly to practices such as skin scarification or the parenteral administration of medicines using unclean instruments. The situation in the U.S. was understood by much of the public to mean that AIDS was not only transmitted through, but also *caused by* certain behaviors—in particular, those of gay men and intravenous drug users. Hence, persons who did not engage in those behaviors could feel self-righteously safe from AIDS.

These views are commonly held by many in the American public to this day. They are the unfortunate result of a misinterpretation—seemingly vindicated by widely held prejudices—of the early concentration of the U.S. cases detected by the CDC AIDS surveillance program in certain generally unpopular groups. Nor was the U.S. public enlightened by official statements; if anything, in essence it heard only that unless someone practiced anal intercourse with a gay man or shared dirty needles with a drug addict, he or she had nothing to worry about at all. Ostensibly because of this misconception, there was no outpouring of funds for research or of compassion for the first victims of AIDS. There was no general mobilization of resources to institute immediate, vigorous, nationwide educational programs to contain the early epidemic. With very few exceptions, America's "spiritual leaders" did not rise in support of those suffering and dying of AIDS. That there are bisexual men, that drug addicts are predominantly heterosexual, and that all these would, eventually, spread the infection through sexual contacts beyond the original "high-risk" groups, was overlooked.

Meanwhile, since 1981, the overall number of AIDS cases reported to the CDC has essentially doubled each year. The mortality rate of AIDS has been very high: 47 percent among adults and 53 percent, or higher, among infants. Its case fatality rate has been 100 percent. Medical science thus far has been totally powerless in preventing either the spread of or death through AIDS.

ETIOLOGY AND EPIDEMIOLOGY

In attempts to identify the cause of AIDS, the possible etiological role of various known viruses and microorganisms was investigated. None could be implicated until May 1983, when a group headed by Dr. Luc Montagnier, working at the Institut Pasteur, in Paris, reported in a scientific publication the isolation of a new virus—a member of the family of retroviruses—from lymphocytes of patients with AIDS-related lymphadenopathy. *In vitro,* this virus could be propagated in—and it eventually killed—human lymphocytes of the T4 type, the very cells found to be depleted in people with AIDS. The authors suggested that this retrovirus, which they called lymphadenopathy-associated virus (LAV), could be the cause of AIDS (Barre-Sinoussi et al. 1983).

One year later, an American research team led by Dr. Robert Gallo, working at the National Institutes of Health, in Bethesda, Maryland, reported that they had repeatedly isolated a similar virus from several patients with AIDS and AIDS-related symptoms. It also killed T4 cells *in vitro* (Popovic et al. 1984). The American group had the good fortune of being able to propagate their virus in a cultured human cell line that could sustain its growth indefinitely without being destroyed by it. They called their virus human T-lymphotropic virus type-III (HTLV-III).

The viruses isolated by Drs. Montagnier and Gallo have since been found to be virtually identical. Although they were originally given different names, recently a subcommittee of the International Committee for the Taxonomy of Viruses recommended that these and other isolates of the same virus all be designated as "human immunodeficiency virus," or HIV (Coffin et al. 1986).

HIV is convincingly implicated as the causitive agent of AIDS because, thanks to the ability to culture it on a very large scale, a test could be developed which detects the antibody that HIV induces in humans (Sarngadharan et al. 1984). This test, the enzyme-linked-immunosorbent-assay, or ELISA test, is based on the principle that purified viral proteins attached to a substrate (either beads or the internal surface of a test tube or microwell) bind specifically to anti-HIV antibody present in human serum. The bound antibody can, in turn, become bound to heterologous antibody, anti-human immunoglobulin (anti-human IgG). When the latter is "tagged" with an enzyme capable of catalyzing a color-generating chemical reaction, the amount of color produced—after removal of excess anti-human IgG—is quantitatively related to the amount of anti-HIV antibody present in the sample of human serum tested. The ELISA test can be very specific. It can also be made to be very sensitive, but at the cost of loss of specificity—and positive ELISA results need to be verified by a second, more elaborate but more specific test, usually the immunoelectrophoretic "Western blot" test that detects antibodies to various viral proteins.

With the use of these two tests, antibody to HIV was found in virtually all patients with AIDS and AIDS-related symptoms—whether AIDS-related complex (ARC) or persistent generalized lymphadenopathy (PGL)—as well as in relatively high proportions of healthy people belonging to the major high-risk groups. In contrast, antibody to HIV was found to be extremely rare in the general population, particularly in areas where AIDS itself was rare or unknown. Since antibody is very specific for the antigen that induces it, the presence of anti-HIV antibody reveals prior infection with HIV. The association of anti-HIV antibody, and hence HIV infection, with AIDS was irrefutable. HIV's clear predilection for T4 lymphocytes and its ability to kill them could explain why HIV-infected individuals showed a progressive loss of such cells. Progressive immune dysfunction in HIV-infected people became understandable in light of the known, all-important role T4 lymphocytes play as "helper-inducer" cells that regulate a multitude of immune functions in the body. Thus, HIV became firmly established as the major cause, if not necessarily the only cause, of AIDS.

The valuable ELISA and "Western blot" tests for the detection of antibody to HIV have been put to other very important uses: they were applied as soon as practicable to the testing of blood donated for either transfusion or the preparation of blood products. Blood donations contributed by individuals who had been exposed to the virus could in this way be eliminated from the national blood supply (Centers for Disease Control 1985). Beginning in early 1985, the testing of blood donations was implemented nationwide. It has made the medical use of whole blood and blood products very much safer than it was prior to such testing.

Since 1984, the ELISA and confirmatory tests have made it also possible, for the first time, to study the prevalence of *HIV infection*—as opposed to AIDS itself—both in various population groups at high or low risk for AIDS and in different geographic areas.

As a result of this testing, many more people were found to be infected with HIV than presented with clinical symptoms. For example, although only 1 percent of all hemophiliacs had been diagnosed with AIDS, almost all of them were found to be positive for antibody to HIV. In New York City, more than one-half of all intravenous (IV) drug users had the antibody, and so did approximately one-half of the gay men who were tested. Furthermore, it was obvious that the infection was not necessarily linked to their lifestyles, because people with similar lifestyles and living elsewhere could show a much lower prevalence of infection or no cases of infection at all. HIV infection was also detected in some individuals, including women, who had had sexual contacts with people in the high-risk groups. Repeated testing of the same groups in certain urban areas showed that the incidence of HIV infection was rising sharply over time. In early 1985, Dr. Anthony Fauci, Director of the National Institute of Allergy and Infectious Diseases, was able to estimate—on the basis of these early, limited surveys—that there were at least one million people already infected with HIV in the U.S. (Curran et al. 1985; Fauci 1986).

These results were supplemented in 1986 by important—and unexpected—information that emerged from a program of screening for HIV antibody imposed by the U.S. Department of Defense on all new military recruits. This mandatory screening revealed that, while prevalence of infection among army recruits varied greatly from region to region of the U.S., it was as high as 2 percent—that is, it affected 1 out of 50—among recruits (aged 18 to 25) coming from New York City's borough of Manhattan. Among these recruits, the ratio of infected men to infected women was 2.5 to 1, which was very different from the 10 to 1 male to female ratio observed in the same city among people with a clinical diagnosis of AIDS (Barnes 1986a). This was a surprisingly high prevalence of infection in what is close to being a cross-section of predominantly heterosexual and non-drug-addicted young Americans. Despite the fact that New York is clearly the epicenter of the AIDS epidemic in the United States, these were sobering figures.

In the course of these studies, the concept emerged that the U.S. epidemic of HIV infection and resulting disease could be represented as a pyramid, or, perhaps more appropriately, an iceberg: At its base is an invisible, or submerged, large pool of asymptomatic infected individuals—now estimated to include from one to three million people. Another large group, estimated to include some 300,000 infected people who have developed mild to serious AIDS-related symptoms (ARC and PGL), occupies the middle range, and at the top of the pyramid—or the tip of the iceberg—is the highly visible but relatively smaller group of cases who meet the CDC clinical criteria for AIDS. At this writing in early 1987, this last group accounts for a cumulative total of over 30,000 AIDS cases—17,000 of which have resulted in death.

Clinical observations confirm that for each person diagnosed with CDC-defined AIDS there are 10 or more people who present with symptoms of ARC or PGL and that a pathological continuum exists between all HIV-infected people. CDC-defined AIDS is only the late, most severe manifestation of a progressive HIV-induced disease (Haverkos et al. 1985; Centers for Disease Control 1986).

What are the dynamic relationships between the visible part of the iceberg—that is, people with AIDS and ARC—and the submerged mass of either less sick or asymptomatic infected people? In other words, what is the fate, in time, of those who are infected but are asymptomatic or do not manifest all the typical symptoms of AIDS? In a group of people with AIDS who acquired HIV infection through blood transfusion—that is, for whom the actual date of infection was known—if was found that an average of some five years elapsed between infection and diagnosis of AIDS. Other groups, mostly antibody-positive but asymptomatic gay men, have been followed longitudinally over various periods of time by different investigators. A composite of the findings shows that infection is usually followed by a very long incubation period during which there occurs a slow but progressive loss of T4 cells accompanied by immune dysfunctions of increasingly severe nature (Biggar 1987). After five years, nearly half of the study subjects showed clinical manifestations of either ARC or AIDS. Although it is still not known whether *all* infected people eventually go on to develop clinical disease, the proportion of those infected who will do so in the long run is now believed to be much higher than was suspected as recently as two years ago (Seale 1985). In addition, HIV can, and frequently does, infect cells of the central nervous system. Neurological and mental disorders often complicate other symptoms of ARC and AIDS and add further gravity to an ominous situation (Snider et al. 1983).

The inescapable conclusion from these findings is that infection with HIV is potentially a most serious condition. In at least half of those infected, it will lead to immunological breakdown and vulnerability to infections and malignant complications. These conditions are rapidly deadly because they are, as yet, medically unmanageable within the context of profound immune deficiency.

Will some of those who have not become ill five or more years after being infected always remain well? Will some develop resistance to HIV? The answer to these questions is simply not known, because the total experience with AIDS and its related conditions is no longer than five years. What is known, though, is not encouraging. Although HIV infection elicits an antibody response—an immune defense reaction that is sufficient in the case of many other viral infections to ensure recovery and future protection—the antibody produced against HIV is, for the most part, of an ineffective kind: it is not "neutralizing" antibody; that is, not one that can eliminate the infectious nature of the virus. Thus, people with even high levels of anti-HIV antibody can still harbor infectious virus. Not only are they incapable of effectively suppressing the spread of the infection within their own organism, but they also remain capable of transmitting infectious virus to others. Infectious virus can be readily and repeatedly isolated from their blood and various body fluids—in fact, more easily so during the asymptomatic or early symptomatic phases of HIV disease than during its most advanced stage, AIDS itself.

There is, nevertheless, a silver lining to the dark cloud of HIV infection: all of the epidemiological studies done to date concur in attributing the transmission of HIV only to infected sperm, infected vaginal secretions, or infected blood. It has been shown convincingly that HIV is *not* transmitted through casual human contacts. Although infectious virus has been isolated from the saliva, urine, and tears of certain antibody-positive individuals, these particular body fluids do not appear to have been responsible for any cases of HIV infection. In addition, the pattern of spread of HIV infection has led scientists to dismiss animal vectors such as blood-feeding insects as a source of infection, at least in the United States (Selwyn 1986).

It is of crucial importance that the public understand that, while there is no reason to fear contacts with people who have either asymptomatic or symptomatic HIV infection, there is now a degree of danger in *any new sexual* encounter. This is particularly true in geographic areas or in social circles where drug abuse is not unknown. It is also important that the public understand that those who suffer from AIDS today can all truly be said to be "innocent victims," having in the vast majority of cases acquired their infection long before the existence of HIV was known and before preventive information about its transmissibility was available (Selwyn 1986).

In the future, however, HIV infection and AIDS will mainly be diseases of, one might say, "consenting adults." This will be the case because, in the light of present knowledge, avoiding HIV infection clearly is under most people's personal control. Limiting the number of one's sexual partners and adopting "safer sex" practices—meaning, essentially, the consistent and proper use of barrier prophylactics (condoms) and of products containing germicidal substances in all sexual relations other than very long-standing and absolutely mutually monogamous ones—can be expected to result in significant risk reduction, perhaps even complete protection from HIV infection. For those who cannot give up illicit drugs, using only sterile syringes and needles, at all times, has life-saving importance.

Regrettably, in the continuing absence of a nationwide AIDS prevention educational program these messages of caution have still not reached many Americans, at least not forcefully enough to provide the motivation necessary for behavior modification. This is especially true for adolescents, who, we know, are sexually active at younger ages than in the past. As a result, it can be expected that HIV infection will continue to spread over the next few years, particularly among drug addicts and their sexual contacts, as well as among unwary heterosexuals, in general, and the children born to them.

AIDS consequently looms on the horizon as an enormous health problem, a pandemic that may significantly surpass in seriousness the influenza pandemic of 1918–1919 that killed 20 million people worldwide. The fact that HIV infection also causes mental and neurological abnormalities and an increased susceptibility to many infections—it has already been held responsible for a recrudescence of tuberculosis in New York and of malaria in the Third World—adds to the extreme gravity and complexity of the problem. The projections made by the CDC for the United States, of a cumulative 270,000 cases of AIDS and 179,000 fatalities by 1991, appear conservative in view of (1) the estimated one to three million Americans already infected, (2) the results of the longitudinal studies of infected people that show close to 50 percent morbidity within five years of infection, and (3) the fact that the spread of the epidemic of HIV infection—far from being under control—is now occurring outside those groups originally identified as being at risk; that is, among the larger non-IV-drug-using heterosexual population and its progeny.

THE HUMAN IMMUNODEFICIENCY VIRUS

Some elementary facts pertaining to the structure and properties of viruses, in general, and to those of HIV, in particular, are useful to a better understanding of the mode of transmission and pathogenesis of AIDS, as well as of the promise—and limitations—of future treatments and preventive measures.

Viruses are tiny particles, much smaller than any bacteria, usually composed of one molecule of nucleic acid that encodes genetic information encased in a capsid, a protective envelope formed by a small number of protein molecules. Viruses are not capable of independent life; an isolated virus particle is merely a small piece of inert organic matter. They become "alive," that is, capable of reproducing their genetic material, only inside living, fully metabolizing cells of higher organisms. They exploit the cells' metabolic machinery for their own purpose, that of forming many new virus particles. Viruses are much more fragile than bacteria and more selective with regard to the animal species and the types of cells they infect. They can only infect cells to which they can attach themselves through particular receptors, and for infection to occur, virus-to-cell attachment must take place in a liquid environment compatible with *cell* survival.

Thus, for HIV to be passed from one person to another and achieve infection in the recipient, very specific conditions must obtain. Intact skin, for example, is an absolute barrier to HIV and other viruses. Because HIV has a particular predilection for infecting T4 lymphocytes, and because these are a type of white blood cell, infection with HIV is probably best achieved when this virus is given direct access to the blood circulation. The current very high prevalence of HIV infection among users of illicit injectable drugs—and hence the rapid early spread of this infection among members of that particular high-risk group—reflects the efficacy of even small amounts of blood carried from one person to another, by shared hypodermic needles, in achieving HIV transmission and infection. HIV can also infect certain white blood cells other than T4 cells. These, as well as T4 cells, can be present in fluids and secretions bathing the internal lining of male or female genital organs. It has recently been reported that HIV may also be capable of infecting and multiplying in the cells lining the lower intestine. All of these cells are readily accessible to HIV during intimate contacts with an infected sexual partner. Unprotected sexual intercourse *of any kind* is therefore capable of realizing the conditions required for HIV transmission and infection; namely, immediate access for virus or virus-producing cells contributed by an infected individual to susceptible live cells, in a fluid physiological environment, of an uninfected partner. As discussed earlier, epidemiological studies have amply confirmed the unique importance of the sexual and blood routes for HIV transmission (Fauci et al. 1985; Curran et al. 1985; Selwyn 1986).

As already mentioned, HIV is a retrovirus. Retroviruses have been so designated because their multiplication requires, first, the "reverse transcription" of their ribonucleic acid (RNA) core molecule, that carries their genetic information, into deoxyribonucleic acid (DNA). Usually, in nature, the "flow" of genetic information goes from DNA to RNA. Once the retroviral genetic information is encoded in DNA, this DNA can become incorporated into, and henceforth remain an integral part of, the genetic material—also composed of DNA—of the human host cell. In its integrated DNA form, the retroviral genetic material is called "provirus." Proviruses are the ultimate parasites; they persist indefinitely in infected cells, ready to act as genetic blueprints for the production of a new retrovirus, so that, once acquired, infection with a retrovirus, including HIV, is acquired for life (Wong-Staal and Gallo 1985).

In addition, HIV can infect a variety of cells and appears capable of establishing various cell-virus interactions. In some cells, such as monocytes/macrophages, HIV may multiply constantly at low levels, while in others, such as T4 lymphocytes, it may remain dormant in a silent proviral form for long periods of time until a specific stimulus triggers its replicative cycle. Normally, immunological stimuli selectively induce T4 lymphocytes to divide, but if the latter harbor HIV proviruses, such stimuli also activate an exceedingly rapid production of a vast number of new retrovirus particles that emerge from their T4 host cells ready to infect other cells. The original T4 host cells are killed in the process. It has also been recently reported that coinfection of cells with both HIV and certain other, DNA-containing viruses can similarly activate HIV proviruses and convert their host cells into retrovirus factories.

Because immune stimulation and coinfection with other viruses are believed to stimulate HIV multiplication in T4 cells, which is followed by T4 cell death, they are also believed to precipitate immunological breakdown and resulting clinical manifestations of ARC or AIDS. This constitutes the rationale for strongly recommending adoption of risk-reduction behavior to *both* uninfected and HIV-infected people. The latter must not only avoid infecting others with HIV, but also avoid acquiring additional infections that may precipitate the progression of HIV disease in themselves.

In addition, because adopting risk-reduction behavior will for several years constitute the only form of primary AIDS prevention available, its importance to everyone cannot be overemphasized. Educational programs aimed at prevention *must* explain to the public how HIV infection is and is not transmitted, and, thus, the rationale for urging widespread modification of contemporary sexual mores and practices. The task remains largely to be done.

TESTING FOR ANTIBODY: ISSUES AND EFFICACY

For those for whom information about HIV and HIV infection is not sufficient alone to motivate behavioral modification, knowledge of antibody status, combined with skillful and, if necessary, long-term counseling, will provide powerful additional incentive. For that reason, the HIV antibody test must be readily available—as a voluntary component of education programs—for the purpose of determining the infectious status of individuals. In order for it to be extensively used, the procedure must be available under conditions that guarantee the protection of confidentiality or, even better, total anonymity—preconditions made necessary by the stigma still attached to positive antibody status and even to merely requesting an antibody test.

On the other hand, *mandatory* antibody testing in any setting, whether general or limited to certain groups, is fraught with pitfalls and is, to date, unjustified (Bayer et al. 1986). Large scale or general screening of the entire U.S. population for antibody to HIV, if feasible at all, would be extravagantly costly in terms of financial and scarce technical manpower resources. Such a program would also constitute a violation of privacy rights and would, for this reason, be widely resented by the public and avoided when at all possible, particularly by those at risk of being infected. It would stigmatize those with positive test results, but would not lead, at this time at least, to any medical intervention that would be of help to them. Because of the devastating psychological effects that can ensue from positive test results, large-scale testing would create an urgent and massive need for expert counseling in order to avoid countless and senseless private tragedies, such as suicides and the breaking up of families. Finally, mandatory testing would not eliminate for anyone the need to adopt risk-reduction behavior; effective prevention would still rest, as now, on the volition of each and every individual, regardless of his or her antibody status.

Consequently, whether the cost to society of any large-scale mandatory testing program is justified must be carefully weighed, particularly in view of the fact that no amount of testing will ever identify all infected persons. Antibody develops slowly, over periods of weeks or months; up to 4 percent of infected individuals register negative for antibody for as long as one year after infection. Further, in most people infected recently, and even months after infection in some people, antibody testing yields "false negative" results. Ascertaining whether a negative result is a false negative or accurately reflects freedom from HIV infection requires that the ELISA test be repeated following a period of several months, during which a possibility of exposure must be excluded, which would require, for example, total sexual abstinence. Even repeated testing would still miss some infected people.

More important, mandatory testing programs would create the illusion that "something is being done" about AIDS and would undoubtedly have a reassuring effect. In view of the many false negative results to be expected among those recently exposed to HIV, such reassurance would be unjustified. Nevertheless, the level of motivation of many people at low risk would be decreased. Any relaxation or abandonment of risk-reduction behavior will lead to accelerated spread of HIV infection, with the end result being that mandatory testing may, in fact, endanger the public health rather than protect it.

Thus, it seems preferable that the antibody test procedure be easily accessible but entirely voluntary and confidential, to be used as a valuable adjunct to competent and supportive counseling. Testing for antibody to HIV also, of course, has a role in confirming a clinical diagnosis in symptomatic individuals. And its use could be encouraged for certain individuals who are at risk but prone to denial, or for others who may be at very low risk but in need of objective reassurance. In this last category, for instance, would be young women who plan to become pregnant in the immediate future.

The cornerstone to behavior modification must, however, remain the provision of the factual, explicit information necessary to an understanding of the essential—and relatively simple—biological facts pertaining to HIV transmission, so that what constitutes "safe" and "hazardous" behavior—under innumerable different sets of personal circumstances—becomes clear to each individual. It is indeed a reality that the moments of decision occur for each person away from the scrutiny of health departments, away from doctors' admonitions, or even peer pressure. Fateful risk-reduction decisions must be made when only one's instinct for self-preservation and one's own conscience can be heard. These speak louder when personal dignity is intact and when true, informed free will can be exercised. Given the two modes of HIV transmission, a public armed with the information necessary to behave intelligently and ethically would have nothing to fear even from some irresponsible individuals in its midst.

BIOMEDICAL RESEARCH TOWARD TREATMENT AND VACCINE

While, thus far, private sector organizations, largely, have been developing, implementing, and evaluating programs of public education on AIDS, biomedical research has been mounting an assault on HIV disease that is gaining momentum as private and federal financial support for such research is increasing.

An intensive basic research effort is under way in order to develop antiviral drugs capable of specifically blocking HIV multiplication in humans and in the study of substances capable of stimulating the production and function of cells of the immune defense system. Meanwhile, control of the spread of infection in the population—that is, primary prevention of AIDS—is being sought through the development of a vaccine against the AIDS virus.

Efforts are also being made toward developing improved treatments for several types of cancers—that include Kaposi's sarcoma, lymphoma, and squamous cell carcinoma—and for the plethora of opportunistic infections that plague severely immunosuppressed people. These cancers and infections are the immediate cause of death in people with advanced HIV disease.

A beginning in the search for rational treatments for AIDS had to await knowledge, first, of the etiology of the disease and, then, of the causative virus's mode of replication. Several drugs have now been identified that are capable of interfering selectively *in vitro* with the replicative cycle of HIV or with its ability to attach to its cellular receptor (de Clerq 1986; Robbins 1986). Some of these drugs are being studied, or soon will be studied, for their possible usefulness in HIV-infected humans. Many of them—such as ribavirin (Virazole), azidothymidine (AZT), and di-deoxy-cytidine, are analogs of the natural building blocks for nucleic acids. They impede the function of the viral enzyme, called reverse transcriptase, to a significantly higher degree than that of the major corresponding cellular enzyme, DNA polymerase α. They also cross the blood-brain barrier and have potential for the treatment of neurological manifestations of HIV infection.

To date, only AZT has been unequivocally shown to have a therapeutic effect in patients with AIDS, whose life it has prolonged and in whom it appears to have both suppressed HIV multiplication and permitted a certain degree of immunological reconstitution, accompanied by much improved well-being. Despite the fact that AZT can also exert an undesirable bone marrow suppressive effect in a certain proportion of patients, it is anticipated that this, and probably other related drugs, will have applications in the treatment of AIDS and AIDS-related conditions. When used prior to the development of profound immune dysfunction, selected nucleoside analogs may in fact be able to retard or prevent the development of full-blown AIDS. Even so, they will not be capable of eliminating proviral DNA from infected cells; therefore, they will not constitute a "cure."

Other drugs under investigation are: sodium phosphonoformate (Foscarnet), first studied in Sweden; antimoniotungstate (HPA-23), studied primarily in France; AL 721, a complex lipid preparation that interferes with viral attachment to cell membranes, studied in Israel and the U.S.; Ansamycin, a derivative of rifamycin; and a synthetic nucleic acid (Ampligen), a non-toxic interferon inducer and amplifier of its antiviral action that has been shown effective against HIV infection *in vitro* (Mitchell and Montefiore 1987).

Combinations of certain antiviral drugs will also soon be studied. Among such combinations, AZT and the commercially available acyclovir (Zovirax), a guanosine analog effective against herpes viruses, have demonstrated marked anti-HIV effectiveness *in vitro*—for reasons not yet well understood. The natural antiviral and immunomodulatory agents, the interferons α and β, are effective *in vitro* against retroviruses and perhaps also against HIV in humans. Their combination with one or more synthetic antiviral agents, such as nucleoside analogs, is attractive because the interferons' mechanism of antiviral action is very different from that of such drugs. These combinations could result in additive or even synergistic therapeutic effects.

Among possible immunorestorative approaches, no single agent tested up to now appears to have sufficient potency. However, certain lymphokines, natural activators of cellular functions, used in succession or in combinations, hold the promise of providing the powerful physiological stimuli necessary to an enhancement of the multiplication of function of immunocompetent cells. Among these, interleukins and interferons are expected to find a role in future immunorestorative therapy. The colony stimulating factors (CSFs)—a family of hormone-like substances produced by activated T-lymphocytes—also show promise. CSFs have the potential to augment certain host defenses and to have an impact on the morbidity and mortality due to opportunistic infections, particularly those caused by protozoans. CSFs may also be capable of enhancing natural defense mechanisms against the malignancies associated with AIDS. Two CSFs have been cloned and can be produced in sufficiently large quantities for clinical trials. One of them is now undergoing early, limited tests in patients with AIDS.

The variety and promise of possible therapeutic approaches augur well for a future ability to slow the progression of HIV disease and to maintain HIV-infected people alive and functioning. AZT alone has already achieved this result in certain AIDS patients, at least over a limited period of observation.

Still, it is difficult to say when effective and safe treatments can be expected to become generally available for people with HIV disease. This will be determined by a number of factors. The pace of advances will depend, for instance, very much on the speed at which the 19 clinical AIDS Treatment Evaluation Units, created by Congressional mandate in 1986 for the development of AIDS therapies, are put to work at maximum capacity. A very large-scale, intensive, and coordinated clinical research effort is urgently needed both within and outside these units. Early accessibility to treatment will also depend on the flexibility of the Food and Drug Administration in releasing new drugs before they can be approved for marketing, but as soon as they become known to be tolerably safe and effective for the treatment of AIDS patients who have no time to wait and no other recourse. Thus far, of the experimental drugs, only AZT has been released on this basis—and only on a very limited scale.

Concurrently, a basic research effort is under way that must be greatly expanded in order to gain a better understanding of HIV's precise pathogenic mechanisms and of the resulting specific immune malfunctions. Only such knowledge can ultimately lead to highly specific and nontoxic therapies.

PROSPECTS FOR A VACCINE

The development of a safe vaccine for the protection of the general public against HIV infection is generally regarded as a very high research priority, but HIV presents unusual difficulties in this respect. The use of the whole virus in either an "attenuated" or "killed" form must be avoided because of the inherent risk that exists in administering any preparation that contains the genetic material of a potentially lethal virus. Modern biotechnology provides many opportunities to develop vaccines composed of only pure whole viral proteins or viral protein subunits (Barnes 1986b). Yet, because HIV displays considerable genetic variability, neutralizing antibody raised against a protein derived from a particular strain of HIV may not neutralize other strains of this same virus.

Several preparations of a relatively large protein component of HIV's envelope have been produced by genetically engineered mammalian cells, bacteria, or even a large virus (vaccinia). In animals, such preparations have all elicited the production of antibody that was capable not only of neutralizing HIV *in vitro*—that is, preventing the infection of susceptible cells and the killing of T4 cells by HIV—but also of doing so for diverse strains of HIV. However, there is still a risk that vaccines made of the whole HIV envelope protein may themselves be immunosuppressive. They may mimic too closely the effects of the virus itself and similarly block the function of T4 lymphocytes. In the case of such preparations, the spectre of liability looms particularly large, at this time, for pharmaceutical companies interested in sponsoring anti-HIV vaccine development. For this reason, subunit vaccine preparations—made of mere fragments of viral proteins—are also being developed using various complex strategies, including outright chemical synthesis. Although carefully devised for probable strong immunogenic properties, subunit vaccines may still be less protective than those made of whole viral envelope protein. It remains to be seen whether the production of high levels of neutralizing antibody can be induced safely in humans with any of these preparations.

The testing of several potential vaccine preparations in chimpanzees—the only other animal species susceptible to infection with HIV—or even directly in humans, is now imminent. Establishing vaccine safety and efficacy in humans will be a time-consuming process because vaccinated humans—unlike chimpanzees—cannot be "challenged" through the deliberate administration of infectious virus in order to assess the vaccine's protective effect. In humans, the spread of naturally acquired infection in vaccinated and unvaccinated groups must be followed over a period of time in people who—for ethical reasons—must also be informed of the precautions they can take to protect themselves from HIV infection. Testing a vaccine's efficacy may therefore require the recruitment of many thousands of suitable—that is, "at risk" but seronegative—volunteers, and these will have to be followed for periods estimated to be as long as from three to eight years. This is necessary because of the expected slow rate of seroconversion and late onset of disease symptoms following infection with HIV. Were the Food and Drug Administration willing to consider, as sufficient proof of a vaccine's effectiveness, certain expected differences in the kinds and amounts of antibody developed by the vaccinated and unvaccinated groups, the period of follow-up required could be much shorter. Whether and when a serologic endpoint to vaccine trials could be acceptable remains, however, to be fully debated.

Despite all of these difficulties and the many still unanswered questions of fundamental importance regarding the possibility of vaccinating humans against HIV infection, cautious optimism is permissible because animals—cats and mice—can be successfully vaccinated against some of their own retroviruses and protected from diseases caused by them.

As for the problem of recruiting volunteers for vaccine trials, it is likely that at least some of those individuals at the highest risk—namely uninfected life partners of HIV-infected people—would be willing to volunteer for such trials, particularly should "safer sex" practices prove unable to provide the very high level of protection everyone would wish them to have.

Many more cases of AIDS, with a progressively higher incidence of disease and death among women and infants, will undoubtedly occur. This will create justified alarm in the general public and a pressing demand for a vaccine. Political pressure favoring the enactment of state and federal legislation for liability protection of biotechnology and pharmaceutical companies engaged in vaccine development will increase considerably. Certain bills that address this issue, some of which have already been introduced in the California State legislature and in the U.S. Congress, will then stand a good chance of being enacted. Therefore, the likelihood that anti-HIV vaccine development will be pursued vigorously is good. In this area, too, the proficiency of the biomedical research enterprise can be expected to be equal to its task.

CONCLUSION

If this society creates the climate in which research and development work can be pursued efficiently, biomedical research can and will develop, relatively soon, methods for AIDS treatment and prevention. This will require not only much greater financial resources than have been committed to date, but a national will to succeed, to focus on solving the scourge of AIDS as a *health* problem and to abandon distracting, futile, and irrelevant moralizing. Success will also require coordinated, cooperative private- and public-sector efforts, and the ingenuity, on the part of all our institutions, to develop innovative, more humane, and faster ways to deal with the enormous challenges faced by the research and the medical care communities. A multitude of economic, legal, and ethical problems will have to be solved in ways that do not destroy the social order and everyone's civil liberties. What character the public policy dimensions of AIDS will assume in the United States in the near future will determine, to a large extent, how soon and how well the biomedical research enterprise can free humanity of one of its worst killers.

REFERENCES

Barnes, D. 1986a. Military statistics on AIDS in the U.S. *Science* 233:283

———. 1986b. Strategies for an AIDS vaccine. In Research News. *Science* 233:1149–1153.

Barre-Sinoussi, F., J. C. Chermann, F. Rey, M. T. Nugeyre, S. Chamaret, J. Gruest, C. Dauguet, C. Axler-Blin, F. Vezinet-Brun, C. Rouzious, W. Rozenbaum, and L. Montagnier. 1983. Isolation of a T-lymphotropic retrovirus from a patient at risk for acquired immune deficiency syndrome (AIDS). *Science* 220:868–871.

Bayer, R., C. Levine, and S. M. Wolf. 1986. HIV antibody screenings: An ethical framework for evaluating proposed programs. *Journal of the American Medical Association* 256: 1768–1774.

Biggar, R. J. 1986. The AIDS problem in Africa. *Lancet* I:79–83.

———. 1987. Epidemiology of human retroviruses and related clinical conditions. In *AIDS: Modern concepts and therapeutic challenges*, ed. S. Broder. New York: Marcel Dekker.

Centers for Disease Control. 1982. Update on Kaposi's sarcoma and opportunistic infections in previously healthy persons—United States. *Morbidity and Mortality Weekly Report* 31:294–301.

———. 1985. Provisional Public Health Service interagency recommendations for screening donated blood and plasma for antibody to the virus causing acquired immunodeficiency syndrome. *Morbidity and Mortality Weekly Report* 34:1–5.

———. 1986. Classification system for human T-lymphotropic virus type III/lymphadeno-pathy-associated virus infection. *Morbidity and Mortality Weekly Report* 35:334–339.

Coffin, J., A. Haase, J. A. Levy, L. Montagnier, S. Oroszlan, N. Teich, H. Temin, K. Toyoshima, H. Varmus, P. Vogt, and R. Weiss. 1986. Letter. *Science* 232:697.

Curran, J. W., W. M. Morgan, A. M. Hardy, H. W. Jaffe, W. W. Darrow, and W. K. Dowdle. 1985. The epidemiology of AIDS: Current status and future prospects. *Science* 229:1352–1357.

de Clerq, E. 1986. Chemotherapeutic approaches to the treatment of the acquired immune deficiency syndrome (AIDS). *Journal of Medical Chemistry* 29:1561–1569.

Fauci, A. S. 1986. Current issues in developing a strategy for dealing with the acquired immunodeficiency syndrome. *Proceedings of the National Academy of Sciences, U.S.A.* 83:9278–9283.

Fauci, A. S., H. Masur, E. P. Gelmann, P. D. Markham, B. H. Hahn, and H. C. Lane. 1985. The acquired immunodeficiency syndrome: An update. *Annals of Internal Medicine* 102:800–813.

Francis, D. P., H. W. Jaffe, P. N. Fultz, J. P. Getchell, J. S. McDougal, and P. M. Feorino. 1985. The natural history of infection with the lymphadenopathy-associated virus/human T-lymphotropic virus type III. *Annals of Internal Medicine* 103:719–722.

Gottlieb, M. S., R. Schroff, H. M. Schanker, J. D. Weisman, P. T. Fan, R. A. Wolf, and A. Saxon. 1981. *Pneumocystis carinii* pneumonia and mucosal candidiasis in previously healthy homosexual men: Evidence of a new acquired cellular immunodeficiency. *The New England Journal of Medicine* 305:1425–1431.

Haverkos, H. W., M. S. Gottlieb, J. Y. Killen, and R. Edelman. 1985. Classification of HTLV-III/LAV-related diseases. Letter. *Journal of Infectious Diseases* 152:1095.

Institute of Medicine, National Academy of Sciences. 1986. Summary and Recommendations. In *Confronting AIDS: Directions for public health, health care, and research.* Washington, D.C.: National Academy Press.

Koop, C. E., 1986. *Surgeon General's report on acquired immune deficiency syndrome.* Washington, D.C.: U.S. Department of Health and Human Services.

Mitchell, W., and D. Montefiore. 1987. Mismatched dsRNA inhibits HIV. *Proceedings of the National Academy of Sciences, U.S.A.* (in press).

Popovic, M., M. G. Sarngadharan, E. Read, and R. C. Gallo. 1984. Detection, isolation, and continuous production of cytopathic retroviruses (HTLV-III) from patients with AIDS and pre-AIDS. *Science* 224:497–500.

Robbins, R. K. 1986. Synthetic antiviral agents. *Chemistry and Engineering* (January 27): 28–40.

Sarngadharan, M. G., M. Popovic, L. Bruch, J. Schupback, and R. C. Gallo. 1984. Antibodies reactive with human T-lymphotropic retroviruses (HTLV-III) in the serum of patients with AIDS. *Science* 224:506–508.

Seale, J. 1985. AIDS virus infection: Prognosis and transmission. *Journal of the Royal Society of Medicine* 78:613–615.

Selwyn, P. A. 1986. AIDS: What is now known. II Epidemiology. *Hospital Practice* (June 15): 127–164.

Snider, W. D., D. M. Simpson, J. W. Gold, C. Metroka, and J. B. Posner. 1983. Neurological complications of acquired immunodeficiency syndrome: Analysis of 50 patients. *Annals of Neurology* 14:403–418.

Wong-Staal, F., and R. C. Gallo. 1985. Human T-lymphotropic retroviruses. *Nature* 317: 395–403.

AIDS
PUBLIC POLICY DIMENSIONS

PART ONE

Overview

AIDS and Health Policy
PHILIP R. LEE
PETER S. ARNO

CHAPTER 1

AIDS and
Health Policy

PHILIP R. LEE
PETER S. ARNO

Because of the catastrophic nature of acquired immune deficiency syndrome (AIDS) and the fear the disease engenders, the AIDS epidemic in the United States poses a unique challenge to policymakers at all levels of government—federal, state, and local. They are challenges that must be met within a federal/intergovernmental system whose foundations are 200 years old.

Since the first cases of AIDS were reported in the United States in 1981, more than 16,000 cases, resulting in 8,220 deaths, have been reported through the end of 1985, and the number is expected to increase to more than 30,000 by the end of 1986 (Boffey 1986). Predictions about the future are difficult, because we do not know the number of people who have been exposed to or infected with the AIDS virus, although it is estimated that between one and two million Americans are already infected (Curran et al. 1985). Of these, between 5 and 30 percent, may ultimately develop AIDS. Another 25 percent may develop AIDS-related complex, an often debilitating syndrome of fever, weight loss, fatigue, lymphadenopathy, and multiple other complications that require prolonged medical care and occasionally prove fatal even without progressing to AIDS.

The costs of the AIDS epidemic rise with each passing day. Total direct costs in the United States were estimated at $837 million during 1985, while the indirect costs due to morbidity and premature mortality were placed at $3.3 billion (Scitovsky et al. 1986).

While the majority of AIDS cases have been reported in New York, California, Florida, New Jersey, Texas, and Illinois, more than a dozen other states have reported more than 100 cases, and at least some cases have now been reported from every state and the District of Columbia. Among the metropolitan areas hardest hit are New York City, San Francisco, Los Angeles, Washington, Miami, Houston, Newark, and Chicago (see Table 1.1).

How the federal government, as well as the state and local governments, has responded to the AIDS epidemic is related to a variety of

3

Table 1.1

AIDS Cases Reported to the Centers for Disease Control,
by Metropolitan Area

METROPOLITAN AREA	AIDS CASES REPORTED*
New York City	4,923
San Francisco	1,730
Los Angeles	1,306
District of Columbia	483
Miami	475
Houston	402
Newark	373
Chicago	323
Philadelphia	284
Dallas	236
Atlanta	223
Boston	221
Jersey City (N.J.)	179
Nassau County (N.Y.)	159
Ft. Lauderdale	153
San Diego	147
Seattle	141
New Orleans	125
West Palm Beach	122
Anaheim	114
Baltimore	114

*Data as of 20 December 1985.
SOURCE: Centers for Disease Control.

political, economic, social, and public health factors. These include:

- the magnitude of the epidemic
- the modes of transmission of the AIDS virus, particularly through sexual activity and intravenous (IV) drug use
- the nature of the groups at highest risk—gay and bisexual men and IV drug users (see Table 1.2)
- the availability or lack of effective treatment strategies

Table 1.2

Distribution by Patient Group of Reported AIDS Cases, United States

PATIENT GROUP	NUMBER*	PERCENT
Adult		
Homosexual/bisexual men not IV drug users	10,600	65.3
Homosexual/bisexual men and IV drug users	1,310	8.1
IV drug users	2,766	17.0
Hemophilia patients	124	0.8
Heterosexual contacts	182	1.1
Transfusion recipients	261	1.6
None of the above/other:		
No identified risks	586	3.6
Born outside U.S. †	398	2.5
SUBTOTAL	16,227	100.0
Pediatric		
Parent with AIDS or at increased risk for AIDS	175	75.8
Hemophilia patients	11	4.8
Transfusion recipients	33	14.3
None of the above/other	12	5.2
SUBTOTAL	231	100.0
TOTAL	16,458	100.0

Note: Percents may not total due to rounding.
*Data as of 13 January 1986.
†Includes persons born in countries in which most AIDS cases have not been associated with known risk factors.
SOURCE: Centers for Disease Control. *Morbidity and Mortality Weekly Report* 35:20.

In this chapter, we will focus on the public policy aspects of the AIDS epidemic within the context of the complex intergovernmental system linking federal, state, and local governments, often described by the term "federalism." In order to set the stage for our consideration of the policy responses to the AIDS epidemic, we will briefly review the changing nature of federalism. We will then examine the responses of the federal, state, and local governments to the epidemic, and conclude with some general observations and recommendations.

THE CHANGING NATURE OF FEDERALISM

Federalism is the term commonly used to describe the relationship between the United States government and the 50 state governments. As originally used in the United States, federalism was purely a legal concept to define the constitutional division of authority and responsibility between the national government and the states (Hale and Palley 1981).

Federalism initially stressed the independence of each level of government from the others, and limited the function assigned to the federal government largely to foreign affairs, national defense, and efforts to stimulate commerce, while other functions, such as police protection and education, became the responsibility of state and local governments. In the early years of the republic, public health and medical care were the responsibility of local governments and the private sector, and responsibility for the payment for medical care rested largely with the individual (Lee and Silver 1972).

The Civil War and the emergence of dual federalism

The role of the federal government in relation to state and local governments remained a limited one until the Civil War, which brought about dramatic changes in the role of the federal government in order to preserve the union. During the Civil War period, the federal government also began a process that has continued to this day—the allocation of federal resources to the states for national purposes. The Morrill Act of 1862, for example, provided grants of federal land to the states to support higher education. Later, cash grants for the establishment of agricultural experiment stations were provided. The federal grants to the states during the Civil War began a revolution in federal-state relations (Hale and Palley 1981).

The New Deal: Cooperative federalism

The next period of great change in federal-state relations occurred during the New Deal in the 1930s. In response to the Great Depression, the role of the federal government was dramatically changed, with a series of actions designed to save the banks, regulate financial institutions, restore consumer confidence, aid the poor and unemployed, provide social security in old age, and provide federal aid to states for public assistance and public health, including maternal and child health. The most significant domestic social program ever enacted by Congress was the Social Security Act of 1935 (Public Law 74-241), which established a new role for the federal government in domestic affairs.

The Great Society: The era of creative federalism

In the 1960s, there was a further transformation in the federal role in domestic social policy. Civil rights, medical care, elementary and secondary education, early childhood development, consumer protection, auto safety regulation, housing and community development, air and water pollution control, and anti-poverty programs were among the areas in which the federal role was expanded.

The traditional federal-state relationship was extended to include direct federal support for cities and counties, nonprofit organizations, and private businesses and corporations in order to carry out a variety of health, education, social service, and community development programs (Reagan and Sanzone 1981). Over 200 separate grant programs were enacted during the Kennedy and Johnson administrations. In health, programs ranged from Medicaid to rat control, from air pollution controls to student loans, and from expanded food and drug regulations to services for the mentally retarded. Among the many new health programs initiated during the 1960s, only Medicare, enacted in 1965 as an amendment to the Social Security Act, was directly administered by the federal government.

"New Federalism" and a diminished federal role

Two major themes were to emerge early in the administration of President Nixon: welfare reform and "New Federalism." President Nixon coined the term New Federalism to describe the efforts of his administration to move away from the federal categorical programs of the Johnson years toward the transfer of federal funds to state and local governments with as few strings attached as possible. This was done through revenue sharing and block grants.

Beginning in 1981, the Reagan administration dramatically accelerated the degree and pace of change in domestic social policy that had begun under the New Federalism policies of President Nixon. To President Reagan, New Federalism meant a diminished role for government, decentralization, deregulation, federal budget cuts, emphasis on the private sector, and competition. The goal was a return to the dual federalism that existed prior to the New Deal (Palmer and Sawhill 1982). Although this goal was not achieved, a number of important policy changes occurred. New Federalism policies were reflected initially in the Omnibus Budget Reconciliation Act of 1981, which consolidated 21 categorical health programs into block grants and extended state discretion over Medicaid policies while reducing the share of federal expenditures (Lee and Estes 1983).

Problems arose for state and local governments as a result of the New Federalism policies, but these paled in comparison to the impact of a federal tax cut that reduced federal revenues dramatically, the increased military spending that was initiated in 1981, and the recession of 1981-1982. The record federal budget deficit that was generated has continued to cast a very long shadow on domestic federal policies since 1982. The Balanced Budget and Emergency Deficit Control Act of 1985, also known as Gramm-Rudman-Hollings, is the legacy of the policy changes initiated in 1981 and 1982.

Yet, despite these dramatic policy changes of 1981 and 1982, the federal government continues to play a major role in domestic social programs. Not only did Social Security, Medicare, and Medicaid remain basically intact but in 1985 the federal government also expended more than $100 billion on 351 grant-in-aid programs to state and local governments. These federal funds represented about one-fifth of all state and local government spending for the year.

THE FEDERAL RESPONSE TO THE AIDS EPIDEMIC

In 1986, there is no more pressing domestic problem facing policymakers at the federal, state and local levels than the AIDS epidemic. The public policy response to AIDS at the federal, state, and local levels is being shaped in a time of transition, when economic issues, rather than social needs, dominate the agenda.

The need to clarify the policy, financing, and administrative responsibilities among the levels of government is evident to both politicians and students of the policy process. The AIDS epidemic provides an opportunity to examine, and, it is hoped, resolve many of these issues. To do so, however, will require a major change in course and a political will that is not yet evident.

Initial responses

The initial federal response to the AIDS epidemic was ambivalent at best. At the onset of the epidemic in 1981, the Reagan administration began to record the growing number of cases at the CDC, initiate intramural research on AIDS in the National Institutes of Health (NIH) and CDC, and provide technical assistance to state and local governments.

Soon after the onset of the epidemic, the U.S. Public Health Service (USPHS) began working with state and local governments, professional associations, and private organizations to develop guidelines to assist public health officials at the state and local levels (Intergovernmental Health Policy Project 1985). To date, guidelines have been issued in three areas:

1. *Protection of the nation's blood supply*, including recommendations for screening donated blood and plasma for HTLV-III/LAV* antibodies after the test was developed and marketed, beginning in March 1985.

2. *School attendance, day care, and foster care for children with AIDS*, including recommendations that most AIDS-infected children be allowed to attend school.

3. *Prevention of AIDS in the workplace*, with an emphasis on health care workers, food handlers, and personal service workers.

In addition, the USPHS, through the CDC, assisted the U.S. Conference of Mayors in establishing an AIDS information exchange.

In 1983, the Secretary of the U.S. Department of Health and Human Services, Margaret Heckler, declared that AIDS was the department's number one health priority (Brandt 1983). Three areas were to receive special emphasis:

1. The identification of the causal agent (the AIDS virus) in NIH laboratories.

2. The development of an antibody test for the AIDS virus.

3. The identification of high-risk groups and the routes of transmission.

In spite of the budgetary limitations placed on the NIH, the CDC, and the Food and Drug Administration (FDA), rapid progress was subsequently made in these areas.

Early funding and financing patient care

In the early years of the epidemic, the Reagan administration requested no new funds for AIDS research, training, or services; instead it transferred funds from other programs to fund these activities. Every year since the epidemic began, Congress has substantially increased the funds requested by the Reagan administration, particularly the funds for biomedical research. In November 1985, the U.S. House of Representatives and the Senate agreed to spend $244 million on federal AIDS programs for fiscal year 1986. This year, however, proposed cuts of $41 million by the Reagan administration and an additional $10 million in cuts resulting from the Gramm-Rudman-Hollings legislation have curtailed funds for biomedical research, education, treatment, and community services for AIDS patients (Congressional Research Service 1986).

---

*Human T-lymphotropic virus type III/lymphadenopathy-associated virus.

The federal financing of care for AIDS patients has attracted relatively little attention on the part of federal policymakers. Currently, five sources of federal funds are potentially available to pay for the care of AIDS patients:

1. The federal tax subsidy for the purchase of private health insurance for employees by employers.

2. The federal share of Medicaid funds.

3. The Veterans Administration.

4. Medicare, to a very limited extent.

5. Funds at the NIH Clinical Center used to support clinical trials of new drugs.

Currently, no data are available that identify these five sources of federal financing for hospital care, physicians' services, home care, or nursing home care for persons with AIDS. The two largest federal contributions are the federal tax subsidy and the share of Medicaid funds used to pay for such care, although only the latter includes a direct expenditure of government funds.

Because there has been no specific federal policy developed to deal with the catastrophic costs often incurred in the care of AIDS patients, most of the burden has been borne by the AIDS patients themselves directly out of pocket, by private health insurance, by state Medicaid programs, and by local governments in cities or counties with large numbers of AIDS patients, that is, New York, San Francisco, and Los Angeles.

Shortfalls in federal funding

Federal funds for the development of a spectrum of community-based health services, such as home health and social services, required by AIDS patients have been extremely limited. The cost of community-based health and social services falls mainly on the afflicted individuals, their families and friends, volunteers, local charitable contributors, and, increasingly, local governments.

The allocation of resources to AIDS-related programs within the USPHS has been heavily weighted toward basic biomedical research, vaccine development, clinical trials, and epidemiological surveillance. The paucity of federal resources devoted to public health education and prevention programs, especially for high-risk groups, is of particular concern.

Although much of the factual information available on high-risk groups, modes of transmission, and strategies to prevent the transmission of the AIDS virus has been developed in cooperation with CDC and NIH, the federal government has played a very limited role in the dissemination of information. For fiscal years 1984 and 1985, for example, less than 4 percent of all USPHS AIDS resources were appropriated for information dissemination and/or public affairs (Office of Technology Assessment 1985).

In lieu of a vaccine, which may be years away, effective public health education is the best known method to curb transmission of AIDS. This should include dissemination of information about safe sexual practices and the dangers of needle sharing—to limit exposure to the AIDS virus— as well as other health-promoting activities that bolster the immune system, such as better nutrition and stress reduction. A study conducted by the U.S. Conference of Mayors (1984) found that one of the greatest needs at the local level was funding for training and technical assistance in community education, particularly on "safe sex" guidelines.

THE STATES' RESPONSES TO THE AIDS EPIDEMIC

Markedly different policy and financing responses have emerged in states with the largest numbers of AIDS cases: New York, California, Florida, New Jersey, and Texas. The AIDS epidemic hit these states at the same time that the burden of financing health care for the poor was being shifted from the federal government to state and local governments and to the private sector.

In order to respond to the added responsibilities related to the financing of health care for the poor, state governments have introduced various methods to attempt simultaneously to contain costs and to ensure access to adequate levels of care. Some states, such as New York, have emphasized a regulatory approach to ensuring access while containing costs. Texas and California, on the other hand, have long favored the competitive approach, with greater cost-sharing by consumers. Other states, such as Florida, have used both policy strategies.

The predominance of different risk groups—gays in California and IV drug users in New Jersey and New York, for example—has influenced the policy response. The liberal traditions in New York and California contrast with a far more conservative attitude in Texas, and these traditions have influenced a particular state's response. The political effectiveness of gay groups in different areas of the country has also been important in shaping the response to AIDS.

AIDS-related legislation

State policymakers were reluctant to examine the possible financial impact of the AIDS epidemic in its early years, and initially the approach focused on the public health aspects of the epidemic. By the end of 1985, nine states had enacted legislation related to the AIDS epidemic (Intergovernmental Health Policy Project 1985). Among the five states with the greatest number of AIDS cases, only Texas has not enacted any legislation to deal with the epidemic. Most AIDS-related legislation addresses one or more of the following areas:

• confidentiality

• medical and psychosocial services

• protection of the blood supply

• public education

• research

In 1983, New York became the first state in the nation to pass AIDS legislation, with the enactment of Chapter 823 establishing the AIDS Institute. Three appropriations were provided by the legislation:

1. $4.5 million for a research program and the administrative costs of the AIDS Institute.

2. $600,000 for educational activities.

3. $150,000 for a public information program.

Additional appropriations for 1984-1985 included $1.2 million for research and $1.6 million for education and services. In 1985-1986, a total of $4.5 million was requested for research, education, and services.

During 1983, California enacted legislation creating an AIDS Advisory Committee within the Department of Health Services and providing funds for education and information programs. In addition, funds were provided to the University of California to support research.

In 1984, both California and Florida enacted legislation designed to protect the public blood supply by requiring antibody testing by all blood banks and plasma centers. Both states also authorized alternative test sites in addition to those at blood banks, and the laws provided means to protect the individuals tested from unauthorized disclosure of their test results.

In 1985, California expanded the scope of its AIDS legislation to include pilot detoxification and treatment programs for IV drug abusers, funds to evaluate the effectiveness of AIDS education and information programs, and funds for a prospective two-year study concerning the medical costs of AIDS (SB No. 1251, 1985). Between 1983 and 1986, AIDS-related spending by the state of California totaled more than $22 million (California AIDS Advisory Committee 1986).

The 1985 legislation also required that the state of California develop a comprehensive plan to cope with the AIDS epidemic. The plan is to include sections on surveillance; prevention and community education; HTLV-III/LAV antibody testing, including issues related to confidentiality; diagnosis and treatment services, including hospital care, outpatient care, home care, and hospice care; research; and AIDS in the state's corrections systems.

According to a recent report by the Intergovernmental Health Policy Project (1985) at George Washington University, since the beginning of 1983, approximately $45 to $50 million in state funds has been spent or obligated specifically for the support of AIDS-related programs. Thirty-three states and the District of Columbia reported spending between $21 and $22 million of these funds on surveillance, laboratory services, education and information, outreach, antibody testing, and administration. Allocations for research accounted for $21.8 million, and the balance of the funds was earmarked for psychosocial support services and treatment. California, New York, New Jersey, and Massachusetts have made the bulk of these expenditures—about $41.5 million of the total.

Data have not been gathered nationally on AIDS in the states' corrections or criminal justice systems, but this is already a major problem for New York and New Jersey, and all states are likely to be forced to address the issues involved.

LOCAL RESPONSES TO THE AIDS EPIDEMIC

The policy, financing, and administrative responses to the AIDS epidemic among the cities and counties affected by the disease have been as markedly different as they have been among the states. Many of the political, economic, and public health factors affecting the policy responses at the federal and state levels have also affected the response of local governments. The task of responding appropriately to an epidemic of unknown potential magnitude is difficult.

Problems of organizing, financing, and providing the spectrum of medical, social, and public health services to deal with the AIDS epidemic are complex, costly, and difficult to resolve in any community. The services required to care for AIDS patients include:

- screening

- inpatient hospital care

- outpatient hospital, clinic, or office-based care

- skilled and intermediate nursing facility care

- home health and homemaker/chore services
- psychosocial support
- hospice care
- housing
- substance abuse—especially IV drug abuse—services

In addition, services are required for the education of high-risk groups, for dissemination of information to the general public, for the protection of the blood supply, for laboratory support, and for epidemiologic surveillance. These services may be provided by public agencies, nonprofit community agencies, volunteers, private practitioners, community hospitals, proprietary home health agencies, and nonprofit or proprietary nursing homes.

New York and San Francisco

New York and San Francisco, two cities that account for more than 40 percent of all reported AIDS cases in the United States, have poured enormous financial resources into coping with the epidemic. It is estimated that AIDS-related expenditures in fiscal year 1986 will total $137 million in New York City and $37 million in San Francisco (Arno and Hughes 1986). However, these are not all local resources. In fact, in New York and San Francisco, respectively, 59 and 30 percent of these expenditures are derived from combined state and federal funds. The remainder is derived principally from local tax levies in each municipality, and through private insurance coverage.

There is a major difference between the cities in how local tax monies have been allocated. It is estimated that more than 90 percent of local New York City AIDS funds are spent on inpatient hospital care, as compared with 25 percent in San Francisco (Comptroller of the State of New York 1985; San Francisco Department of Public Health 1985). This is due largely to New York City's 25 percent share of Medicaid expenditures and a direct subsidy to the municipal and voluntary hospitals providing care to AIDS patients. But it is also a result of a greater level of hospitalization in New York. The average length of hospital stay for an AIDS patient in New York is 25 days as compared with 12 days in San Francisco (Sencer and Botnick 1985; West Bay Hospital Conference 1985).

Government support for community-based services for persons with AIDS illustrates a key difference in the local policy response between New York City and San Francisco. These community-based services include crisis intervention and counseling, basic home care, hospice care, legal services, entitlements advocacy, group therapy, and education. In 1984, the Gay Men's Health Crisis (GMHC) provided the bulk of these services in New York, using primarily private (64 percent) and state (33 percent) funds. Only 3 percent of the funds was provided by New York City. In sharp contrast, the three largest organizations providing these services in San Francisco—the Shanti Project, the San Francisco AIDS Foundation, and Hospice of San Francisco—received 62 percent of their financial resources from the City and County of San Francisco, 30 percent from private sources, 4 percent from the state, and 4 percent from the federal government (Arno 1986).

A highly significant contribution is made to these groups by voluntary workers. Except for Hospice of San Francisco, all of these community groups rely heavily on donated labor. Approximately 130,000 volunteer hours were contributed to GMHC in New York City during 1984. This is comparable to the total hours donated to community groups in San Francisco. The funding mechanisms vividly illustrate the process by which the burden of dealing with a national public health crisis is continually shifted from the federal to the state level, then to local government, and finally to individuals, either AIDS patients or volunteers.

What of the rest of the country? A survey by the U.S. Conference of Mayors in 1984 assembled information from 55 local governments about their AIDS efforts (U.S. Conference of Mayors 1984). Of these, 40 percent of cities with populations greater than 200,000 and almost 25 percent of those with populations less than 200,000 reported some AIDS-related local public spending. Two-thirds of the larger cities had established task forces on AIDS by late 1984. However, the majority of cities and states in both high- and low-incidence areas have not been able to generate the level of support necessary to create service agencies, education programs, and comprehensive approaches to the health needs of people with AIDS.

The need for a wide-ranging, community-based approach to public education and prevention efforts, as well as an integrated health care service delivery system for persons with AIDS, will intensify across the country as the epidemic spreads, particularly among the high-risk populations. With total—direct and indirect—cost estimates already in the billions of dollars, the burden of medical care and social services can no longer rest solely on local governments and voluntary groups. To meet the needs of the growing number of AIDS patients in communities throughout the country, both states and the federal government will have to respond far more effectively. It is critical that the issue of paying for the care of AIDS patients be faced openly at all levels of government.

PAYING FOR CARE

Financing for hospital and physician care and community-based social services for AIDS patients has been provided by a mixture of private health insurance, Medicaid, direct out-of-pocket payments by patients, charity, and local governments. Providers, whether they are public, non-profit, or for-profit, cannot provide services without the necessary funds. The costs of paying for the care of AIDS patients are substantial and have to come from local tax funds that must also be used to meet a variety of other community needs, including a growing number of needs in health care. Costs have been a barrier to the development of comprehensive services in many communities.

A recent report from the Comptroller of the State of New York (1985) suggests the problems ahead for state and local governments in the financing of inpatient hospital care, as well as other needed medical and social services. According to the report, "If present trends continue, New York City could find itself spending over $500 million a year for treatment of AIDS by 1989."

For many AIDS patients, the disease means loss of job, loss of health insurance, catastrophic medical care costs, and social isolation, in addition to the burden of a debilitating and eventually fatal illness. Those who lack private health insurance or have inadequate coverage must pay for very expensive care directly out of pocket, or turn to local physicians, hospitals, and community agencies for charity care, to public assistance through Medicaid, or to local municipal hospitals for publicly provided care. These choices are not unique to AIDS patients but reflect a generic and growing problem in our health and long-term care systems, namely, the inability of the current system of fragmented financing for acute care and long-term care to ensure access to needed services.

In a political climate where it is becoming increasingly difficult to differentiate between cost containment and national health policy, an estimated 27 to 35 million Americans are without any health insurance for acute hospital care and physician services. The number rises to 50 million when the underinsured are added to those who do not have any third-party coverage (Swartz 1984; Monheit et al. 1984; Davis and Rowland 1983).

Should national health policy leave the fate of AIDS patients to the vagaries of private health insurance, Medicaid, local governments, and the pocketbook of the individual AIDS patient? Although private health insurance coverage has been crucial for many AIDS patients, for others it has been inadequate or unaffordable. At best, the public sector has responded in some states and in some communities to ensure provision of and to cover the costs of necessary care. Both California and New York have

Medicaid programs that are more liberal in their eligibility requirements and in the scope of their benefits than those of most other states. San Francisco has responded with public funds to meet the continuum of care needs of AIDS patients, while New York, Los Angeles, and other communities have relied upon hospitals or volunteers to provide needed care. In other states, needed outpatient and community-based services have been lacking, and AIDS patients have remained hospitalized for prolonged periods. It remains to be seen whether these other communities will respond as generously as the epidemic continues to spread.

The availability and accessibility of outpatient and community-based care in San Francisco, and the relatively low charges per admission at San Francisco General Hospital, as compared with those elsewhere (see Chapter 21), may give policymakers an important clue to the direction they should follow in the development of policy for the care of AIDS patients. Local funding in San Francisco, particularly from the Department of Public Health and private donations, has been critical for the development of educational, social, psychological, home care, and hospice services in that city. Although these services are essential for the adequate care of AIDS patients, virtually none of them is funded by private health insurance.

WIDER IMPLICATIONS OF AIDS POLICY ISSUES

What are the respective responsiblilities of federal, state, and local governments in dealing with the AIDS epidemic? Is AIDS a national problem or only a series of local problems? Is the federal role limited primarily to biomedical research, disease surveillance, and technical assistance to state and local governments? What is the federal role in financing health care for AIDS patients? What is the role of the private sector? Of state and local governments?

How the country chooses to answer these questions with respect to the financing of care for AIDS patients may have a profound influence on the future direction of health care financing policies affecting all those— not only AIDS patients—who are uninsured or underinsured for health care costs in the United States. The current federal emphasis on competition and deregulation, and the reliance in the United States on a hodgepodge of financing mechanisms, including private health insurance provided through employment, Medicare, 50 different state Medicaid programs, a variety of different local (usually county) government programs, payment directly out of pocket by patients, and private charity, has produced a system of health care that is inequitable and very costly in relation to what other countries, such as Canada, receive for their health care dollars.

The Committee on Federalism and National Purpose (1985) clearly identified three basic functions of government:

1. The policy function—determining the goals and the standards of a program.

2. The financial function—providing funding for the program and deciding how much is provided.

3. The administrative function—delivering a government service and deciding on the delivery system.

The overriding concern of those who question the federal strategies of decentralization, deregulation, and competition in health care is the adequacy of resources at the state and local levels to assume full responsibility for health care delivery programs, including the costs that have been transferred to state and local governments, or to individuals, by the federal government.

The failure of the federal government to meet its responsibilities does not eliminate the costs of acute health care or of the spectrum of community-based long-term care services required by AIDS patients. Rather, it simply shifts those costs to other levels of government or to the private sector and to the individual citizen. In the past, the bill could also be shunted to private health insurers through cost shifting within the hospitals, but this is less and less the case in those states, such as California, that have stressed competition rather than regulation to control costs.

The day will soon be upon us when this broader health care issue of equity in sharing responsibilities will have to be addressed by policymakers at the federal and state levels, as well as in the private sector.

CONCLUSION

The AIDS epidemic has sharply delineated the current issues in both intergovernmental relations and health policy. In fact, if it does nothing else, the epidemic underscores the urgent need for an adequate and equitable national system of health care financing. Such a system can include a significant role for states and the private sector, but the foundation for such a system must be a strong federal role in policy and financing.

Although pressing issues in the AIDS epidemic appear to be in health care financing, policymakers must continue to give a high priority to biomedical, epidemiological, behavioral, and social science research; to community education programs; to the control of IV drug use and other measures designed to reduce the risk of AIDS and to slow its spread; and to the development of nonhospital services, such as hospice care, in-home services, psychological counseling, social services, and other office- or clinic-based physician and nursing services.

Finally, the AIDS epidemic must make us all—policymakers, program managers, health professionals, advocates—reexamine our values and our roles as citizens. The emphasis that the current dominant ideology places on individualism and the private role of the individual citizen in the United States has had devastating consequences. The example that has been set for us by the AIDS patients themselves and by those who have volunteered to care for them can point the way to the rebirth of the concept of our public responsiblilities and our community obligations as citizens, as well as our private privileges.

REFERENCES

Arno, P. S. 1986. The non-profit sector's response to the AIDS epidemic: Community-based services in San Francisco. *American Journal of Public Health* 76:1325-30.

Arno, P. S., and R. G. Hughes. 1986. Local policy response to the AIDS epidemic: New York and San Francisco. Unpublished paper. Institute for Health Policy Studies, Institute for Health and Aging, University of California, San Francisco; June.

Boffey, P. M. 1986. AIDS in the future. *New York Times,* 14 January.

Brandt, E. 1983. Federal Response to AIDS. Testimony at hearing. U.S. House of Representatives Subcommittee on Intergovernmental Relations and Human Resources, 1-2 August.

California AIDS Advisory Committee. 1986. State of California. Unpublished data.

Committee on Federalism and National Purpose. 1985. *To form a more perfect union.* Washington, DC: National Conference on Social Welfare.

Comptroller of the State of New York. 1985. *Review of New York City's proposed financial plan for fiscal years 1986 through 1989.* Report No. 30-86. Albany, NY: Office of the State Comptroller, 11 December.

Congressional Research Service. 1986. Unpublished data.

Curran, J. W., W. M. Morgan, A. Hardy, W. H. Jaffe, W. W. Darrow, and W. R. Dowdle. 1985. The epidemiology of AIDS: Current status and future prospects. *Science* 229:1353-57.

Davis, K., and D. Rowland. 1983. Uninsured and underserved: Inequities in health care in the United States. *Milbank Memorial Fund Quarterly/Health and Society* 62(2):149-76.

Hale, G. E., and M. L. Palley. 1981. *The politics of federal grants.* Washington, DC: Congressional Quarterly Press.

Intergovernmental Health Policy Project. 1985. *A review of state and local government initiatives affecting AIDS.* Washington, DC: George Washington University.

Lee, P. R., and C. L. Estes. 1983. New federalism and health policy. *Annals of the American Academy of Political and Social Science* 468:88-102.

Lee, P. R., and G. A. Silver. 1972. Health planning—A view from the top with specific reference to the USA. In J. Fry and W. A. J. Farndale (eds), *International Medical Care.* Oxford, England: Medical and Technical Publishing Co., Ltd., 284-314.

Monheit, A. M., M. Berk, and G. Wilensky. 1984. *Unemployment, health insurance and medical care utilization.* Washington, DC: National Center for Health Services Research.

Palmer, J. L., and I. V. Sawhill (eds). 1982. *The Reagan experiment.* Washington, DC: Urban Institute.

Reagan, M. D., and J. G. Sanzone. 1981. *The new federalism* (2nd ed). New York: Oxford University Press, 7.

San Francisco Department of Public Health. 1985. *San Francisco's response to AIDS: Status update.* City and County of San Francisco, 8 October.

Scitovsky, A. A., D. Rice, J. Showstack, and P. R. Lee. 1986. *The direct and indirect economic costs of acquired immune deficiency syndrome 1985, 1986 and 1990.* Final report prepared for the Centers for Disease Control, task order 282-85-0061, #2. Atlanta: Centers for Disease Control.

Sencer, D. J., and V. E. Botnick. 1985. *Report to the mayor: New York City's response to the AIDS crisis.* New York: Office of the Mayor, December.

Swartz, K. 1984. Statement before the Subcommittee on Health, Committee on Finance, United States Senate. 27 April.

U.S. Conference of Mayors. 1984. *Local responses to acquired immune deficiency syndrome (AIDS): A report of 55 cities.* Washington, DC: U.S. Conference of Mayors.

Office of Technology Assessment, U.S. Congress. 1985. *Review of the Public Health Service's response to AIDS* (OTA-TM-H-24). Washington, DC: Government Printing Office.

West Bay Hospital Conference. 1985. Monthly AIDS hospitalization utilization report. San Francisco, CA. 25 October.

PART TWO

The
Politics
of
AIDS

CHAPTER 2

The Politics of AIDS

DENNIS ALTMAN

In an end-of-the-year readers' survey, the news magazine *U.S. News and World Report* (1985) posed the question: "Which of the following problems concern you the most?" Readers were given four alternatives: crime, recession, nuclear war, and AIDS (acquired immune deficiency syndrome). This represents an interesting measure of the extent to which fear and loathing about AIDS, to borrow a phrase coined for another event (Thompson 1971), has entered the American consciousness. I use this phrase to emphasize the reality that the most common discourse about AIDS involves panic, even hysteria, about its transmission, rather than any sign of genuine compassion for those who are suffering and dying from the illness.

To look at the politics of AIDS is a broad mandate; few illnesses have been so politicized. Politics, in the most conventional sense of the word, have played a central role in the ways in which AIDS has been conceptualized, constructed, researched, treated, and mystified, and there is room for a great deal of discussion about the role of ideology and politics in both the social construction of illness and the control and direction of medical research. I shall restrict my remarks, however, to the role of the press and of certain interest groups in the conceptualization of the disease, and to a discussion of the response of governments to the epidemic.

In this chapter, I want to examine three interconnected points of public policy, all of which I think illustrate the failings of governments to adequately deal with the challenge of AIDS. These are

- the provision and the financing of health care

- the use of the AIDS virus antibody test

- the provision of preventive education

THE CONCEPTUALIZATION OF AIDS

AIDS was first conceptualized by both scientists and the media as a disease of homosexuals, and for a time was known popularly as "GRID" or "gay-related immune deficiency" (Altman, *AIDS*, 1986). Scientists abandoned this characterization as it became clear that there was no inherent or necessary connection between AIDS and homosexuality, but neither the media nor most politicians have been as quick to do so. At best, there has been some recognition that other groups are affected by AIDS, but in the public imagination, AIDS remains an illness defined by the groups it most afflicts and, therefore, an illness of "The Other."

The most pernicious example of this view of AIDS is the use by the media of the term "innocent victims," which is applied to those other than gay men and intravenous (IV) drug users suffering from AIDS, with the clear corollary that if you belong to these two groups and contract AIDS you are somehow guilty. This view persists despite the fact that over one-third of AIDS cases in New York City, the epicenter of the disease in the United States, are not found among gay men, and this proportion is increasing (New York City Department of Health 1986). Additionally, in Europe, the second largest number of cases is among patients not belonging to any of the major risk groups, and in Belgium, Greece, Italy, and Spain, and in Central Africa, the majority of AIDS cases are not found among gay men (Centers for Disease Control 1986; Clumeck 1985). As AIDS becomes a global problem, there are fewer and fewer reasons to think of it as, in the phrase still used by some journalists, "the gay plague."

Despite this, there has been resistance on the part of most politicians and journalists to see AIDS as a public health crisis rather than as the disease of promiscuous homosexuals, who somehow infect innocent victims with the illness. The public image of AIDS is linked to white male homosexuals, while in reality the disease is increasingly affecting nonwhites and nongays. As New York Assemblyman Roger Green pointed out recently: "Of the 77 children who were reported to have AIDS in our city in 1985, 68 were Black and Latino. . . . Thus an inappropriate response to AIDS interconnects with the general decline of public health" (Green 1986).

"Guilt" and "innocence" are irrelevant terms when one speaks of an epidemic disease. No one sets out to get sick or to infect others. I do not blame the CIA, KGB, CDC, Haitians, Zairians, Cuban mercenaries, or promiscuous gay men, although you can find someone who at some time has pointed his finger at one of these groups as the culprit.

THE RESPONSE OF GOVERNMENTS

Guilt and innocence become meaningful concepts when one examines the response of governments to the AIDS epidemic. And it is not only reasonable but necessary to ask whether governments have done everything that could reasonably be done to save lives and to prevent both the spread of AIDS and unnecessary panic about it. Even in this era of budget reductions and shrinking government assistance, no one has seriously argued that the state does not have a responsibility to safeguard the health of its citizens. Nor have we yet reached a point where anyone of consequence is calling for the abolition of the Centers for Disease Control and the National Institutes of Health.

There are many, however, who would slash the budgets of those agencies, and one of the more unfortunate aspects of the AIDS epidemic is that it has coincided with a determined attempt by the federal administration to cut back on domestic spending, including that related to health. In fact, the failure of the Reagan administration to respond promptly and adequately to the emergence of a new epidemic disease has been well documented (Office of Technology Assessment 1985). It took considerable congressional pressure on a resistant administration before substantial monies were made available for AIDS research, and too often that money has come at the expense of other programs of health research and surveillance (Lee 1986).

Most of us would accept that, ultimately, governments have the responsiblility to support and facilitate the research, prevention, and treatment programs required by a new lethal and epidemic disease. If this is so, the governments of the United States, with a few honorable exceptions—such as the San Francisco city and county government—have failed dismally. Overall, the official response to AIDS in the United States and most other countries has been a mixture of hysteria and neglect, in which the desire of politicians and bureaucrats to look good to a frequently necrophiliac media has too often overshadowed their interest in sensible and rational public health policies.

As Philip Lee and Peter Arno emphasize in Chapter 1, much of the failure to deal with AIDS results from a federal structure that too often facilitates buck-passing. When I visited southern Florida in 1985, for example, I was struck by the ingenuity whereby the city of Miami, Dade County, the state health department, and Governor Robert D. Graham all refused to accept responsibility for doing anything constructive about AIDS.* Examples of inadequate health care, woeful support services, and negligible attempts to provide public education and information are unfortunately the rule across the United States, and, in the majority of places, only volunteer efforts by community groups—largely based in the gay community—have provided support services for the sick and preventive education for those most at risk.

In one sense, the virtues of the American system—the division of powers, the strength of interest groups, the reliance on free enterprise—all

*The best coverage of AIDS in Florida is found in Steve Sternberg's articles in the *Miami Herald.*

help explain the failures of the system to respond adequately to the AIDS crisis. Even more distressing, demands for governments to "do something" seem increasingly to be demands for punitive types of action—quarantine, tattooing, exclusion from schools and employment, and bathhouse closures—rather than for measures that might actually help those who are sick and those most at risk of infection. As Jonathan Lieberson observed in the *New York Review of Books* (1986), "The continued reluctance of so many people to give up unwarranted apprehensions about AIDS seems at times almost as compulsive and driven as the behavior of those drug abusers and bathhouse patrons who are accused of spreading the illness."

THE FAILURE OF THE AMERICAN HEALTH CARE DELIVERY SYSTEM

Since the beginning of the AIDS epidemic, I have been struck—and I think this is particularly so for those of us who are not Americans—by the way in which the epidemic so clearly underlines the defects of the American health care system. Above all, the linkage of health insurance to employment, which is a feature almost unique to the United States, means that a disproportionate percentage of those people afflicted with AIDS will find themselves in a situation where their health insurance runs out, through no fault of their own, when they become too ill to work.

The consequences of such a situation, both for the person with AIDS and for service providers, need not be dealt with at length here. Without private insurance to pay for the treatment of catastrophic illness, for instance, many Americans are left with no alternative but to try to negotiate the horrendous patchwork of laws and restrictions related to eligibility for Social Security or other government assistance, which is for many people a living—and, unfortunately, dying—nightmare, when they are afflicted with AIDS. It is important to stress, however, that in the United States there is a whole dimension to dealing with this epidemic that we in Australia and people in Western Europe do not face: Nobody in Australia, or the Netherlands, or France, who gets AIDS faces the possibility that he or she will lose health insurance as a consequence, or faces the possibility of being forced to sell off assets in order to qualify for some meager form of government support which is both inadequate and demeaning.

I emphasize this because it is essential that AIDS be understood within a larger context, namely, the failure of the American health care delivery system. One of my great regrets is that the AIDS advocacy groups by and large have not made that connection, and have not reached out to other groups in the United States, particularly minority and labor groups and representatives of the elderly, who are committed to pressing for a more equitable and better system of health care. It is ironic, in fact, that discussions about improving health care delivery seem to have moved off the political agenda just at a time when AIDS makes the topic all the more relevant.

ANTIBODY TESTING AND ITS RAMIFICATIONS

The general problem of providing adequate health insurance acquires additional complexity with the availability of a test for the presence of antibodies to the AIDS virus—identified as human T-lymphotropic virus type III/lymphadenopathy-associated virus (HTLV-III/LAV). Insurers have been quick to see the opportunity of using the test to screen applicants for AIDS risk and thereby limiting their liability by declining to insure—or cancelling coverage for—persons whose tests are positive for antibodies to HTLV-III/LAV. Earlier this year, for instance, there was a discussion on an early morning television news program in which representatives from some of the major life insurance companies justified the use of the antibody test in screening applicants for insurance.

At this stage, I do not think that any health insurer has required people to be tested and to show themselves as antibody-negative in order to purchase health coverage. However, there is no question that, as time goes on, this is going to be a major problem. If one talks to people who sell health insurance, one will find that all sorts of measures are already under way to make it more difficult for single men who are presumed to be gay to get adequate health care coverage. In an article in the *Washington Monthly*, Steven Waldman (1986) reports a spokesman for the Health Insurance Association of America as saying that a halfway intelligent insurer will find some way to deny coverage if he suspects the candidate is in a high-risk group.

In several states, legislators have addressed, for better and worse, such practices. In 1985, for example, California and Wisconsin enacted legislation banning insurers' use of blood tests for HTLV-III/LAV antibody; however, Wisconsin later modified its law, in November 1985, to permit the test to be used for insurance purposes if the state epidemiologist and insurance commissioner both certified its reliability. Legislation proposed in early 1986 by New York Governor Mario Cuomo would prohibit insurance companies from requiring the antibody test or from asking whether an applicant had taken it (Carroll 1986). Meanwhile, in Michigan, HB 5272, a bill pending in that state in early 1986, would allow insurers to screen potential customers by asking them AIDS-related questions and requiring them to submit to an examination to detect the virus (Merritt and Toff 1986).

Testing may lead to discrimination

Because of the potential use of the test as a screening tool for employment and/or insurance, widespread antibody testing—an issue that comes up in most discussions about AIDS—is extremely difficult to advocate. Some public health officials argue that it desirable to encourage as many people as possible who are at risk for AIDS to be tested for the HTLV-III/LAV antibodies (Altman, "U.S. urges test," 1986). Medical opinion is divided on this—in Australia, for example, there is fierce debate over the usefulness of such tests—but the present reality is that the social, economic, and political consequences of testing are such that it is very difficult to argue for it. We face the specter of hundreds of thousands of thus far healthy people, distinguished only by their exposure to HTLV-III/LAV, being "marginalized"—fired or refused jobs, excluded from the military (as is already the case), denied insurance—and living in constant fear of what new restrictions hostile legislators and an uninformed hysterical public might impose upon them. Otis Bowen, the U.S. Secretary for Health and Human Services, for example, is reported to have called for antibody screening for all prospective immigrants to the United States (*Advocate* 1986). And the proposal by conservative columnist William F. Buckley, Jr. (1986) that persons in the United States who test positive for HTLV-III/LAV be tattooed on the upper forearm and buttocks for purposes of "identification" as AIDS "carriers" is a further case in point.

In Australia, where medical insurance, at least, is not at risk, the head of the Anti-Discrimination Board in New South Wales, the state where the greatest number of AIDS cases has been reported, tells me that she foresees enormous discrimination and difficulties with widespread testing (Carmen Niland, interview with author, 1985). If this is true in New South Wales, can anybody argue that it will not be of even more concern in Texas, or South Carolina, or Oklahoma? There is already discrimination against whole groups—drug users, gays, Haitians, hemophiliacs—who are seen as carriers of the so-called AIDS virus. And only in a few localities, particularly in California, have politicians been prepared to try to use legislation to protect both groups and individuals from discrimination based on the assumption that they somehow present a risk to the general population (City of Los Angeles 1985).

PROVIDING PREVENTIVE EDUCATION

These issues lead into the last major area of public policy that I want to discuss: namely, the question of preventive education. It has become a cliche to observe that the only effective means of preventing the spread of AIDS are programs designed to dissuade people from sharing needles and from engaging in high-risk sex. Almost everybody in the AIDS business subscribes to this point of view. Almost nobody in government is prepared to do anything about it.

Again, with the exception of the city and county of San Francisco and the partial exception of other localities in California, city, county, and state governments have been too scared of seeming to condone homosexuality or drug use to provide either funding or other resources for the sort of large-scale educational campaigns that are needed to supplement work already being done by community groups.

One of the ironies surrounding the AIDS epidemic is that there is a paradoxical attitude among governments, particularly the federal government. On the one hand, they refuse to recognize the gay community as a legitimate entity, but then they turn around and say that they can look after AIDS education themselves—a classic case of governments wanting to have their cake and eat it too. An adequate information and education program requires cooperation between governments and community groups.

The need for such programs is immense, although not all of our politicians may agree. The mayor of New York, Edward I. Koch, for example, has said he is convinced that almost everybody in New York City is aware of the ways in which AIDS can be transmitted (Koch 1986a). This assertion is belied by the mayor in his own book, *Politics*, published early this year. In the last section of his book, Mayor Koch tells the story of how Mother Teresa came to New York to establish a hospice for people dying from AIDS (Koch 1986b). According to the mayor's account, when he and his officials were meeting with Mother Teresa, she said,

> "If we open the hospice, I want to see every one of you washing and brushing the floors."
> I thought to myself, Mother, they say AIDS can't be contracted by casual contact. But it will be a long time before I would be willing to brush and wash the floors. That seemed to be the opinion shared by all of us in the room. We are not saints.

Now, it may be, of course, that the mayor was merely offended by the suggestion that he should wash and brush floors. It is difficult to imagine that happening. But I think the mayor is suggesting that by scrubbing floors he would run the risk of catching AIDS, which merely reinforces what is probably the single most dangerous misapprehension and myth about AIDS: casual contact with an AIDS patient or with someone who is antibody-positive results in infection.

Information deficiency

If we think not only about those people who worry that if they come into Manhattan and go a restaurant where the waiter is gay they will break out in ulcerous sores on their way back home but also about those people who really are at risk—because of their sexual practices or because of their use of shared needles—then, as a gay man who has access to places that many other people are not able or would not feel free to go, I can testify that there is less information being made available to people in New York about the transmission of AIDS than in my own home city of Melbourne, which has had, so far, 21 cases.

No one can claim to know how we can change behavior most effectively, particularly in terms of sharing needles, but there is a strange morality around that seems to accept that it is better not to do something that might check the spread of AIDS than to openly discuss the acts that lead to its spread. I know that the decision-makers at the Centers for Disease Control, undoubtedly under great pressure from their superiors, have procrastinated over the last few months in providing money for preventive education programs. They are now offering to make money available, but with strings attached that, according to people working in the two largest community AIDS information organizations in the United States, would make current programs unworkable (Freiberg 1986). That is, organizations will be granted government funds to go out and tell people to have safe sex, but only as long as they don't actually tell people what safe sex entails.

One of the most striking aspects of the AIDS epidemic to date is that very rarely have we heard a word of compassion or sympathy from American political and religious leaders for the more than 9,000 Americans who have died from AIDS thus far. We have seen President Reagan appear on television and shed tears for one child who needs a liver transplant, but only the death of a Hollywood star who was a personal friend of the President elicited any sign that the man in the White House was aware of a new and lethal disease in the United States.

VOLUNTARISM IN ACTION

What is striking, in contrast to the government's response, is how much has been done for AIDS victims by volunteer groups, largely—but not entirely—based in the gay community, and how little credit they have been given by a federal administration that claims to support voluntarism and community groups. Indeed, there is perhaps a need to gently chide some of the AIDS community groups for too easily accepting the Reagan administration policy that leaves to individuals and charity groups the responsibility for providing the basic support services that anyone who is seriously ill should surely expect to be provided by any decent, civilized government.

Too often, in fact, sections of the gay movement itself have failed to focus on the right targets. When the leading gay newspaper in New York City viciously attacks people such as Dr. Mathilde Krim as "homophobic" (*New York Native* 1985) while endorsing Mayor Koch for reelection, or when self-proclaimed gay leaders attack the Centers for Disease Control for procrastinating in research but seem unaware of the reasons that researchers have been starved for funds, one can only conclude that some of the gay movement is as uncritical of Reaganism as are those who actually benefit from current government policies.

WHAT CAN BE DONE?

Governments cannot be blamed because there is as yet no cure or an immediate prospect of a vaccine for AIDS. They could, however, handle the present crisis more humanely, more intelligently, and in ways that are more likely to save both lives and money than is the present patchwork of panic and neglect. For a start, the president could take seriously the proclamations of his own Public Health Service that this is a major emergency and appoint a top-level task force to advise him on all possible means to combat the epidemic. There are already bills pending in Congress that would help relieve some of the extraordinary burdens this disease is placing on certain local governments and individuals. Moreover, a call from the president for compassion for those who are dying and for an end to the ugly scapegoating of people who are sick and suffering would be a major psychological boost for those who are most deeply affected by this disease. The governor of New York State and the mayor of New York City could also commit themselves to a real program of preventive education rather than to the selective closures of bathhouses that, while perhaps politically satisfying, have little real benefit for the public health.

In addition, the media could begin analyzing in some detail the response of governments to this crisis instead of playing on the fears and panic of so many people who still believe, against all scientific evidence to the contrary, that AIDS can be transmitted by casual contact. A contributing editor of *Commentary* magazine, for example, wrote a diatribe, published in the *Wall Street Journal*, in which he somehow used AIDS to prove that pornography should be banned (Himmelfarb 1986). But the *Wall Street Journal* does not make that sort of space available to people who, whether they are medical experts or are working with community-based groups, actually have some real knowledge and experience about how to deal with the spread of this disease.

CONCLUSION

Finally, I want to ask a question that I find most perplexing when I think about the politics of AIDS: Why has it been so difficult to focus attention on the failure of government to adequately respond to the AIDS epidemic, and so easy, instead, to focus on the people who are themselves sick? If there has ever been a case of scapegoating the victim, then I think the AIDS epidemic is going to rank high as an example in the annals of the sociology of deviance for a long time to come.

When I was in San Francisco at the end of 1985, I went to United Nations Plaza, where a group was holding a vigil outside the San Francisco offices of the U.S. Department of Health and Human Services. Some people with AIDS-related conditions had chained themselves to a railing outside the office and said that they would not move until the federal government met their demands. Without going into the details of their specific demands, I want to point to the degree of anger and bitterness and fear and alienation that leads sick people to lie in the winter cold, day after day, outside the Federal Building because they feel their government has failed them. (It is also true that they were only doing this in San Francisco because, at least in San Francisco, there has been a reaction not only from the gay community but also from the whole city that suggests that a humane and civilized response to AIDS is possible.) Indeed, one of the saddest things about that vigil was that when I arrived in New York almost no one was aware that that demonstration was taking place. Yet, I have no doubt that if some third-rate bit player on "Dynasty" or "Dallas" were to say that 12 years ago she was kissed by Rock Hudson, the news would be trumpeted on every television and radio talk show in the United States.

Meanwhile, that people are dying from this disease, that the governments at most levels are not responding to their needs, and that no words of compassion or sympathy are being heard from the people who claim moral and political leadership are apparently not deemed worthy stories. And I want to express and share, as my conclusion, my feeling of exasperation and anger and sadness at seeing sick and gaunt men in the San Francisco winter winds, in the richest country in the world—one that President Reagan tells us over and over again is a beacon of freedom and a bastion of liberty and hope—forced to take such measures to call attention to the fact that the most elementary aspects of civilized health care are not being made available to them.

REFERENCES

Advocate. 1986. Reagan administration proposes AIDS screening for immigrants. 18 March.

Altman, D. 1986. *AIDS in the mind of America.* New York: Doubleday.

Altman, L. K. 1986. U.S. urges test for all at high risk of AIDS. *New York Times,* 14 March.

Buckley, W. F., Jr. 1986. Identify all the carriers. *New York Times,* 18 March.

Carroll, M. 1986. Revised bill would limit AIDS test use. *New York Times,* 24 February.

Centers for Disease Control. Update: Acquired immunodeficiency syndrome—Europe. 1986. *Morbidity and Mortality Weekly Report* 35:35–46.

City of Los Angeles 1985. Municipal Ordinance. No. 160289. AIDS discrimination. City of Los Angeles, California.

Clumeck, N. 1985. Overview of the AIDS epidemic and its African connection. Paper presented at the International Symposium on African AIDS, Brussels, 22-23 November.

Freiberg, P. 1986. CDC puts AIDS education funds 'on hold'. *Advocate,* 7 January.

Green, R. 1986. End the cutbacks. *Villiage Voice,* 14 January.

Himmelfarb, M. 1986. Porn, AIDS and the public health. *Wall Street Journal,* 13 January.

Koch, E. I. 1986a. AIDS: Public Policy Dimensions. Speech at conference. United Hospital Fund of New York-Institute for Health Policy Studies, University of California, San Francisco. New York City, 16 January.

———. 1986b. *Politics.* New York: Simon & Schuster, 245–46.

Lee, P. R. 1986. AIDS: Allocating resources for research and patient care. *Issues in Science and Technology,* winter.

Lieberson, J. 1986. The reality of AIDS. *New York Review of Books* 32 (16 January): 43–48.

Merritt, R., and G. Toff. 1986. AIDS: A raft of new bills. *Nation's Health,* March, 6.

New York City Department of Health. 1986. AIDS—Surveillance update(s). Monthly data.

New York Native. 1985. Waltzing with Mathilde, 3–16 June.

Office of Technology Assessment, U.S. Congress. 1985. *Review of the Public Health Service's response to AIDS.* Washington, DC: Government Printing Office.

Thompson, H. 1971. Fear and loathing in Las Vegas. *Rolling Stone,* 11 November.

U.S. News and World Report. 1985. 1986 readers' survey. 30 December, 134.

Waldman, S. 1986. The other AIDS crisis: Who pays for the treatment? *Washington Monthly,* January.

CHAPTER 3

Five Dimensions to the Politics of AIDS

RONALD BAYER

When we discuss the politics of AIDS, we need to be aware that there are really five dimensions to the issue. Each of the dimensions needs to be examined independently if we are to understand the totality of the political aspects of the AIDS epidemic. Each also raises questions for our society that go beyond AIDS issues themselves. These five dimensions are:

- the politics of equity
- the politics of liberty
- the politics of constituency
- the politics of culture
- the politics of science

THE POLITICS OF EQUITY

What does justice demand of a society that is confronted with the need to distribute the burdens of caring for the sick? How ought those burdens to be shared? Will they be broadly shared by the community as a whole, or will they be borne privately and individually?

In the United States, we have not yet answered these questions. On the level of political rhetoric, at least, there is a commitment to sharing the burden of caring for the sick. In practice, however, we display a unique willingness to tolerate the consequences of forcing individuals to pay for their own health care. Our failure, in this country, to make a serious commitment to equity takes on striking features as we confront the AIDS epidemic.

It is important to recognize that there are millions of Americans who have no health insurance at all, and millions more who have health insurance that is inadequate. It is also important to recognize that the problem of the uninsured and the underinsured is not a problem of AIDS sufferers alone: It is a problem for men, women, and children across the country (Davis and Rowland 1983; Feder et al. 1985).

It is not surprising, therefore, that we seem perplexed about how to mobilize health care services and protection for those with AIDS. After all, we have not done so very effectively for the poor and near-poor, either. In the United States, we have determined that health insurance will be available through the point of employment, and now, ironically, there is the threat that the HTLV-III/LAV antibody test will be used to deny people at risk for AIDS both employment *and* health insurance because they *may* become sick.

In the context of the question of equity, it is important to keep in mind the attitudes that may emerge and influence the way health care for AIDS victims is made available and is delivered. An indication of one possible attitude came in a statement by one public official that there are two kinds of AIDS patients, dead ones and dying ones; therefore, the expenditure of large sums of money on the health care of such individuals is ill-considered. Instead, it was asserted, that money should be available for research. It has also been publicly suggested that the chronically ill elderly have a duty to die, instead of using up resources that might be needed by younger, healthier people.

In the face of an almost single-minded focus on cost containment, and given the virtual disappearance of the issue of justice from public discussions of health care, it is not surprising that the most vulnerable members of society become, for some, a potential source of savings.

THE POLITICS OF LIBERTY

The issue of civil liberties is one that has confronted the gay community and public health officials again and again over the past several years. The ultimate question, given the inevitable emphasis on communal good at the expense of individual privacy, is, How will the demands and needs of public health be brought into balance with the principles of liberty that place great restrictions on what public health officials can do? I believe that there is an essential tension between the commitment to liberty and the commitments to public health, and that this tension must be confronted openly and carefully. The soothing notion offered by some that we can have a vital and effective public health strategy that in no way poses a challenge to individual privacy in our society is both foolish and dangerous.

It has become something of a convention at conferences about AIDS to speak critically about panic and hysteria. Actually, over the past five years since the AIDS epidemic began in this country, the level of public passion and unreason has been relatively controlled, especially given the nature of the disease with which we are confronted and the generally despised character of those groups at highest risk. Of course, there have been moments of outrage and outbursts of unreason, but by and large wrathful homophobia and narcophobia have been surprisingly rare.

It is not insignificant, I think, that the New York Times (1985) wrote one of its strongest editorials, entitled "AIDS and the New Apartheid," on the issue of AIDS panic. It is not an accident that Newsweek ran a several-page spread in the fall of 1985 debunking all the myths about the ways in which AIDS is spread. I think the media that are concerned with order in society are terribly concerned about panic. Big insitutions do not like panic, wherever the panic comes from, and they most likely see the pros-pects of AIDS-related panic as potentially disruptive. As a consequence, these media have, I believe, quite consciously sought to bring some sem-blance of reason to the public discussion of AIDS.

I am not talking about the yellow press, but it seems to me that when the New York Times, Newsweek, Time, and the major television networks all begin to talk about the dangers of panic, something important has oc-curred. It is entirely possible, however, that as the number of AIDS cases mount, and they certainly will, unreason, panic, and hysteria may take on new dimensions.

Before we must face such unpleasant possibilities, we should be clear about the terrible consequences that could follow from the unreasonable demands for quarantine and mass screening that have been voiced in some quarters. We also ought to recognize that there are intellectual excesses on the side of liberty, too: those that suggest, for example, that the problem of AIDS transmission is simply a problem among consenting adults and that, consequently, the public and state have no reason or obligation to inter-vene. None of these sweeping generalizations speaks to a balance of weighing the priorities of public health against the rights of individuals to certain, and general, civil liberties, but such a balance clearly must be sought.

THE POLITICS OF CONSTITUENCY

When the command over and access to limited resources is the outgrowth of the mobilization of interest groups in a pluralistic give-and-take, what happens to the disorganized and the voiceless?

Through its enormous efforts, the gay community has been able to provide a range of extraordinary social services to those afflicted by AIDS—and not only to gays. By dint of their hard work, gay organizations have brought the issue of AIDS to the halls of Congress and to the state legislatures. Their demand has been for "more"—more research, more education programs, more aid for AIDS patients—and rightfully so.

After homosexual men, the group at second greatest risk for AIDS in the United States is intravenous (IV) drug users. Unlike the homosexual AIDS sufferers, however, IV drug users have no "voice"; they are both despised and disorganized. Furthermore, the professionals who work with them have been slow to respond to the AIDS threat and, as a result, the needs of IV drug users with AIDS—and these are special and in some ways very different from the needs of gay men with AIDS—have received less attention from both the health care community and the media. For their sakes and the sake of our entire society, this must begin to change. In short, in facing the public issues of AIDS, we must transcend the limits of pluralistic politics.

THE POLITICS OF CULTURE

How does a disease either underscore or subvert the cultural predilections of various groups?

We know that AIDS has buttressed members of the fundamentalist religious right in their hatred of homosexuality, their hatred of sexual license, and their hatred of liberty in sexual matters in general (Altman 1986). However, there is a different kind of cultural politics surrounding AIDS: the cultural politics within the gay community itself, where the AIDS epidemic has sparked an important controversy about the nature of sexuality and the nature of human relationships. This cultural politics has also demonstrated that unreason is the not the monopoly only of reactionary social forces; it also may affect those who have borne the brunt of the disease and its consequences.

There are, for example, some in the gay community, although not among its leadership, who object to advisories that people should alter their sexual behavior in any fashion because of AIDS. This posture seems to be based on an attitude that advice against indiscriminate sexual encounters amounts to an attack on gay sexual freedom in general. Warnings that persons who continue to engage in anonymous multiple-partner sexual activities are dancing on the edge of the abyss are construed as an attempt to push gays back into the proverbial closet from which they have only recently emerged. Such unreason has been reflected in the *New York Native* (Ortleb 1985, 1986), a gay-community newspaper whose writers have suggested that to speak of the "public" health is to be a standard-bearer for totalitarianism. Such a reaction is also part of the culture of illness.

THE POLITICS OF SCIENCE

Another dimension of the politics of disease that often goes unnoticed, by observers and participants alike, is the politics of science. Consider, for example, the debate over the role of female transmission of the AIDS virus in the demographics of the epidemic.

Some researchers have argued that the epidemiological data in the United States indicate that women play a small and insignificant role in the transmission of the AIDS virus except to their babies during pregancy or birth. Female-to-male sexual transmission, some have asserted, seems unlikely (Polk 1985; Centers for Disease Control 1984). Others have suggested that if one looks across the world, and at Africa in particular, the situation is very different, and it becomes clear that women may play an important role in the transmission of AIDS beyond the known high-risk groups of today (Haverkos and Edelman 1985; Centers for Disease Control 1985). In addition, at least one well-studied example of such apparent transmission has been reported in the United States (Calabrese and Gopalakrishna 1986).

What is remarkable about this debate is that, although it appears to be a debate about science and epidemiology, it is really a political debate. Those who seek to de-homosexualize AIDS tend to emphasize both the possibility of female-to-male transmission and the accidental nature of the epidemiology of AIDS in the United States. Those who seek to control panic tend to stress the fact that AIDS stays within the known risk groups, and, indeed, has stayed within the known risk groups for the past six years.

In general, it is the "keep calm" party that has stressed the inefficiency of transmission by women. A ready example of this approach can be found in an article by Jonathan Leiberson in the *New York Review of Books* (1986). In his essay, Mr. Lieberson dismissed every single suggestion that AIDS might be transmitted by women, while citing but one source to buttress his position. On the other hand, the party of "alarm" in our society has tended to overemphasize the risks associated with female transmission. Since the data in the United States are still ambiguous, it becomes clear, I think, that politics and social issues are driving this particular debate, rather than science alone.

CONCLUSION

Any consideration of the politics of the AIDS epidemic requires, finally, a sobering glance backward through the general history of epidemics. In the nineteenth century, for example, there was an enormous dispute over whether certain diseases were contagious. The debate occurred in the era before the germ theory was fully developed. Those who argued that cholera and yellow fever were contagious diseases were committed to the use of quarantine; they were not threatened by the prospect of bureaucratic interactions in society. They supported the role of the interventionist state. Those persons who tended to oppose the theory of contagion were often liberals seeking to lift what they viewed as the deadening hand of the state from society. They sought to eliminate bureaucratic control and, fundamentally for our purposes, they opposed quarantine as unscientific, as a regrettable medieval heritage.

As it turned out in this particular case, the liberals were wrong about science and the reactionaries were right. That is a lesson I think we should consider, but not because I want to hold high the banner of reaction. It is important because when we confront the issue of how to structure a health policy that is both humane and effective, we should be keenly aware of the ways in which our social and political predilections may blind us to hard, and not always pleasant, facts.

REFERENCES

Altman, D. 1896. *AIDS in the mind of America.* New York: Anchor Press/Doubleday, 25, 65-68.

Calabrese, L. H., and K. V. Gopalakrishna. 1986. Transmission of HTLV-III infection from man to woman to man. *New England Journal of Medicine* 314:987.

Centers for Disease Control. 1984. Acquired immunodeficiency syndrome (AIDS)—United States. *Morbidity and Mortality Weekly Report* 33:661.

_____. 1985. Heterosexual transmission of human T-lymphotropic virus type III/lymphadenopathy-associated virus. *Morbidity and Mortality Weekly Report* 33:561-63.

Davis, K., and D. Rowland. 1983. Uninsured and underserved: inequities in health care in the United States. *Milbank Memorial Fund Quarterly/Health and Society* 61:149-76.

Feder, J., J. Hadley, and R. M. Mullner. 1985. Falling through the cracks: Poverty, insurance coverage, and hospitals' care to the poor, 1980 and 1982. In *Hospitals and the uninsured poor,* S. Rogers, A.M. Rousseau, and S. Nesbitt (eds.). New York: United Hospital Fund, 3-30.

Haverkos, H. W., and R. Edelman. 1985. Female-to-male transmission of AIDS. *Journal of the American Medical Association* 254:1035-36.

Lieberson, J. 1986. The reality of AIDS. *New York Review of Books* 33 (16 January): 43-48.

New York Times. 1985. AIDS and the new apartheid. Editorial. 7 October.

Newsweek. 1985. The AIDS conflict. 23 September, 20-21.

Ortleb, C. 1985. The AIDS prophet of doom. *New York Native,* 14-20 October.

_____. 1986. Heil Bayer!! *New York Native,* 2 June.

Polk, B. F. 1985. Female-to-male transmission of AIDS. *Journal of the American Medical Association* 254:3177-78.

CHAPTER 4

"Your Own Kind": AIDS and the Communitarian Ethic

EMILY FRIEDMAN

A few years ago, I visited Dade County, Florida, where today, as Dennis Altman has noted in Chapter 2, public authorities are reluctant to take responsibility for the care of the AIDS patient population. I was there conducting research on health care for another partly disenfranchised group: Haitian immigrants who had entered the United States through unapproved channels. It is interesting that this group is now also associated with AIDS.

At the time, I was studying Haitians in Florida for an article I was writing on health care for refugees and immigrants in the United States (Friedman 1982a). I was fascinated then, as Dennis Altman was more recently, by the two-step being performed by the various government agencies in Florida in order to avoid having to take responsibility for the health care of this large group of people. They were a high-risk population, particularly in terms of maternal and child health, and they were sapping the resources of Jackson Memorial Hospital, a fine facility in Miami, while everyone passed the proverbial buck up and down the state.

An illuminating sidelight of the situation there is that when some federal money did finally come through to help Jackson Memorial Hospital, it apparently came by way of the Medicaid program (which is one way a special health grant can be made from the federal government to a state). I was told that the state of Florida responded to this largesse by deleting an equal amount from its Medicaid budget for that year. This is, however, hearsay for which I did not seek validation, since I had finished my article by then.

What is more germane to the politics of AIDS is an occurrence that took place one day when I visited Camp Krome, outside Miami, where Haitian immigrants of uncertain status were being kept in a detention camp until their fate could be decided. It was camp policy that men and women, including married couples, be totally segregated in different parts of the camp. This was apparently to prevent the conception and birth of babies who might be considered American citizens by dint of being born on American soil, which would have complicated any attempts to deport their parents.

40

I was a guest of the U.S. Public Health Service (USPHS) staff at Camp Krome, who were doing a yeoman's job, by the way, and were not to blame for the situation in which they were working. As lunchtime approached, they asked if I would like to have lunch with them and the internees. I said I would be glad to.

The camp did not allow people of different sexes to eat together, either. So there we were: me, a half-dozen staff people, a few detainees from other cultures, and about 800 Haitians, all of them men. I was the *only* woman in that gigantic mess hall, and because of that—not because of my charm or good looks—I was the object of a certain amount of attention from the internees. As a result, I felt rather strange.

After a while, I turned to one of my hosts and said, "Gee, I feel a little bit isolated." He replied, "Oh, you shouldn't. See? There are a couple of white guys over there."

The point is that people tend to stick to their own kind in this country. However, our definition of who constitutes "our own kind" is driven as much by politics, social values, and chance as it is by objective data or anthropology. And in the context of the politics of AIDS, what sticking with one's own kind means is that there are grave questions, when all the clumping is finished, as to who is going to be on which side of the wall of internment.

YUPPIE ETHICS

This brings me to the science I recently founded: Yuppie Ethics. Now, I know people do not take this science very seriously yet. When I remarked to my friend Judy, for example, that I was going to New York to talk about Yuppie Ethics, she replied, "That'll be a short speech."

There are those who even suggest that the phrase "Yuppie Ethics" might be a contradiction in terms. So it is necessary to define it: *Yuppie Ethics is the study of what happens with allocation of a limited resource when a large and politically powerful subgroup of those eligible for that resource decide that they are entitled to a disproportionate share of it.*

This new branch of ethics has many rubrics and corollaries, but it is necessary to relate only two of them here. Friedman's First Corollary of Yuppie Ethics is that the level of deservingness of the poor and other vulnerable groups varies in direct proportion to the amount of resources available. The Second Corollary is that if one cannot free up enough resources by disenfranchising the obvious groups, then someone else has to become undeserving. And if there ever was a group made to order for that role, it is the populations at high risk of contracting AIDS.

The politics of the United States should have taught us that fact. The language of Medicare and Medicaid, for example, is very instructive in this regard: Of the approximately 30 million Medicare clients, about 26 million are the politically powerful elderly. In the literature, Medicare eligibles are referred to as "beneficiaries," just as in private insurance. On the other hand, the approximately 20 million Medicaid clients—the vast majority of whom are low-income mothers and children—are referred to as "recipients," just as in welfare.

Our politicians have traditionally behaved as though everyone on Medicare were white and everyone on Medicaid were black. What I find interesting is that, in the current health care cost-containment climate, the elderly are beginning to change color. The politically sacrosanct Medicare population is facing, for the first time, significant client-focused cuts. And if the elderly, who are powerful and who have the highest voting rate of any population group in the country, are beginning to be vulnerable in terms of *their* access to affordable health care, then what can we expect for a group that is *perceived* as being composed largely of promiscuous male homosexuals, drug abusers, prostitutes, and low-income nonwhites?

The hemophiliac population does not lend itself so easily to political unpopularity and accusations that they brought AIDS on themselves, but there *is* a genetic factor in the disease of hemophilia. Perhaps, then, we can blame their parents for having children and develop a sins-of-the-father model, so that hemophiliacs, too, can be subject to the blaming-the-victim mentality that is so much a part of Yuppie Ethics. In any event, aside from the latter group, the AIDS population is so fragile politically that if we could find a way to include low-income women and the mentally ill in it, we would have a clean sweep of those least likely to succeed in American society.

DESERVINGNESS AND DISCRIMINATION

Looking at the situation in that rather dismal light, I am not surprised at the behavior of the political powers in response to AIDS. To complain about their abandoning a helpless, terminally ill population is admirable and necessary, but to be surprised is naive. After all, politics flows toward those who hold power and resources. And Yuppie Ethics tells us that the most convenient and morally undisturbing way to get hold of a resource is to convince yourself that the people who have the resource you want are not deserving of it.

One of the ways in which these grim ethics are expressed is in the realm of insurance. In the first place, we have always discriminated in the provision and pricing of both health and life insurance in this country. Three groups that can be characterized as high-risk, and thus more expensive to insure, can be identified:

1. People who are at risk through no fault of their own.

2. People who incurred health problems through their own actions, but who are only partly to blame for having done so.

3. People who are truly responsible for placing themselves and others at risk.

The group that suffers the least discrimination comprises those whose problem is seen as not being their fault at all. If, for example, you bought a house on Love Canal, or if you came into contact with dioxin at your place of employment, you are at higher risk of serious illness than is the rest of the population, but that is not seen as your own fault. The second group includes people who smoked before the Surgeon General's warnings about the health hazards of cigarettes—or who are, in the view of some, just as addicted to cigarettes as others are to the more fashionable cocaine—and people who engaged in other habits that turned out to be not so good for them. Our view of these people is that, although they might have suspected that something was amiss, although some of this behavior expressed more stubbornness than common sense, and although many other people have been able to walk away from the practices and conditions that have trapped this group, we still cannot view their problems solely as the result of direct irresponsibility and, thus, culpability.

The third group, who are guilty even in my bleeding-heart mind, are the truly culpable, the truly undeserving. These people almost go out of their way to be irresponsible. Although I view alcoholism as a disease and its victims as members of the second or even the first group, people who drink and drive clearly belong in the third group. However, the people who best illustrate this type of behavior are those who, with blind courage in the face of sanity, refuse to wear seat belts, as an expression of their Americanism and rugged individualism, thereby helping us all to pay a great deal more for health insurance and contributing to some 43,000 highway deaths and more than two million traumatic injuries every year. As Jean Forster (1982) of the University of North Carolina pointed out in a brilliant article several years ago, none of these fools is taking much of a risk on a per capita basis because the risk of accident is only 1 in 100,000 automobile trips. However, their behavior is the societal equivalent of yelling "Fire!" in a crowded theater, and should be understood as dangerous and antisocial, despite the fact that it appears to be private and harmless.

No matter how you decide who belongs in which high-risk group, the deservingness of each is different in the public mind, and that is expressed in the amount of health resources we are willing to give them—and at what price.

AIDS AS A PARADIGM

If that is true, then AIDS is more than a terrible disease. It is a paradigm for many other conditions, and, more important, its victims are a paradigm for many other people, because the situation is this: With AIDS, we have the combination of a *perceived* resource shortage in health care (I do not think it is a *real* resource shortage, but I do not want to digress onto the topic of distributive justice), a classic dread disease that is somewhat communicable under certain circumstances, a spreading plague mentality, very high financial stakes, and a politically unattractive at-risk population.

That accidental combination of events is occurring in a political climate that will allow some interests to simply wipe out any distinctions we make between the guilty and the innocent. As we have long tried, fruitlessly, in this society to distinguish between the deserving and the undeserving poor, thus we may now creep to the other end of the spectrum and say, "If you have this disease, you are guilty."

That should raise an alarm in all our minds, because AIDS is not an anomaly. Tragic as it is, it is not a freak occurrence, a one-time-only nightmare, or an isolated case. It could represent the future of us all. It is *our* health, *our* insurance, *our* social contract that is on the line. For in a highly monetaristic, socially narcissistic culture, I find it very difficult to believe that, once it has started, the process of disenfranchisement by disease is going to stop with AIDS.

Because of the politics around AIDS, those who wish to disenfranchise certain groups have already been allowed to get a foot in the door. The movement of some insurance companies to deny coverage not only to persons who test positive for AIDS-virus antibodies but even to *all* single men in certain age groups who live in certain ZIP code areas of New York or San Francisco, for example, is a case in point. And I would ask a question: If we had a test that proved a person's predisposition not to AIDS, but to cancer, when the entire population of the United States would be at risk, how would we view such a test then?

Half the insurance at twice the price?

We know what we would say. But if we have allowed the communitarian ethic on which public programs and responsibility and private insurance have been based to unravel because the AIDS population was vulnerable, who will listen to us? If we have allowed that process to start, will we be able to stop it when it is our own necks on the block? Mark Siegler, a physician and ethicist at the University of Chicago, has said that, at this rate, we will soon be pricing health insurance out of the reach of everyone who is poor, near-poor, old, sick, or at risk of anything for which we have a test (Siegler 1984). Next, we'll price it out of the reach of people who ski, windsurf, hang-glide, or run. In no time at all, we could have half the insurance at twice the price. But by then, the payers will have the bit in their teeth.

I wrote a few years ago, mostly in jest, that we were on the road, in this country, to having half of the health care provider capacity idle while half of the population was unable to get health care (Friedman 1982b). If you look at some of the statistics from my home state of California, you can see that, at least for the low-income population, that may be exactly what has transpired. Physicians are leaving California because they cannot make a living, and hospital occupancy is about 60 percent (California Hospital Association 1986), if that, but some medically indigent Californians have died of hypertensive disease because of an inability to get either care or medicine (Lurie et al. 1984). Will the fatal misallocation of resources stop with them?

Fighting on the margins

Fred Friendly pointed out years ago that the major battles over Constitutional rights, such as freedom of speech and of the press, are not fought in the mainstream: They are fought in the rather seedy areas of libel, pornography, and scandal (Friendly 1981). Similarly, it is unlikely that we will fight our battles over enfranchisement and health care entitlements in the suburbs with computer executives at the center of the struggle. We will fight them on the margins. The AIDS population, being marginal, is therefore becoming a paradigm for the entire future of our societal obligation to each other.

For that reason, I have some optimism. If we can understand—and help others to understand—that this is simply a first skirmish and not an isolated situation, and that the insurance—public or private—that people save may be their own, society may step back from the brink. Similarly, we must bring about a general understanding that the lives we save through supporting research, information, education, and public health initiatives—for AIDS victims and others—also may be, ultimately, our own.

THE REAL COMMUNITY

If we can accomplish that, we may yet win, because we can harness the narcissism of this age to the fact that the basis of community, the basis of communitarian ethics, is not some sucker being duped into taking on a responsibility that he need not shoulder. Communitarianism, rather, represents a recognition that at one time or another, in one arena or another, each of us is in some way vulnerable. As Robert Sigmond, adviser on hospital affairs to the Blue Cross and Blue Shield Association, has said, "At some spend-down level, we are all medically indigent" (Friedman 1986).

In an essay on AIDS and other epidemics that visit the vulnerable, Gerald Weissman, M.D. (1983), writes about the attention given to AIDS while elderly low-income Americans continue to die silently in their overheated homes in the South every summer. In pleading the cause of both sets of victims, he quotes Proust, who in turn quotes a wealthy duchess, who said, "How can one do good to people one doesn't understand? Besides, one doesn't know which people to do good to. One always tries to do good to the wrong people."

Whether it is the elderly who die of hyperthermia in their own homes, or the tragic population victimized by AIDS, these pariahs—old and new—are not, in fact, the "wrong people." That honor will be reserved for us, if we fail them.

REFERENCES

California Hospital Association. 1986. *Hospital fact book 1985*. Sacramento: California Hospital Association.

Forster, J. L. 1982. A communitarian ethical model for public health interventions: An alternative to individual behavior change strategies. *Journal of Public Health Policy* 3 (June): 150.

Friedman, E. 1982a. Health care on the immigrant trail. *Hospitals* 56 (1 October): 82-93.

_____. 1982b. Serving the poor and elderly in tough times. *Hospitals* 56 (1 December): 83-90.

_____.1986. Report on care of the medically indigent for the American Hospital Association Society for Hospital Marketing and Planning, Chicago.

Friendly, F. 1981. *Minnesota rag*. New York: Random House.

Lurie, N., et al. 1984. Termination from Medi-Cal: Does it affect health? *New England Journal of Medicine* 311:480-84.

Siegler, M. 1984. Speech at annual convention, Utah Hospital Association, Salt Lake City, 30 March.

Weissman, G. 1983. AIDS and heat. *Hospital Practice* 18 (October): 136.

CHAPTER 5

AIDS and the Political Process: A Federal Perspective

TIMOTHY WESTMORELAND

As one who has been involved with the politics of AIDS since 1981, perhaps longer than almost anyone, I agree to a large extent with Dennis Altman's observations on the politics of AIDS (see Chapter 2). I would quickly add, however, that my own experience has been only at the federal level.

With more than 16,000 cases of AIDS already diagnosed in the United States, with estimates of the number of cases of AIDS-related complex (ARC) running as high as 150,000, and at the rate the epidemic is currently progressing, by the time of the next Presidential election, more Americans will have died of AIDS than died in Vietnam. In view of the magnitude of this disease, there is little doubt that, to date, all levels of government in America, with few exceptions, have indeed failed in their response to AIDS.

There are, however, pockets of exemplary effort, particularly on the part of those scientists and others in the U.S. Public Health Service (USPHS), working under the weight of the Office of Management and Budget (OMB). They—like a number of scientists who are not a part of USPHS—have done remarkable work under often difficult circumstances. Although its record may not match that of the USPHS, the U.S. Congress has initiated and sustained funding for AIDS research and treatment and directed attention to the epidemic, largely in the face of a great deal of apathy from both the Reagan administration and the public at large.

APATHY, IRONY, AND THE POLITICS OF THE FEDERAL BUDGET

If we are losing the war against AIDS, it is because the present administration is allowing us to lose it, and because, by and large, a good many of the press, the professionals in health care and in the health care industry, and the public are allowing the administration to allow us to lose. As Dr. June Osborn, Dean of the School of Public Health at the University of

47

Michigan, very eloquently observed at the Institute of Medicine's 1985 annual meeting, it would be hard to imagine that the Greek gods could have given us a more cruel irony than this epidemic, during this administration, at this time in this culture (Osborn 1985, 1986).

Consider a few of the juxtapostitions for a moment: We have a budget-cutting—and, literally in some cases, budget-ending—administration, and a budget-busting epidemic on all fronts. We have a federal government that will not teach heterosexuals about birth control but that is now being forced to teach homosexual men about mutual masturbation. We have media that five years ago could not use the word "lover" in print or say that someone was "gay" in a newspaper, that are now having daily to describe anal intercourse to the general public. We have a medical and scientific community that has long considered itself above politics that is now being thrashed by the Left, Right, and Center on issues involving schools, bathhouses, and, indeed, its own research protocols. And we have a gay community, which for years wanted only to be left alone by the government, that has a crying need for the government that it has come to fear now more than ever.

We are losing the war against AIDS because of the Reagan administration, because of the politics of the budget, and because of the politics of sex. The budget issue is generic. I have to tell gay men day after day that they are not being singled out by the Reagan administration for budgetary cutbacks. The administration sends USPHS scientists, otherwise very credible people, day after day to commit virtual perjury before Congress on issues ranging from AIDS funding to childhood immunization and beyond. These scientists testify that administration budgets are adequate, and that all is being done that can be done. Then, these same officials go back and write desperate memoranda to the OMB about what will happen if they don't have more personnel or greater access to funds.

Much of public health is chronically underfunded, but the effect of underfunding for AIDS is potentially worse than for many other chronically underfunded public health agendas. If screening for childhood lead poisoning is not continued after this year, we'll have a finite level of increase of lead poisoning in children next year and the year after next. But if AIDS is not researched and treated, during this next year we will almost certainly have double, perhaps triple, perhaps even quadruple the number of cases. And the Gramm-Rudman-Hollings deficit reduction process that has already been adopted will only exacerbate this problem. The administration is already proposing, in response to Gramm-Rudman-Hollings, a reduction of $51 million—over 20 percent—in budget allocations for AIDS. The incidence of the disease can only go up as the budget dollars come down.

THE POLITICS OF SEX

The politics of sex have also affected the response of this administration to AIDS. Consider the current predominance of homosexual men among people with AIDS, and then consider that it was the Reagan administration's Director of White House Communications, Patrick Buchanan (1983), who postulated in print that AIDS is nature's revenge on homosexual men. Keep in mind that this is an administration whose New Right fundraisers have in many ways, both publicly and by mass mailings, raised money by campaigning against homosexuals and homosexual rights.

The administration's trouble with the politics of sex has also affected its attitude toward what needs to be done in the war against AIDS. It has been repeatedly pointed out that, with neither an effective treatment nor a vaccine against AIDS on the horizon, prevention of person-to-person AIDS virus transmission is currently the only way to stop its spread. And prevention is largely a matter of public education about how to prevent transmission. The effectiveness of education about AIDS and the potential of education and information programs to change the personal behaviors that facilitate transmission are demonstrated by facts such as the unprecedented decline in venereal disease rates among gay men over the past two years in communities where education and information programs have been implemented—usually, I might add, by the gay communities themselves, who have disseminated information about "safe sex." However, we have a federal administration that does not want to be seen or perceived as "condoning" homosexuality, and it does not want to talk about condoms to either gay or straight people, so federal education programs for AIDS prevention have not been forthcoming.

THE FAILURE OF THE MEDIA

It is also important to understand, I think, that the media have been at least unwitting accomplices in the Reagan administration's failure to respond adequately to the AIDS epidemic. In answer to Dennis Altman's question, in Chapter 2, about how this situation is allowed to go on, about how people—the administration, in particular—can remain silent, and why attention has not been focused on this failure, I would point out that it was not until 1985 that President Reagan was ever asked a direct question about AIDS by the media (Presidential Press Conference 1985).

Of course, AIDS had not been ignored until then. AIDS had already become a big issue in 1983. It was on the covers of all the major newsmagazines, and interest peaked. Then, in April 1984, Margaret Heckler, Secretary of the Department of Health and Human Services, announced not only that the AIDS virus had been identified but also that we would have a treatment for the disease within two years—a period that has come and gone with no actual effective treatment. As a result of that announcement, media pressure went down, public confidence went up, and, for a time, there was a false sense of security.

It was not until August 1985, with the diagnosis of Rock Hudson's AIDS, that the media began to take the issue to the public again. By that time, however, it was already very late, and even the administration had begun to recommend increased funding for AIDS research and treatment, albeit under the threat of a Congressional subpoena of budget documents.

THE FAILURE OF THE HEALTH CARE COMMUNITY

I would also point out that professionals in the health care community and the health insurance industry have done little to help move the administration. They have been slow to recognize the politics of the situation, and they have been slower still to pressure the Congress and the administration. The issues of funding for AIDS research, treatment, prevention, and education have been left, for the most part, to AIDS-specific groups and the gay community alone. Where were those health and life insurance companies and their spokespersons, who now want to use the HTLV-III/LAV antibody test to screen out their underwriting risks, when AIDS prevention and research funding was being debated in the Congress? The sort of credibility that those groups could bring would have helped enormously, and only now are they beginning to realize that their lack of action then will likely cost them billions of dollars over the next few years.

Where was the American Medical Association when confidentiality of antibody test results began to become an issue two years ago? Where were the hospital administrators and the American Hospital Association when treatment costs became an unquenchable sponge soaking up ever larger sums of public money? And where are they now, when these issues are still being debated in the Congress?

THE LOBBYING ROLE OF THE GAY COMMUNITY

The only people who come to Washington directly lobbying on these points and issues are gay groups and members of other AIDS risk groups. The insurance and health organizations, that have millions and billions of dollars, and in some cases, in fact, the solvency of their industry to worry about, have not begun a concentrated effort on AIDS lobbying.

However, the gay community, too, must assume some responsibility for allowing the administration to fail in its response to AIDS. While this group has been exemplary in its struggle for research and education funding, and its lobbying for AIDS-related appropriations has produced amazing results for a usually disenfranchised group, it also has suffered from a failure of synthesis of thought, as both Dennis Altman, and, in Chapter 4, Emily Friedman have pointed out.

The first reaction of many of the gay people to whom I have spoken about AIDS is, "This sort of thing with the government is not supposed to happen to me. I'm white, I'm male, I'm affluent. The government works for my benefit." It is with a great deal of displeasure that I have to point out to these people that an administration that would cut funds for childhood polio immunization, that allows infant mortality to rise around the country, and that discharges elderly people from the hospital while they are still sick will not turn to gay people as the first group to whom they will suddenly show compassion. And gays who continue to look for AIDS funding while supporting the President's economic plan for higher military spending and lower taxes simply are not paying attention to what is going on in Congress.

AIDS ISSUES IN A BROADER CONTEXT

Medicaid, for instance, is an AIDS issue now. It has been found to be an AIDS issue through hard experience over the past few years. Social Security is becoming an AIDS issue, as well. Medicare will become an AIDS issue very soon. And, as I have pointed out for a long time to gay community leaders, Medicare is already a gay issue. Who, for example, are those people who reach age 65 without extended families on whom they can depend for support when they are chronically ill or disabled? Those people are in many cases single. And even though AIDS patients have not suddenly become a major drain on the Medicare budget, gay people should be greatly concerned that the Medicare program is also being gutted by this administration.

WHAT NEEDS TO BE DONE? WHO SHOULD DO IT?

So what can be done? Clearly, AIDS education is needed in the halls of Congress as much as in the streets of New York City's Lower East Side. At the national level, health care organizations, medical and hospital associations, and insurance companies can make it known that AIDS is something that affects political districts other than Manhattan, West Hollywood, San Francisco, Miami, and Houston. Then, the Congress will begin to respond, because for a long time it has looked at AIDS as a problem of limited geographical impact rather than one of national import. For instance, many people in Congress have yet to understand that large-scale health insurers are going to experience AIDS in terms of financial difficulties that may affect their fiscal stability.

However, lobbying should not be left entirely to the specialists in Washington. The easiest and most effective way for Americans to communicate these concerns about AIDS to their representatives in Congress is through professional associations and personal contact at the local level. Congressional district offices are the most underutilized resource in the American political system: People who come to Washington to get two minutes of a representative's time are wasting their efforts. An infectious disease specialist in Portland, Maine, for example, can be much more effective by spending 40 minutes with a district-office staff person, who will then communicate to the member of Congress that someone in Portland, Maine, actually cares what is happening in regard to AIDS and that it is not an issue of concern only to Manhattanites.

CONCLUSION

I must say that, unfortunately, I think the politics of AIDS are only going to become worse. The medical McCarthyites are already gearing up for what they are going to do with AIDS as a campaign issue. Major journalists are telling politicians of all stripes that AIDS is the undiscovered election issue of 1986 and 1988. The political problems—the substantive issues of insurance, hospital costs, antibody testing, quarantine, and so forth—are not going away; they will grow in prominence right along with the census of AIDS patients. Futhermore, as such widely diverse works as Daniel DeFoe's *A Journal of the Plague Year* ([1722] 1984) and Allan Brandt's *No Magic Bullet* (1985) make clear, we may never be very far removed from hysteria and overreaction in the political arena where epidemics are concerned.

Finally, the overriding question for health care policymakers, community leaders, social workers, people with or at risk for AIDS—indeed, for all of us—is, quite simply, How can we move those people who are in charge to honestly, compassionately, and fearlessly care and work to make the American system of government effectively confront the AIDS epidemic and diminish the suffering and social dislocation in its wake.

REFERENCES

Brandt, A. 1985. *No magic bullet: A social history of venereal disease in the United States since 1880.* New York: Oxford University Press.

Buchanan, P. 1983. AIDS disease: It's nature striking back. *New York Post,* 24 May.

DeFoe, D. [1722] 1984. *A journal of the plague year.* reprint. New York: New American Library.

Osborn, J. E. 1985. Speech at conference, Mobilizing Against AIDS: The Unfinished Story of a Virus, sponsored by the Institute of Medicine, National Academy of Sciences, Washington, DC, 16-17 October.

_____. 1986. The AIDS epidemic: Multidisciplinary trouble. *New England Journal of Medicine* 314:779-82.

Presidential Press Conference, 1985. Ronald Reagan, at the White House, 17 September. *Weekly Compilation of Presidential Documents.* Washington, DC: U.S. Office of the Federal Register, 23 September, 1105.

PART THREE

AIDS
and the
Schools

CHAPTER 6

Public Policy and Risk Assessment in the AIDS Epidemic

DAVID J. ROTHMAN

No single issue better frames the central concerns of public policy and risk assessment in the acquired immune deficiency syndrome (AIDS) epidemic than the controversy over the presence in the public schools of students with the illness. To some observers, the attempt by groups of parents to have students—and staff—with AIDS excluded from the schools is the clearest indication of public hysteria. To others, the protests seem entirely understandable and justifiable. As one angry, but puzzled, parent asked a representative of the New York City Department of Health, "If a child has lice you send him home immediately. If a child has AIDS you keep him in the classroom. How can that be?"

AIDS AND THE UNKNOWN

AIDS has many unique and unprecedented features. Too young to remember the summer scares about polio in the early 1950s, not to mention the deep concern about tuberculosis in earlier decades, no one under the age of 45 in the United States has any firsthand experience with a deadly and transmissible disease. Nevertheless, this is hardly the first time that policy decisions must be made when the number of unknowns is high and the potential injury significant. In the debate about appropriate responses to AIDS, as in many other controversies, the dispute comes down to judgments of how far one will allow potential negative consequences to determine social policy. What is the appropriate degree of risk tolerance as against risk aversion? Are policy decisions to be made on the basis of the best-case or the worst-case scenario? Are all the many unknowns to be put in the favorable or unfavorable outcome column?

Although the literature on risk analysis is substantial—with findings available on how individuals will balance future losses against immediate gains, or sacrifice small gains to minimize the possibility of greater losses—we know very little about how one or another public issue ends up in the risk-maximizing or risk-minimizing category (Covello 1983). In

57

some areas, public policy tends to adopt apocalyptic thinking and do everything possible to avoid a negative outcome, even if the probability of that outcome is judged to be quite low. In other instances, apocalyptic thinking seems very foreign to policy considerations and day-to-day decisions are made with little regard for potential disaster.

Before attempting to analyze where AIDS fits into this framework, let us briefly examine one or two other cases, for they will demonstrate that no obvious reasons determine how distinctions are made. The common-sense notion, for example, that the greater the possible risk, the more likely that apocalyptic visions will abound and that everything possible will be done to avert the disaster, turns out not to be a useful predictor of policy directions.

APOCALYPTIC THINKING

There are two classic instances in which apocalyptic thinking dominates much, although certainly not all, policy consideration. The most obvious one is nuclear war; the other is nuclear energy. In both cases, debate and decision-making are in deep dialogue with the possibility of catastrophe. Those who would block the development of nuclear energy, for example, point to the potential failure of plant safety mechanisms and insist that the benefits of nuclear power are far outweighed by the risks, even if the risks are relatively low. They repeatedly cite the 1979 incident at the Three Mile Island nuclear facility near Harrisburg, Pennsylvania; indeed, it is not difficult to imagine how much more heated their rhetoric would be had even one or two deaths occurred there. In any event, when it comes to issues involving nuclear power, the debate is often framed in apocalyptic terms.

Yet, there are other potential disasters that could be almost as devastating as what would follow from nuclear power plant failures that do not raise such specters. The injuries that would follow from the collapse of a dam are not necessarily fewer than those that would result from the malfunction of a nuclear power plant, but the public concern about regulation of dam safety or the location of dams in areas with a high likelihood of earthquakes certainly does not rise to the level evoked by nuclear energy. Somehow, death from drowning is not perceived to be as terrifying as death from radiation.

So too, significant health damage from pesticides is probably more real and extensive at the moment than damage from nuclear power plants, but, by comparison, the level of agitation is low. And, to cite examples from the area of drugs and medical innovations, it is clear that apocalyptic visions are not allowed to keep new therapies out of the marketplace. We do not, as a matter of course, test all drugs for safety to the children of the users, although we have no way of knowing when we may be creating a second diethylstilbestrol (DES) incident. By the same token, no restrictions are being placed on *in vitro* fertilization programs, despite the imaginable possibility of some grave defect in the children or grandchildren of those born from test tube procedures. In brief, the willingness to maximize an unknown risk is not spread evenly among policy debates; the gravity of the risk is not by itself determinative of the public response. At times, we are prepared to run the risk of danger to gain benefits; at other times, we are not, and where an issue will appear on this scale is not easily predicted.

APOCALYPTIC THINKING AND PUBLIC HEALTH

From this perspective, let us move directly into the field of public health. Here, one finds a tradition of maximizing the degree of risk and taking all measures that seem necessary to counter it. Public health practitioners generally tend to act upon apocalyptic visions, to treat unknowns as unfavorable outcomes. When in doubt, they assume that the risks are maximal and they will recommend doing everything possible to avert them.

The great swine flu disaster of 1976

The example that best demonstrates this mind-set in action is the 1976 swine flu incident (Neustadt and Feinberg 1977). After some American soldiers were diagnosed as harboring an influenza virus that was antigenically related to the influenza virus of the 1918–1919 epidemic, the Centers for Disease Control (CDC) had to confront the question of the likelihood of the spread of the disease to the general population, and to determine what precautionary steps, if any, should be taken. The CDC's subsequent decision to recommend vaccinating the entire population of the United States clearly reflected the triumph of apocalyptic thinking.

At the time, there was no consensus among public health experts on the likelihood of a swine flu epidemic. A significant body of opinion held that the CDC should do nothing. However, this group lost out in the debate precisely because it could not demonstrate that the epidemic would *not* occur. The burden of proof fell on those who would minimize the potential risk; they had to prove conclusively that the disaster would not happen. In other words, the operating assumption was that those who predicted disaster were right until proven wrong. As long as no one could conclusively demonstrate that the untoward event would *not* take place, health policy assumed that it *would* occur, and moved to counteract it. When risks cannot be ruled out, they must be ruled in. In the field of public health, a virus or its carrier is guilty until proven innocent.

In the end, of course, the swine flu epidemic did not materialize, but a number of vaccine recipients developed Guillain-Barré syndrome. The effects of the vaccination policy were costly not only in terms of energy and fiscal resources but also in actual harm done. Thus, it must be remembered that acting on the worst-possible-case scenario is not a neutral decision or without costs of its own. The actions taken can and often do have important negative consequences.

The case of hepatitis B in the classroom

Another example of the public health readiness to maximize risks—and one that is even more immediately relevant to the AIDS controversy—involved a consideration of the threat that hepatitis B carriers posed to their classmates and teachers in New York public schools (Rothman and Rothman 1984). A 1975 consent decree called for the return to the community of some 5,400 severely and profoundly retarded residents at the Willowbrook State School on Staten Island. Hepatitis B had been endemic at the institution, so endemic, in fact, that pediatrician-researcher Dr. Saul Krugman felt justified in purposefully injecting the virus into new arrivals in order to study the etiology of the disease. Not surprisingly, about 40 of those residents released to the community, and who subsequently attended public schools, were hepatitis B carriers.

After an incident in September 1977, in which a Staten Island teacher of the retarded came down with hepatitis (at first thought to be hepatitis B but which turned out to be hepatitis A), the Board of Education and the Department of Health became concerned about the possibility of contagion. The Department of Health sent two staff members to observe the carriers in their classrooms and they reported an epidemiological nightmare: the carriers hugged, kissed, drooled over, and shared food and drink with their susceptible classmates. After convening a task force of hepatitis B researchers and other public health professionals, the Department of Health recommended segregating the carriers in their own classrooms, on the grounds that the risk of contagion was great. One new case of hepatitis B was one case too many, and, given the risks of the spread of disease, the carriers had to be isolated from day-to-day contact with susceptible students. Upon receiving this recommendation, the Board of Education went a step beyond the Department of Health's advice and summarily expelled the carriers from the schools.

Civil liberties versus public health

Since the Willowbrook deinstitutionalization effort had been spearheaded and supervised by a group of civil libertarian lawyers, the Board of Education's action was immediately contested. Attorneys for the ex-Willowbrook residents moved to enjoin the expulsion, and the federal courtroom became the setting for a fascinating and revealing conflict between a public health outlook and a civil libertarian point of view.

The public health representatives argued that, because the carriers were so likely to transmit hepatitis B through blood or saliva contact with susceptible persons, it was appropriate to adopt preventive measures such as carrier segregation. Since no one could demonstrate that the carriers would not seed the classrooms with the hepatitis B virus, the carriers had to be isolated. The civil libertarians, on the other hand, insisted that the students could not be penalized in advance of any demonstrable evidence of contagion. They maintained that, since there was no documented case of any student in a classroom with a carrier contracting hepatitis B, the carriers should not be deprived of their right to an education in the least restrictive setting. The carriers were, according to the civil libertarian view, innocent until proven guilty, and predictions of dangerousness were not dispositive.

After hearing this dispute, the court ruled in favor of the civil libertarians: Judges are not in the habit of penalizing anyone without proof of guilt. The conflict did not end there, however; the Department of Health next tested the blood of all the classmates of the carriers and discovered that six of them had antibodies to the hepatitis B virus, a finding that the Department of Health presented as evidence of contagion and a justification for isolation. The civil libertarian attorneys countered that, since this was the first time that the classmates had been tested, there was no way of knowing whether the change in antibody status had occurred before the carriers entered the classrooms, or was the result of contact in some other, non-classroom setting. Again, there was a difference in the evidence that a public health specialist found conclusive, as compared to an attorney. The public health professional is trained to act on suspicion; the civil libertarian lawyer represents a tradition in which suspicions are not enough. Not surprisingly, the court adopted the civil libertarian perspective: It was unwilling to penalize anyone—whether a carrier or an accused felon—without firm evidence; it wanted a smoking gun, not a statistical probability.

A ruling with relevance to AIDS

One final consideration led the court to rule against the Board of Education and the Department of Health, a consideration that also has direct relevance to the AIDS issue. The Department of Health offered recommendations for policy toward mentally retarded hepatitis B carriers but not toward any other group of carriers. Its proposals did not affect hepatitis B carriers who might be surgeons or dentists or gays or persons of Chinese origin or dialysis patients, all groups with abnormally high percentages of carriers. In fact, it was the reluctance of the Department of Health to write a general code about hepatitis B carriers that kept it in a posture of recommending actions but not promulgating binding regulations, and the court took this distinction very seriously. It appeared that the retarded were being singled out for special, discriminatory treatment. If this were not so, then why had the Department of Health failed to follow its own established procedures and issued a binding and general administrative ruling?

APOCALYPTIC THINKING AND AIDS

Judged against the background of the swine flu and hepatitis B incidents, one would have anticipated that both the societal and public health responses to the AIDS crisis would be quintessentially apocalyptic. The disease is deadly; it makes hepatitis B seem trivial by comparison. The groups most affected, male gays and intravenous (IV) drug users, are stigmatized and considered socially deviant. Indeed, among the gays, it is thought that the most sexually active or "promiscuous" are at greatest risk and disproportionately affected. Here, then, is a disease that victims seem to bring on themselves, and hence any risk that they pose to others might well be defined as too great. Some proponents of such a position argue that the moral culpability of the victims, their blameworthiness, justifies measures that would protect others from the possibility of contagion; others in this camp avoid moral judgments but fault the AIDS victims for not adopting safer sexual or drug habits. In either case, the thinking goes, "the rest of us" should not run the risk of danger because "they" behaved badly or imprudently. Thus, if ever incentives existed to put all the unknowns into the dismal outcome column, for considering the risks to be maximal rather than minimal, surely AIDS is that case.

Predictably, there are groups that have adopted and urged this very approach, and segments of the media have encouraged and supported it. Even among those not prone to define gays as blameworthy or culpable, the risk of contagion seems to justify an exclusionary response. Some of the parents who have wanted to remove AIDS-afflicted students and teachers—and even those who only test positive for AIDS virus antibodies—from their children's classrooms are not responding to AIDS hysteria so much as to the lessons of good health care that have been learned

over the years. These parents have been trained to believe that lice is sufficient grounds for keeping a child out of school and that youngsters with
sore throats should be kept home so as to minimize contagion. Without
belaboring the point, American society tends to be obsessive in matters of
health. So how unreasonable would it be to conclude that, if saccharine
can be banned because megadoses fed to mice proved to be carcinogenic,
then, in a crisis situation, surely a student with AIDS can be excluded
from a classroom?

Notions of catastrophe have not dominated

Despite the seeming likelihood of apocalyptic thinking, the extent to
which the AIDS threat has been met with reasoned, sane, and non-
exclusionary responses is remarkable. Had someone 20 years ago described an epidemic like AIDS and predicted the public response, surely
findings would have been in the direction of massive hysteria and extraordinary sanctions. However, to date, apocalyptic thinking has not marked
the general reaction, although, with little difficulty, one could sketch an
apocalyptic ending to this epidemic. In fact, several leading AIDS researchers, including Harvard University's William Haseltine and Myron
Essex, have begun to draw this very picture. "The dire predictions of those
who have cried doom ever since AIDS appeared," Essex told the *New York
Times Magazine*, "haven't been far off the mark" (Hunt 1986). Haseltine
informed a Senate subcommittee that "for every case of reported AIDS in
the United States there are about 100 or more carriers . . . Once infected,
infected for life. . . . We see a wave of devastating disease approaching"
(Hunt). To date, however, notions of impending catastrophe have not been
the dominant theme of scientists' statements.

By the same token, many of the leading daily newspapers and weekly
magazines have been educative, not inflammatory, in their editorials and
news coverage of AIDS, and have taken the minimal-risk side in policy
arguments. The editorial page of the *New York Times* (1985), for example,
has more consistently adopted a civil libertarian stance on AIDS matters
than on the rights of the homeless or the mentally ill. Nor have the public
health professionals been as unanimous or aggressive in this case, as they
have been in others, in staking out a guilty-until-proven-innocent position. The posture of the New York City Department of Health regarding
AIDS, for example, is far more risk tolerant than it was with hepatitis B.

The situation is volatile

To be sure, the situation is volatile and hysteria can be contagious. Incidents of rank discrimination have certainly occurred; one would probably want to include on this side of the ledger the recent attempts to shut

down a few bathhouses, not to mention hearings held in the state of Texas on the right to quarantine persons with AIDS. Generally, though, in the conflict between a public health "guilty-till-proven-innocent" stance and the civil libertarian "innocent-until-proven-guilty" attitude, the AIDS victims and potential victims have been spared many imaginable sanctions and reprisals. Compulsory testing for HTLV-III/LAV* antibodies or the virus is not the rule, outside the armed forces at least, and boards of health are not carrying out massive screening efforts. Neither universities in general nor medical schools in particular are revising application procedures to screen out gays; neither are they asking students to take blood tests. Attempts by insurance companies to discriminate against gays are being contested, with some success. Calling for the massive segregation or quarantine of people with AIDS has so far been a fringe effort. School-children with AIDS appear more often than not to be able to keep their places in classrooms. All of this suggests that what needs explaining most is why, to date, the civil libertarian perspective, rather than the traditional public health one, has dominated.

THE ROLE OF POLITICS

Some of the answer may rest in politics. By happenstance, the majority of people with AIDS live in the two states with the highest number of electoral votes, California and New York. So, Congressional pressure for earmarking funds for AIDS research, and the administration's approval, however grudging and inadequate, points to the importance of not alienating a large bloc of voters. By the same token, people with AIDS cluster in the two cities and states whose political leaders have been relatively enlightened on gay rights in general and, now, on AIDS in particular. Gays are a much stronger political force than, for example, the retarded, and hence AIDS victims are being dealt with in ways that the hepatitis B carriers were not.

There is no doubt that part of the reason for the more tolerant response to people with AIDS reflects the continuing strength in the 1980s of a minority rights orientation. Following the civil rights agitation of the 1960s, the gays won their place as a minority group, and penalizing them is often viewed on a par with penalizing women, blacks, or the mentally handicapped. In a very real way, the court victory that the hepatitis B carriers won in 1978 works to the benefit of AIDS victims in 1986, making it all the more likely that measures that claim to be advancing the public health will be judged by civil libertarian, rather than public health, stan-

---

*Human T-lymphotropic virus type III/lymphadenopathy-associated virus.

dards, and that, when the conflict between the two is acute, civil liberties will prevail.

THE ROLE OF HEALTH CARE PROFESSIONALS

The part that physicians and other health care professionals have played in reassuring the public should not be minimized. They have explained that the virus does not appear to be easily transmitted—one physician has called it a "pathogenic weakling" (Osborn 1986)—and that, absent intimate and sustained contact, the risks of contagion are very low. Perhaps their stance would have been different had even a handful of health professionals not in known risk groups succumbed to the disease in the course of diagnosing it or treating it. Standard precautions in handling blood, however, have proved completely efficacious for health care workers, and research findings have been able to demonstrate why this is so. Still, in and of itself, this message might not have been heard, and the fright around AIDS could have been so great as to render the public incapable of grasping the information.

It is also possible that public health professionals have learned some lessons from past actions. The head of the New York City Department of Health through 1985, David Sencer, headed the CDC during the swine flu scare, and the criticism leveled at him in that affair may have influenced him to adopt a very different strategy with regard to AIDS. So too, the Department of Health may have learned something from the hepatitis B litigation and decided this time to proceed more cautiously.

A COURT TEST OF AIDS PUBLIC HEALTH POLICY

That disputes about AIDS frequently end up in the courtroom has helped ensure an equitable response, as evidenced by the New York Supreme Court decision, in February 1986, on the rights of students with AIDS to attend public school (*District 27 Community School Board* v. *The Board of Education of the City of New York*; Supreme Court, Queens County; 11 February 1986; Index No. 14940/85). In the fall of 1985, the New York City Board of Education adopted a policy that children with AIDS would not be automatically excluded from the schools; instead, each case would be reviewed individually. The review that followed permitted the admission of a child with AIDS to a Queens County school, whereupon two local community school boards and the parent of a public school child went to court to obtain a permanent injunction against the admission of pupils with AIDS. A five-week trial ensued, attracting wide press coverage. Many of those who participated in the proceedings, noting the ways in which the issues were framed and considering the asides and questions of the judge, predicted that the court would grant the injunction.

To the contrary, however, the judge upheld the child's admission to school, and his decision in many ways echoed the federal court's findings in the Willowbrook case. Again, uncertainty was not allowed to become the basis for penalties. According to the ruling by Judge Harold Hyman, "Although this court certainly empathizes with the fears and concerns of parents . . . at the same time it is duty bound to objectively evaluate the issue of automatic exclusion according to the evidence gathered and not be influenced by unsubstantiated fears of catastrophe." Again, the court would not allow one group to be singled out for what seemed to be discriminatory action: "It is difficult to conceive of a rational justification imposing a discriminatory burden on known [AIDS] carriers . . . while untested and unidentified carriers still remain in the classroom where they pose the same theoretical (though undocumented) risks of transmitting the virus to normal children." In the end, the courts are not likely to allow sanctions to be imposed on vulnerable groups because they pose a "theoretical" risk.

QUARANTINE: INAPPROPRIATE AND INEFFECTIVE

It may be, too, that circumspection has outbalanced panic because, in truth, there is really very little that can be done on a grand scale to prevent the spread of AIDS. The traditional mechanisms by which early modern communities combatted the spread of epidemics are irrelevant. It makes no sense to talk of sealing one's borders to keep out gays, IV drug users, or AIDS patients in particular. The other major weapon, quarantine, is equally ineffective. On the one hand, it is probably too late; on the other, the logistics of quarantining no fewer than one million people are truly daunting.

Moreover, exploring the history of plagues and epidemics reveals a record of the failure of quarantines. In seventeenth-century Tuscany, for example, there were constant struggles between the authorities and the townspeople over such orders, and the authorities generally lost. They would appoint watchmen to make certain that the co-residents of a plague victim did not leave their quarters, and the residents would then proceed to bribe the watchmen and sneak out at night. So, too, disputes over the costs involved in maintaining the quarantine were bitter. Every family confined was a family that had to be fed, and the towns vigorously protested the expense (Cipolla 1980; Defoe [1722] 1984).

The historical precedents suggest only a few of the problems that would face any contemporary effort to quarantine (Mills et al. 1986). Imagine trying to select those who would be forced into an encampment: Would the gays be expected to identify themselves? Would there be hearings in cases of a protest of misidentification? Imagine keeping people inside the encampment: Would it have barbed wire? Imagine trying to care for those in the encampment: Would the food be prison fare? Would the inmates be expected to keep internal order? Even so brief an exercise makes clear how utterly fantastic notions of quarantine are.

CONCLUSION

None of this is to suggest that the story is over or that less extreme, but nevertheless important, discriminatory measures are unlikely. The possibility that gays will be deprived of the opportunity to purchase life or health insurance is strong, and so is the potential for job discrimination. If, as is expected, the number of AIDS cases climbs—with the number of new cases in 1986 equaling the total of all previous cases—then the possibilities for discrimination in jobs, housing, and even in access to health care services will be greater. And if female-to-male transmission becomes frequent, the public—and public health—attitude could change markedly.

Aware of all that may happen, however, it still remains impressive that, thus far, civil liberties concerns have been more influential than traditional public health orientations, and that the representatives of public health, the media, and a large segment of the public have been more sensitive to civil liberties issues in this crisis than in others. Not that the conflict between the two orientations is, in theory, any less severe. Rather, the initial responses have tilted more to the civil liberties side.

In this same spirit, we have allowed the existing data, not the possibility of catastrophic events, to set the basis for policy: Children with AIDS are being allowed in public classrooms. In fact, a poll of adult Americans, conducted by the Gallup Organization in March 1986, indicated not only that 98 percent of the respondents were aware of AIDS but also that two-thirds of them would permit their children to attend school with an AIDS-afflicted student (*New York Times* 1986). Although it is possible that all that we have seen so far is the sore throat before the flu strikes, fears of catastrophe have not become the foundation for public policy or, by and large, other reactions. In sum, apocalyptic visions have not carried the day, a fact that is one more astonishing feature of this astonishing epidemic.

REFERENCES

Cipolla, C. M. 1980. *Faith, reason, and the plague in 17th century Tuscany.* Trans. M. Kittel. Ithaca, NY: Cornell University Press.

Covello, V. 1983. The perception of technological risks: A literature review. *Technological Forecasting and Social Change* 23:285–97.

Defoe, D. [1722] 1984. *A journal of the plague year.* Reprint. New York: New American Library.

Hunt, M. 1986. Teaming up against AIDS. *New York Times Magazine,* 2 March, 42, 81–82.

Mills, M., C. B. Wofsy, and J. Mills. 1986. The acquired immunodeficiency syndrome: Infection control and public health law. *New England Journal of Medicine* 314:931–36.

Neustadt, R., and H. Feinberg. 1977. The epidemic that never was: Policy making and the swine flu scare. In *Influenza in America 1918–1976: History, science, and politics,* ed. J. Osborn. Canton, MA: Neale Watson Academic Publications.

New York Times. 1985. AIDS and the new apartheid. Editorial. 7 October.

New York Times. 1986. Poll finds support for pupils with AIDS. 17 April.

Osborn, J. E. 1986. The AIDS epidemic: Multidisciplinary trouble. *New England Journal of Medicine* 314:779–82.

Rothman, D. J., and S. M. Rothman. 1984. *The Willowbrook wars: A decade of struggle for social justice.* New York: Harper & Row, Chap. 11.

CHAPTER 7

District 27 v. Board of Education

ROBERT G. SULLIVAN

In Chapter 6, David Rothman speaks of hysteria over the issue of students with AIDS in public schools. If there was any hysteria about AIDS in the schools in New York City in 1985, it was manifested by my clients, the parents and local school board who went to court to challenge the New York City Board of Education's decision to place an anonymous seven-year-old child with AIDS in a public school classroom in the Borough of Queens. I know that that is not a popular position as far as the medical and health policymaking professions are concerned, nor is it a popular position with the City of New York. However, I want to explain that hysteria and examine its context. The point is that this sort of hysteria should not have had to happen. It should not have happened in New York; it should not happen in other cities.

I want to examine how public health officials dealt with the issue of AIDS in the schools in the City of New York, and, in doing that, I must say at the outset that I am not going to have anything good to say about the City of New York, the Department of Health of the City of New York, or the Board of Education of the City of New York.

AIDS IN THE SCHOOLS: TWO POLICY APPROACHES

New York City

How did New York handle the problem of AIDS in the public classroom? I want to begin by comparing how this issue has been handled in two neighboring geographic areas: New York and Connecticut. In 1984, New York City Schools Chancellor Nathan Quinones recognized the impending problem of school-aged children with AIDS and wrote to the city's Department of Health. He pointed out that, in September 1985, the city was going to be confronted with the problem of AIDS in schools, and asked, what should we do? He asked the Department of Health for some guidelines. That was a year ahead of time. And that was a very responsible thing for Chancellor Quinones to do. Unfortunately, he got no response, and apparently did little to get a response.

The State of Connecticut

Compare that result with what happened in Connecticut, which did not really have a significant AIDS problem. At the same time that Chancellor Quinones asked the New York City Department of Health for guidelines, the Department of Education in Connecticut also was looking for guidance. They brought together 35 experts—pediatricians, neurologists, nurses, psychologists, attorneys, educators, social workers, parents—and they publicized who they were, and they had open hearings throughout the state. In March 1985, six months before school opened in the state of Connecticut, they published a document. It answers all the questions about AIDS in the schools; it tells what the guidelines are; it tells who drew it all up. And these guidelines were published months before the new school year began.

Waiting for guidelines in New York City

Meanwhile, what happened in New York? Nothing. On August 15, 1985, Chancellor Quinones wrote a letter to the New York City Deputy Mayor: He had asked for guidelines, he told the Deputy Mayor. School is going to open in two weeks and he still did not have any guidelines.

Five days before school was scheduled to begin, New York City appointed a panel: one doctor, one educator, one social worker, one parent. The panel held one meeting and, 36 hours before the school doors were scheduled to open, its members announced that they were going to put children with AIDS in the New York City public school classrooms. And there it was, in all the newspapers and on television, right after the Rock Hudson episode, just when public awareness of AIDS was at a peak. There had been no hearings, an inadequate panel, and an important public policy announced only 36 hours before it was going to be implemented. And there were protests. The parents wanted to know what was going on; in the Borough of Queens, a school boycott was organized. What did New York City officials expect?

Compare how well Connecticut's public health department handled this problem with how poorly New York City's public health officials responded. Consider that during that entire 15 months from the time Chancellor Quinones first asked for guidelines until school opened—and beyond—there was no education about AIDS—no education of the public, and, more importantly, no education of the teachers. Thus it was not only the public that was unprepared for this situation; the teachers were not prepared, either. A teacher who is going to school on Monday morning finds out on Saturday night that he or she might have an AIDS child in the classroom, with no guidelines about how to handle the situation. No wonder a group of parents in the Borough of Queens, represented by their district school board and me, went to court.

POLICY AT THE BAR: WHAT THE TRIAL REVEALED

The parents and District Board 27 went to court to stop the city from placing a child with AIDS in public classrooms. We did not go into court to prove that AIDS is transmitted by casual contact; we all understand that it is not. However, not all the scientific facts on AIDS are in, and we did believe that a child with AIDS could pose a potential risk to other children because of the way children—especially young children—naturally behave. They may bite and scratch each other, and blood contact can occur, with a risk of virus transmission. This was not our hysterical fantasy; our expert witnesses were qualified people. We brought in, for example, Dr. Arye Rubinstein, the leading pediatric AIDS expert in the world.

What did the trial reveal? It revealed why the citizens of New York City lacked confidence in their public health officials—and public confidence is an important matter in public health. The City had said that those four appointed panelists made the decision to place a child with AIDS in a public classroom. At the trial, however, Dr. David Sencer, then New York City's Health Commissioner, testified that, no, he had made the decision, and he had made it weeks before the panel was even convened. Faced with that kind of revelation, how can the public have confidence in the next panel that comes along?

A communications gap

We also brought out in the trial that Chancellor Quinones had known all along—for eight months, in fact—that there were food handlers and workers with AIDS in the school system, and that apparently he had never told the Board of Health, never asked for advice about that AIDS matter from the Board of Health, and never even informed the board that the situation existed.

At the same time, when we went to trial, the plaintiffs all thought there was one child with AIDS in the schools, but, during the trial, a representative of the Department of Health reported that they estimated there were 300 children with AIDS virus in the New York City school system. Had the Department of Health informed the Board of Education about its estimate? No—not until the trial.

Apparently the Department of Health and the Board of Education do not talk to each other in New York City. There are food handlers with AIDS that the Board of Education knows about, but it does not tell the Department of Health. Meanwhile, the Department of Health knows about 300 students with the AIDS virus, but it does not tell the Board of Education. How can the Board of Education formulate policy and take safety precautions if it does not even know how many students with AIDS are attending school?

The Department of Health also asked us not to bring out the fact that health care workers had contracted the AIDS virus from needle-stick injuries, because it had not been widely publicized at the time (Centers for Disease Control 1985). This revelation, it was claimed, would cause hysteria among health care workers, and they would walk off the job when they learned about it. In actuality, that unhappy event did not come to pass, and about two weeks after we disclosed this information at the trial, it was published in a journal (Weiss, Saxinger, Rechtman, et al. 1985), and was the subject of a lecture at a conference in Minneapolis (Weiss, Rechtman, Saxinger, et al. 1985). Nevertheless, people did not panic, and health care workers did not walk off their jobs. The social reaction was calm.

THE MAYOR'S NEW PANEL

More importantly, during the trial, Edward Koch, Mayor of New York City, for whom I have great respect, saw what had transpired with that four-person panel—or, more accurately, what had not transpired—and put together a new panel of seven experts to consider the problem and what to do about it. These seven doctors, including two from among our expert witnesses, were asked to do two things:

1. Review the condition of the child in question.

2. Formulate safety guidelines to be implemented in New York City's school system.

Let's examine how the new panel—and these were very qualified people, the City's own people—disposed of its charge. The first thing they told us was that, although the City had said that the child had AIDS, the child actually had the AIDS *virus*. There is a difference. We understand that, but the virus is still infectious. And when do the people get a straight answer from their public health officials? On that aspect of the case, the new panel was totally wrong.

On the second charge, we were going to get safety guidelines to be implemented. During the trial, in a period of frustration one night, on television, I said that it will take them months to implement the guidelines. That's why we feel the child should be out of school, just for this school year. Draw up new guidelines. Come September of 1986, the new school year, rethink your position. Meanwhile, educate the AIDS child at home.

The City said no. They said we'll implement those safety precautions in weeks. And I said, it takes them months just to get chalk. Perhaps I should not have said that, but, now, in the middle of January 1986, let us look back on the City's assertion that it would take weeks: The panel was convened in the first week of October 1985; in November, they issued a release saying that the child did not have AIDS. What about the recommendations, the guidelines? On that, the panel would report further. In effect, "we'll get back to you."

Three and a half months later, there is still no report: there is still no policy; there are still no guidelines. We have Connecticut's. We do not have New York's. Connecticut does not have the problem; New York does. We said it would take months to implement the guidelines; the City said we would have them in weeks. Three and a half months later, we are still waiting for the panel's recommendations. What are we supposed to do? Schools cannot implement recommendations until they receive them.

WEIGHING THE UNCERTAINTIES

A personal reaction

It comes down to this: How do I, the attorney for the plaintiffs, feel about the subject? I spent five weeks in court arguing that the child should be out of the classroom. Someone had to take the position. I do not know whether the city's lawyer, Corporation Counsel Frederick A. O. Schwarz, Jr., believed fully what he was saying, and I know that I was not completely in agreement with the position I was representing in court. It was a public issue. We were not getting paid; we were trying to bring out the facts. Somebody had to take the legal position.

As for my personal feelings: Forty percent of the time, I think the child should be in the classroom; 40 percent of the time, I think the child should not be in the classroom. And 20 percent of the time, I do not know what I think.

What about the people and the experts who say that 100 percent of the time they are absolutely sure that the child should be in the classroom? I do not buy that. I do not buy that, and they scare me. Especially when we recall what happened with swine flu. First, we are told that a panel deliberated and made the decision to put a child with AIDS in the classroom; then we find out that, no, the decision really was made by one man, and kept a secret. And who is that one man? The same man who ran the federal swine flu program: Dr. David Sencer. You have to ask yourself questions.

ASSESSING THE RISKS

A question of choice

Consider the following: If a person chooses to go to a bathhouse, if a person chooses to go to a singles bar, if a person chooses to go to a restaurant, if a person chooses to work somewhere, or if a person chooses to get a blood transfusion, those are his or her choices, freely made. Why do we have to treat the school issue differently? Because we legislate that children *must* attend school; New York State law requires attendance from age 6 through 16. We do not require that anyone go to a restaurant, where he or she might worry about a food handler, but we legislate that children must go to school. Should we not also make it safe for them?

Furthermore, this was a seven-year-old child among seven-year-old children that we were talking about in this particular case. They are not responsible for their actions, as adults are. Who makes the decisions for these seven-year-old children? In addition, there is also the issue of protecting the AIDS-infected—and presumably immunologically deficient—child, whose health and welfare may be threatened by exposure to illnesses or normally harmless microbes carried by classmates. That is another problem that has to be raised and that should be considered when the question of sending children with AIDS into public classrooms is discussed.

We, the plaintiffs in this case, would err on the side of caution. And that is the first thing the mayor himself said back in August 1985. He thinks we, society, that is, should err on the side of caution. We agree; we would have educated the child at home. The New York City Board of Education says no, the child should be in the public school. There is no decision yet from the judge [as of January 16, 1986], but it is expected during the week of January 27.

THE ISSUE OF CONFIDENTIALITY IN THE CLASSROOM

I respect someone who says that the child should be in the classroom. As I indicated earlier, I feel that way 40 percent of the time. However, we believe the teacher, the principal, or the school nurse, on a confidential basis, at least, should know the child's identity—not to spread it around, but in the event of a problem. Connecticut agrees with that policy; it is written in their guidelines. Other states have done likewise. In fact, New York is the only city where nobody in the school system knows who the AIDS children are. So if the seven-year-old child gets a bloody nose, bleeds profusely, or bites someone and draws blood, no one knows whether there is a risk of spreading infection. If my seven-year-old child is sitting next to that child and something happens, do I have a right to know, so that I can have my child tested and, if necessary, monitor his or her health? I think so, but if the teacher in the classroom does not know who the AIDS child is, no one will ever know.

We recognize, of course, that in the event of some incident, if the child with AIDS bites another child, for example, and draws blood or otherwise exposes the other child to potential infection with AIDS virus, confidentiality may be blown when the second child's parents are informed of the risk encounter. However, the AIDS child and his or her parents are simply going to have to recognize the risk to confidentiality if such an event occurs, because the alternative is to have another child exposed to AIDS and do nothing about it. It is important, I think, to educate the child with AIDS, and the child's parents, and emphasize as much as possible that behavior that risks virus transmission should not take place. Once an incident happens, though, I think that the parents of the healthy child who may have been exposed to AIDS have a right to know.

By and large, I think we have to have confidence in the teachers to handle these matters discreetly. They are, after all, professionals. We keep hearing concern about hysteria. The hysteria from the people in Queens has come and gone. It was expectable under the circumstances, and it was not too bad. The health care workers did not walk off the job when they found out about a couple of needle-stick incidents. There was no hysteria there. We can educate the teachers, too. It should have been done in New York, as it was in Connecticut, before there was a crisis. And if teachers were adequately educated about AIDS, if they understood AIDS as health care professionals understand it, there is no doubt they would accept AIDS students in the classroom and handle them discreetly, but be aware of the risks if a situation arises.

CONCLUSION

In New York City we did not get the sort of studied, planned, and publicly-arrived-at approach to the problem of AIDS in the schools that is reflected in the way the state of Connecticut handled the question. And there was some hysteria, but the public, after all, has a right to know. It does not pay anymore, in this day and age, to lie to the public. Authorities should tell the public the truth and then treat the public intelligently. Above all, people in other cities should not wait until AIDS gets to their schools; they should follow Connecticut's example. They should send for Connecticut's guidelines, which are excellent.

As for New York, when someone gets New York City's guidelines on how we are going to deal with AIDS in the schools, please send them to me. I think it is a shame that they still do not exist. And I also think that public health officials in New York City could have prevented all the hysteria in Queens. The public will respond sensibly if you give them something sensible to which they can respond. However, do not wait until Saturday night, and then announce, "Hey, we're sending kids with AIDS to school on Monday morning."

EDITOR'S NOTE: In the case of *District 27 Community School Board* v. *The Board of Education of the City of New York* (Supreme Court, Queens County, Index No. 14940/85), discussed in this chapter by Mr. Sullivan, the attorney for the plaintiffs, New York State Supreme Court Justice Harold Hyman ruled on February 11, 1986, that children with AIDS could not automatically be excluded from regular classes in New York City public schools. Although Justice Hyman upheld the city's policy of determining on a case-by-case basis whether children with AIDS should attend normal classes, he also declared that city officials had arrived at their policy "behind the cloak of secrecy," and "perhaps unwittingly, let loose the forces of anxiety and fear." In addition, according to a report in the *New York Times* (Fried 1986), Justice Hyman also criticized unidentified "members of the medical community" who, he said, had "exacerbated the fears and fueled the passions" by their "professionally irresponsible and baseless characterizations" of AIDS as "a plague."

REFERENCES

Centers for Disease Control. 1985. Update: Evaluation of human T-lymphotropic virus type III/lymphadenopathy-associated virus infection in health-care personnel—United States. *Morbidity and Mortality Weekly Report* 34:575-77.

Fried, J. P. 1986. Judge backs AIDS policy of schools. *New York Times,* 11 February.

State of Connecticut. 1985. *Prevention of disease transmission in schools: Acquired immune deficiency syndrome (AIDS).* Hartford, CT: Department of Education and Department of Health Services.

Weiss, S. H., W. C. Saxinger, D. Rechtman, et al. 1985. HTLV-III infection among health care workers: Association with needle-stick injuries. *Journal of the American Medical Association* 254:2089-93.

Weiss, S. H., D. J. Rechtman, W. C. Saxinger, et al. 1985. HTLV-III seropositivity in health care workers. Abstract. 25th Interscience Conference on Antimicrobial Agents and Chemotherapy, American Society for Microbiology, Minneapolis, MN, 30 September-2 October.

CHAPTER 8

AIDS and "Otherness"

RALPH C. JOHNSTON, JR.

Those who strive to reduce the irrational fears surrounding AIDS frequently call for the disease to be responded to strictly on the basis of its implications for public health. In reality, however, AIDS is more than a public health issue: While it is obviously a disease syndrome whose parameters can be described and whose etiology is thought to be known, AIDS is also a symbol upon which have been projected several of the cultural anxieties of late twentieth-century America.

Only a few of these cultural anxieties, perhaps the most prominent, can be enumerated here. The first is probably the most obvious: AIDS is an occasion for cultural expressions of anxiety about sexuality in general and homosexuality in particular. The second anxiety involves attitudes about drug abuse; stereotypes about intravenous (IV) drug abusers also are projected onto people with AIDS. The perceived cultural marginality of both gay and bisexual males, as well as of IV drug abusers, creates, in the minds of many, a conception of AIDS as a disease of "The Other."

Such categories of "otherness" include, of course, the racial "other," and one of the neglected tragedies of AIDS is the extent to which "people of color" are affected. In the United States (leaving aside the scope of the epidemic in Central Africa), 25 percent of AIDS cases have occurred among blacks. Since blacks constitute only about 12.5 percent of the nation's population, there are twice as many AIDS cases among blacks as might be expected in a random racial distribution. Table 8.1, indicates the distribution of AIDS cases in the United States by racial and ethnic groups. The disproportion of black victims is even greater in pediatric AIDS, with 56 percent of those cases reported in the United States through September 30, 1985, occurring among black children (Boffey 1985).

Other minorities are also reflected among the numbers of people with AIDS. Hispanics, for example, compose 14 percent of the cases. In fact, "people of color" account for fully 39 percent of American AIDS cases nationwide, and in New York City they account for more than 50 percent. The public policy implications of this fact should seize the attention of educators, health care and social services providers, and others concerned with the quality of urban life, especially in those areas where most of these cases are found.

77

Table 8.1

Reported Cases of AIDS by Race/Ethnic Group,
United States, 1981 through 6 January 1986

RACE/ETHNIC GROUP	NUMBER	PERCENTAGE OF TOTAL
White	9,611	60
Black	4,041	25
Hispanic	2,287	14
Other/Unknown	199	1
TOTAL	16,138	100

SOURCE: Centers for Disease Control.

An additional factor involved in the cultural anxieties that have been projected onto AIDS is the public's seeming lack of confidence in modern medicine and, as Robert Sullivan has pointed out in Chapter 7, in those government bureaucracies whose responsibility it is to deal with public health.

Finally, there are, understandably, intense fears of death associated with AIDS. In Chapter 6, Professor Rothman mentions the issue of nuclearism. Both the threat of nuclear holocaust and the threat of AIDS present late-twentieth-century America with two realities which are ultimately fatal and for which, at present, there seem to be no cures. In a culture that has relied so heavily on technology for answers to many of its problems, these two grinning skulls—AIDS and nuclear war—represent our real inability to solve the issue of our mortality with any "magic bullet."

AIDS AND APOCALYPTIC THINKING

Professor Rothman contends that, by and large, the response of the public health departments has been a considered response rather than an apocalyptic one. I would concur in that judgment as far as public health officials in New York and San Francisco are concerned. In light of the cultural anxieties I have outlined above, however, I am not at all sure that we will not see somewhere an exhibition of the catastrophic dimensions of apocalyptic thinking on the part of some of the institutions responsible for the establishment of public policy in America.

Consider, for example, that in Houston in the fall of 1985 a group of candidates styling themselves "the straight slate" in a city council election campaign proposed that all local food handlers, day-care workers, and blood-bank employees be required to take AIDS virus antibody tests and carry health cards as a condition of employment (*Wall Street Journal* 1985). A bill submitted in the Florida legislature would require that students with AIDS be separated from the rest of the school population, that any teacher infected with AIDS be dismissed, and that students and teachers submit to an antibody test if there were probable cause to suspect infection (Merritt and Toff 1986). And an AIDS cover story in a recent issue of a health care publication was illustrated with a bomb with a burning fuse (*Hospitals* 1986).

Segments of the general public have been beating the apocalyptic drum, too. Religious leaders of the fundamentalist right have been in the vanguard, with the media close at hand. Newscaster Chuck Scarborough, for example, anchored a series entitled, "Is God Punishing Us?" on WNBC-TV News, in New York City, not too long ago, during which AIDS was cited as one of the realities that stimulated the question (Scarborough 1984). As one who is involved in AIDS education within this cultural context, I would like to respond to the issue of AIDS and apocalyptic thinking that Professor Rothman has raised.

In Greek, apokalypsis means "to uncover." In Judaism and early Christianity it was claimed that God had revealed to one person the secret of the imminent end of the world; that anonymous writer had been given a message that was to be proclaimed to society at large. It is important to realize that the apocalyptist was both a child of hope and a child of despair: a child of hope in the invincible power of God in the world, and a child of despair of the present course of human history in the world. The crux was a conviction that God would act in a climactic moment to change things utterly and forever for the good. Following a period of worldly trial and tribulation, in a cataclysmic triumph of good over evil, the wicked would be scourged and the virtuous lifted up to bask in the glory of the all-powerful deity.

What we have seen in much of the religious language used to describe the AIDS crisis in apocalyptic terms is a preoccupation with despair. Unfortunately, the secularized version of the concept is also unmindful of the hopeful conviction that accompanied the despair in the full apocalyptic concept. Without getting involved in the metaphysical and religious implications of language such as, "God acting," I would like to take on the role of an apocalyptic child of hope in suggesting some ideas that may provide counterpoint to the drums of apocalyptic AIDS despair.

THE CONCEPT OF COMMUNITY

The crisis created by the issue of children with AIDS in the public schools may be in part a product of the unfortunate polarity of "individual liberty" versus "the public good." This artificially bifurcated view of human life has created difficulties for public policy at many levels. It is interesting that scholars in several different disciplines are converging on other concepts that may lead to a synthesis in which this bifurcation can be avoided. The focus is on the concept of community. It is this concept which may be the glimmer of hope that may lead us out of the apocalyptic dread that is characteristic of so much of contemporary American life.

The concept of community is being explored from several different directions. Several examples come immediately to mind: the sociological study, *Habits of the Heart: Individualism and Commitment in American Life*, by Robert Bellah et al.; ethicist Don Beauchamp's "Community: The Neglected Tradition of Public Health," in the *Hasting Center Report*; and two theological works, John Koenig's *New Testament Hospitality: Partnership with Strangers as Promise and Mission* and Thomas Ogletree's *Hospitality to the Stranger: Dimensions of Moral Understanding*.

The thesis of Bellah et al. (1985) is that the primary cultural language or tradition of moral discourse in contemporary American life is that of individualism. The primary focus is on individual liberties and rights. Without discounting that primary language, Bellah et al. raise two secondary languages, also rooted in American culture, which can limit and qualify the scope and consequences of political individualism. These secondary languages of community stem from the republican and biblical traditions.

Beauchamp (1985) seeks to point public health to the second language, republicanism, which reminds us that "we are not only individuals" but also "a community and a body politic, and that we have shared commitments to one another and promises to keep." This is a move away from the dominant discourse of political individualism, which relies either on the harm principle or a narrow paternalism justified on grounds of self-protection alone. Republican language reminds us that the public, as well as the community itself, has a reality apart from the individual citizens who compose it. When the communal nature of life is emphasized, concern becomes focused on the well-being of the community as a whole and not just on the well-being of a particular person.

AIDS AND THE CONCEPT OF HOSPITALITY

And what of the tradition of biblical language in American public life? Can it add any understanding of the way in which we can deal with the problem of AIDS in the public schools and, for that matter, elsewhere?

The emphasis on individual autonomy, which we have noted, often results in inhospitality to the stranger. Inhospitality may be manifested in competition, prejudice, ostracism, and aggression. These attitudes are in contrast to the ancient Judeo-Christian traditions involving a transcendent bond between hosts and guests (Koenig 1985). According to this tradition, which has virtually disappeared from contemporary Western culture, hospitality is seen as one of the pillars of morality upon which the universe stands. When guests or hosts violate their obligations to one another, the entire world trembles and retribution follows.

The ethicist Thomas Ogletree (1985) has rightly noted that close encounters with "The Other" usually tend to disorient us. But despite a possibly painful disorientation of our comfortable world view, an understanding of "The Other" can be an occasion for personal growth. It calls our own self-centeredness into question and teaches us to take "The Other" into account. "The Other" confronts "me" with an appeal to take into account another center of meaning in one's own understanding of the world. Thus, the question arises, how should one respond to "otherness?"

We can and often do resist "The Other's" resistance to us, which results in competition, prejudice, and ostracism. We can aggressively reassert our own sovereignity over and against the alien claim of "The Other." We can seek to annul the plurality of the world, or, we can move toward personal and moral growth by another response: a readiness to welcome "The Other," to show hospitality to the stranger.

CONCLUSION

The challenge posed to us by "The Other" is to develop a concept of public virtue that moves beyond the present cultural withdrawal into private life. Sociologist Bellah describes this withdrawal as characterized by "associating with people who share one's own standards of decency, with familiar others uncorrupted by the public world."

At present, many people get involved in public life only to protect their own health and home and their own decent friends and neighbors from the evils of a mysterious, threatening, and complicated society, composed of shadowy, sinister, and immoral strangers. There is no rationale here, says Bellah, for developing public responses that would tolerate this diversity of a large, heterogeneous society or for nurturing common standards of justice and civility among its members.

AIDS education that takes into consideration some of these psychosocial issues may help one to see one's similarity to certain persons who may belong to groups at risk for AIDS, rather than remaining fixated in a negative, threatened way upon their "otherness." And one may also come to see one's own differences and, instead of responding with revulsion to such "others," respond to that "otherness " as an opportunity to learn, through hospitality, what the world looks like to that "other," that "stranger." By returning to such a communitarian ethic, we may come to a deeper understanding of the ways in which AIDS is not merely a disease of "The Other" but, rather, one that affects us all.

REFERENCES

Hospitals. 1986. AIDS: A time bomb at hospitals' door. 60 (5 January): 54.

Beauchamp, D. E. 1985. Community: The neglected tradition of public health. *Hastings Center Report* 15 (December): 28-35.

Bellah, R. N., R. Madsen, W. M. Sullivan, A. Swidler, and S. M. Tipton. 1985. *Habits of the heart.* Berkeley: University of California Press.

Boffey, P. M. 1985. Rate of AIDS for blacks called disproportionate. *New York Times,* 23 October.

Koenig, J. 1985. *New Testament hospitality: Partnership with strangers as promise and mission.* Philadelphia: Fortress Press.

Merritt, R., and G. Toff. 1986. AIDS: A raft of new bills. *Nation's Health,* March, 6.

Ogletree, T. W. 1985. *Hospitality to the stranger: Dimensions of moral understanding.* Philadelphia: Fortress Press.

Scarborough, C. 1984. Is God punishing us? News report. News 4 New York, WNBC-TV, New York City, November.

Wall Street Journal. 1985. AIDS costs: Employers and insurers have reasons to fear expensive epidemic. 18 October.

PART FOUR

AIDS and the Blood Supply

CHAPTER 9

AIDS and the
Blood Service System

JOHANNA PINDYCK

The blood service system in the United States is that arm of the health care system which provides, to more than 3 million patients annually, whole blood, blood components—that is, red cells and platelets—and plasma derivatives, such as factor 8 for hemophiliacs. Whole blood and blood components are obtained almost entirely from volunteer donors; 90 percent is collected by blood centers, and 10 percent by hospitals. Plasma for derivative manufacture comes primarily from paid donors under the auspices of for-profit agencies.

THE THREAT OF AIDS

In 1982, it became apparent that a new disease, acquired immune deficiency syndrome (AIDS), presented a threat to the safety of the nation's blood supply. Epidemiologic data gathered by the federal Centers for Disease Control (CDC) indicated that AIDS was caused by a then-unidentified transmissible agent that could be spread not only by sexual contact among homosexual men, the group in which the disease was first identified, but also by infected blood to intravenous (IV) drug users and transfusion recipients. As of December 30, 1985, the CDC had reported 252 cases of transfusion-associated AIDS in blood recipients and 123 cases in hemophiliacs, contributing 3 percent of the total 15,948 AIDS cases in the United States (Centers for Disease Control 1985a).

A need to protect the safety of the blood supply for transfusion recipients was recognized and accepted as an important public health policy priority. Parallels were rapidly drawn between AIDS and hepatitis B, a sexually transmissible disease which can be spread by inoculation with infected blood. Measures useful in curtailing the spread of AIDS by transfusion were delineated and recommended by public health authorities in an effort to contain its spread by this route (Centers for Disease Control 1983; Office of Biologics 1983). Thus, the blood service system

became the first area in which a concerted national effort was made to prevent the spread of AIDS.

Evaluating disease control policies

Four central questions must be addressed in generating and evaluating
public health policies to control disease spread:

1. What public health measures will be effective in controlling spread of
the disease?

2. What is the impact of the measures on individual rights and freedoms?

3. How should individual rights and freedoms be respected and, it is
hoped, protected?

4. Will the public health measures actually work, if implemented?

The issues posed by these questions are of such a nature that the
answers to them are often socially and politically controversial. This article focuses on how these questions were addressed in relation to three
approaches to control the spread of AIDS by transfusion:

• exclusion of members of groups at risk for AIDS as blood donors

• testing of all donated blood for evidence of infection with the virus that
causes AIDS

• selection of blood donors by recipients (that is, designated donations)

EXCLUSION OF AIDS RISK-GROUP
MEMBERS AS BLOOD DONORS

This public health measure was introduced in March 1983. It was considered likely to be effective because it would remove potentially infected
individuals from the donor base. The first defense against transmission of
disease by transfusion has been the application of epidemiologic and
medical criteria to donor selection to screen out donors at high risk of
transmitting infection. An example of this is the exclusion of individual
donors who have a past history of hepatitis or who are in groups at higher
risk of having been exposed to it, such as IV drug abusers and persons who
work in renal dialysis units. Thus, when AIDS was found to be transmitted by transfusion, it became necessary to extend restrictions on blood
donation to members of groups identified on epidemiologic grounds to be
at high risk of developing AIDS.

Groups at high risk for AIDS

The exclusion criteria denied the right of individuals in groups at high risk for AIDS to give blood. As currently defined (Office of Biologics 1984, 1985), these include:

• Haitians who have entered the United States since 1977

• all men who have had sexual contact with another man since 1977

• intravenous drug users, either past or present

• patients with hemophilia

• anyone who has had intimate (sexual) contact with persons in the above categories

• anyone who has had intimate (sexual) contact with a person who has AIDS

Exclusion policies and the right to privacy

Members of some of these groups are socially stigmatized, particularly gay and bisexual men and IV drug users, and the right to privacy of information about membership in these risk groups could be compromised by donor exclusion policies. Public health officials and blood service system staff appreciated that protection of the right to privacy would be of great importance to risk group members because of possible repercussions with respect to employment, social status, family relationships, or threat of legal action.

The implementation approach that evolved respects the donor's privacy. It is based on three key elements:

1. Donor education.

2. Individual decision-making.

3. The opportunity for private compliance.

In an important break with the past practice of directly eliciting information about exposure to disease, specific historical information with respect to sexual preference was not elicited at the time of donor screening.

Specific approaches to donor screening

Blood collection agencies adopted the following specific approaches to donor screening:

• Prospective donors are informed of the groups at high risk for AIDS, and of the risks of transmitting this disease to transfusion recipients.

- Persons in risk groups are requested not to give blood.

- Prospective high-risk donors offered an additional option: They give blood but confidentially exclude it from the blood supply by means of a special form given to all donors.

This last, and novel, approach was pioneered at the New York Blood Center. The form asks persons in apparent good health whether their blood may be used for transfusions or should, because of possible AIDS risk, be used only for laboratory studies.

Leaders of the gay community, who participated in deliberations on the implementation approaches, endorsed the steps and communicated them through publications and meetings directed at community members. Donor group sponsors and donors accepted the steps and embraced them. The news media also reported the information, thus disseminating it widely and, in most instances, responsibly.

Evidence of risk group compliance

Although evidence suggests that these educational efforts have been successful, it is impossible to determine the relative importance of the several communication routes in effecting behavior change. Furthermore, it is difficult, by the nature of the intervention, to establish its impact in a direct manner. Nevertheless, several facts indicate that risk group members have complied with the public health recommendations by excluding themselves as donors.

First, blood donations by males declined precipitously, particularly in areas in which large numbers of high-risk group members were known to reside. For example, New York City reported a significant 6 percent decrease in male donors during the first two months of the intervention; at the same time, donations by females increased by 1.5 percent (Pindyck et al. 1985). This change in the proportion of males to females giving blood has been sustained. Similar data have been reported from Philadelphia (Dahlke 1984).

Second, analysis of data on donors exercising the option to give blood but designate its use for laboratory studies only indicates that 2 percent of New York City donors, mostly males, exercised this option. Those who give "for studies only" have now been found to include a significantly greater proportion of individuals positive for antibody to human T-lymphotropic virus type III/lymphadenopathy-associated virus (HTLV-III/LAV): up to 40 times higher than "for transfusion" donors (Pindyck 1986). Additional indirect data supporting the effectiveness of the exclusion approaches are provided by the fact that, as of mid-1985, only two transfusion-associated AIDS cases were traced to donations given after institution of the educational campaign directed to restricting donations by risk group members (Osborn 1986).

TESTING OF ALL DONATED BLOOD

Another major step that has been taken to protect the blood supply has been the introduction of blood testing of all donated blood for evidence of donor infection with the virus that causes AIDS. Units of blood that indicate the possible presence of such infection are removed from the blood supply.

Testing was introduced because past experience with prevention of transmission of other diseases by transfusion had shown it to be effective. For example, since 1972 all donated blood has been tested for evidence of hepatitis B virus infection in the donor. This has contributed to the control of the spread of hepatitis B by transfusion.

The HTLV-III/LAV antibody test

Blood testing became possible subsequent to the discovery in 1983 and 1984, by French and American workers, of HTLV-III/LAV, the virus that causes AIDS. The U.S. Department of Health and Human Services declared the development of suitable test systems for donor testing a health priority. In a remarkable cooperative effort, the Food and Drug Administration and the pharmaceutical industry mobilized for action, and by March 1985 the first licensed test system for screening donated blood became available. This was accompanied by myriad new problems and opportunities.

The impact of testing on donor rights and freedoms

In planning the introduction of testing, it was recognized that this step would have a major impact on the rights and freedoms of blood donors. It was also realized that the potential impact could only be partially discerned at the time of test introduction. It was not clear then, nor is it clear now, how information derived from the test, except for withdrawal of blood units from the blood supply to protect recipients, should best be used, or how, in a society stricken with fear of AIDS, it might be misused.

The issues which have had to be faced by officials of the blood service system, in concert with public health authorities, members of groups at risk for AIDS, ethicists, attorneys, and other concerned individuals, include the following:

1. In order to donate blood, one gives up the right not to be tested for infection with HTLV-III/LAV. How should the loss of this right be handled?

2. Being tested generates records of test results, and there is concern about their confidentiality. How should these records be treated by the testing agency, since it is feared that inappropriate use of test results could occur, such as to restrict employment or to limit insurability?

3. Should or would the test results be reportable to public health agencies, and should the donor be advised about this?

4. Since the finding of a positive test result may have importance to the person's health, should he or she be informed of the finding? If so, what advice should be given, and how? Many people have expressed serious concern that this information would generate severe anxiety in the individual, and that, since uncertainty exists as to the actual meaning of a positive test result to the person, its communication might not be of value or might do harm.

5. Since the finding of a positive test result indicates that the person may be infectious to others, does he or she have the right *not* to be informed of it? If not, what behavioral restrictions does this information impose and how should the imposition of these restrictions be accomplished?

Informed consent

Introduction of testing required the development of socially acceptable responses to these questions to serve as the basis for implementation policies, and many groups played a role in this effort. The policies that evolved attempt to balance individuals' rights and society's rights.

Central to the implementation approach is informed consent. It protects the donor's freedom to decide whether to accept being tested when giving blood. Blood collection agencies have introduced or expanded their informed consent procedures to include information for donors that their blood will be tested for antibody to HTLV-III/LAV and what this implies. Individuals can choose whether or not they wish to give blood, but they are aware that, once blood is donated, the test will be performed.

I believe that the informed consent approach has set an important precedent in dealing with the potential risks of being tested for infection with HTLV-III/LAV. Specific consent for a laboratory test has not usually been obtained. Other agencies, such as hospitals, will need to address the issue of a special consent if the test is introduced for diagnostic or for selected screening purposes, as is currently advocated by the medical and public health communities (Centers for Disease Control 1986).

Confidentiality of test results

Prospective donors elect not to be tested by not giving blood. The pros and cons of whether or not to be tested will be more complex in other health care settings, and in other situations in which the test may or will be applied. As an example, as many as 75 insurance companies already require testing of applicants for anti-HTLV-III/LAV in order to determine acceptability for insurance (Kristof 1985). In this situation, there are risks whether one is tested or not. This is especially true if a testing policy were to be adopted more widely by the insurance industry. These risks should be clearly defined to the person being tested. One risk of great concern to many persons being tested is the confidentiality of the HTLV-III/LAV antibody test result.

In order to protect the donor's right to privacy of test information, strict confidentiality procedures have been encouraged as public policy by federal and local public health agencies. In some states, such as New York, New Jersey, and California, strict confidentiality procedures have been mandated as public health law (Carroll 1986). Blood collection agencies have been required to undertake an intense review of internal record-keeping procedures, and changes in internal protocols to safeguard the information have been necessary.

Reportability of test results

Closely related to the confidentiality of test results is the policy currently in place with respect to reportability. At present, public health laws in most states do not require the reporting of positive HTLV-III/LAV antibody test results. However, the state of Colorado has recently made reporting a requirement (Council of Community Blood Centers 1985). There is uncertainty as to whether other states or the federal government will take similar action. Since notification of public health authorities may in the future be required by public health law, some blood service institutions have chosen to inform the donor of this fact. It is important to recognize that, out of respect for concerns about confidentiality of test results, there is anonymous testing available through local public health channels.

I think that public health policies providing for anonymous testing may preclude required reporting of test results obtained by other agencies to public health authorities. To require reporting of positive test results on blood donors, while permitting anonymous testing through satellite facilities, would discriminate against blood donors. It is anticipated that, in the foreseeable future, public health officials will address the scientific justification for reporting test results. It would appear that this will become a socially acceptable step in efforts to effect and enhance disease containment only if the public safety indications for this are overwhelming and new legislative protections are accorded to HTLV-III/LAV antibody-positive individuals.

BLOOD SERVICE DONOR NOTIFICATION POLICY

Regardless of whether or not testing is done anonymously, policies have had to be generated to deal with reporting test results to individuals who have been tested. The two paramount considerations in developing policies for donor notification have been:

- the potential importance of the information with respect to the donor's health, and his or her right to receive it

- the importance of the information to the health and safety of others, because of the potential infectivity of HTLV-III/LAV antibody-positive persons

Conflict exists between these two considerations.

Despite the potential importance of information about being HTLV-III/LAV antibody-positive, little or nothing can be done, at present, to affect the course of infection; therefore, the benefit to the donor of receiving the information is presently limited to an improved ability of the donor's physician to diagnose secondary effects of infection, should they occur. On the other hand, negative effects of notification are likely because of the fear surrounding AIDS and the anxiety created by knowledge of infection.

The problem of false-positives

Further complicating donor notification is the importance of distinguishing positive screening tests—resulting from the actual presence of antibody to HTLV-III/LAV—from tests which are "falsely positive." A conservative policy has been adopted for removal of blood units from the blood supply: Units from donors showing reactive screening tests are removed. However, the question of whether to advise donors of screening test results which may be falsely positive has been controversial, and policy varies. The Western blot, which permits detection of antibodies to individual viral proteins, has helped distinguish false-positive screening tests from those positives actually due to antibody to the AIDS virus but has not completely resolved this problem to date.

The social, ethical, and legal ramifications relating to advisement of individuals of results of false-positive tests for anti-HTLV-III/LAV are serious. Criteria for interpretation of test results need to be established and agreed upon by the public health, medical, and scientific communities. As testing is expanded to other populations, this issue will confront all institutions performing anti-HTLV-III/LAV testing. This will be especially important if the person tested does not have the right not to be advised of a positive result.

Donor notification

In most medical situations, the patient has the right to decide whether or not to be told the results of medical procedures and laboratory tests. This right is denied to blood donors. The policy that has been adopted by blood services requires notification of individuals whose test results are positive for anti-HTLV-III/LAV. This policy is consistent with public health recommendations that test-positive persons be so advised. Because donors will be advised of positive results, this is often included in their informed consent. I believe this policy is consistent with an individual's right to know information of public health importance, and to be aware of the recommendations attendant to this knowledge. It is likely that the policy of advisement of test-positive persons will apply in other clinical situations in which the test is applied because of the overriding need to protect the public safety occasioned by the potential infectivity of the individual. Having determined that donors would be advised of positive test results, approaches to accomplish this have been developed.

Positive-test donor advisement procedures

In all cases, the need to maintain confidentiality of the test results has been respected, but the manner in which information is transmitted has varied between two extremes: Some blood collecting agencies have elected to notify individuals of test results by special direct mail; others have preferred to request that test-positive persons come to the agency for personal notification and counseling by a physician or trained staff member.

In either case, owing to the fact that the finding is not reportable in most states, and is confidential, notification has devolved on the testing agency. Because of concerns about the impact of notification on the donor's psychological well-being, some states, such as New York, have mandated personal notification and counseling. In my opinion, this approach is sensible and respectful of the responsibility to protect the HTLV-III/LAV antibody-positive person from harm occasioned by improper receipt of the information.

The importance of a personal notification session

Persons need to be reassured that positive test results do not mean that they have AIDS or will necessarily develop it. In fact, some estimates are that only 1 to 10 percent of infected individuals will ultimately develop

AIDS, although a larger proportion may develop conditions related to AIDS (Centers for Disease Control 1985b). A personal notification session also provides an important opportunity to help the person understand that current evidence suggests that, even if he or she is in good health, there is a high likelihood of current infection with the virus. The manner in which the virus is spread should be discussed, as well as how to prevent spread by these routes. This information requires that the person consider lifestyle adjustments. Some of these are minor and rather simple to carry out, such as not sharing razors or toothbrushes because of the possibility they will be contaminated with blood. Others require major changes in sexual and reproductive behavior. Personal notification is consistent with the goal of protecting the safety of others.

Because of the public health importance of the information and the desire to gain the person's cooperation in achieving the goal of transmission prevention, the information needs to be presented in a systematic manner, sensitive to the deep-seated fears which such information generates and which may compete with assimilation of the information. These fears relate not only to the person's own future health and plans but also to how he or she may be viewed by and relate to others. Most importantly, it must be appreciated that the person will ultimately decide whether to modify his or her lifestyle according to the recommendations. Making this a desirable goal requires education, support, and understanding. Without a vaccine or treatment to prevent the spread of infection, enlistment of the cooperation of those currently infected in this disease control effort is an important public health priority. The success of these efforts may, in the long run, provide the most important protection to the rights and freedoms of members of our society, by maintaining the freedom of choice as efforts at disease control expand. As with all measures which have been or will be introduced, evaluation of their effectiveness will be of critical importance to future planning.

THE EFFECTIVENESS OF HTLV-III/LAV ANTIBODY TESTING

It is too early to directly evaluate the effectiveness of the introduction of HTLV-III/LAV antibody testing of the blood supply in preventing the transmission of AIDS by transfusion. However, important data are already available. It can be estimated that between 8 and 9 million blood donors have already been tested. The licensed tests have been shown to be eminently suitable for donor screening. Additional Western blot studies have provided information which may help resolve the issue of false-positive test results. Culture of donated blood for HTLV-III/LAV has shown that Western blot–positive units are usually positive for virus, whereas other units are virus-negative. Furthermore, false-negative results in blood donors appear to be extraordinarily rare, and can be estimated to be in the range of 1 in 250,000 donations. This information is reassuring, and indicates that infectious units are being detected.

Donor cooperation has been excellent

Donor cooperation with informed consent has been excellent and significant donor losses clearly attributable to the introduction of testing have not been documented. Most risk group members comply with donor exclusion, including confidential designation of blood for studies only. Anonymous testing at alternate test sites is being utilized by risk group members, although to a relatively small extent (Forstein et al. 1985).

At the New York Blood Center, the donor notification program is part of a research study funded by the National Heart, Lung and Blood Institute of the National Institutes of Health. We have found that most donors are responsive to notification and counseling. New insights are being gained from this experience. Persons who give either "for transfusion" or "for studies only" are being notified of positive anti-HTLV-III/LAV tests. Some test-positive persons in the "for transfusion" population are not members of groups recognized at risk for AIDS, even after in-depth interviewing to determine the likely mode of exposure to the virus. For these persons, the discovery of anti-HTLV-III/LAV positivity is more stressful than for risk group members, who, on the whole, seem better prepared to receive the information.

Early findings indicate changes in sexual behavior

An important early finding of the study is self-reported cooperation with public health recommendations, particularly changes in sexual behavior. Risk group members often report that they have already changed sexual behavior. This finding is consistent with both reported survey research on the sexual behavior of gay men in San Francisco and the decline in the number of cases of gonorrhea observed in males at clinics for sexually transmitted diseases (McKusick et al. 1985; Centers for Disease Control 1984, 1985c).

The majority of persons who do not appear to know how they were exposed to the AIDS virus have reported changes in sexual behavior on follow-up visits. They have often been desirous of assistance in communicating the information of anti-HTLV-III/LAV positivity to significant others, such as a wife, husband, mother, or boyfriend. This indicates the strength of their commitment to working successfully toward coping with the information, and their need for help in achieving recommended behavior change. Educational programs have been identified as a primary preventive measure in controlling the spread of AIDS. Data are urgently needed on how to make such programs effective and what resources they will require.

The effect of donor testing on AIDS transmission

The Centers for Disease Control has stated that the testing of donated blood has added significantly to the protection of the blood supply, and that transmission of AIDS by transfusion has been effectively controlled (Centers for Disease Control 1985d). Further research and data on the development of post-tranfusion AIDS in patients transfused subsequent to the implementation of testing for anti-HTLV-III/LAV will be needed to prove this point, and are being collected by the CDC.

SELECTION OF BLOOD DONORS BY RECIPIENTS

Designated donors

Another method that has received significant attention as a means of pre- venting transmission of HTLV-III/LAV by blood transfusion relates to the selection of "designated donors" to serve as the blood source for individual recipients. Unlike the previous measures discussed here, the impetus for this approach to protecting of the blood supply has arisen not from the public health or blood bank community, but from fears continuing in the minds of some members of the public that the community blood supply is unsafe. These fears persist despite both evidence indicating the low risk of acquiring transfusion-transmitted AIDS and the implementation of meas- ures to protect the blood supply from future AIDS transmission by this route. As a result of these fears, some individual prospective transfusion recipients and a few special interest groups have demanded the right to have their friends and family serve as donors for their personal needs, on the grounds that this source of supply is safer and will protect them from acquiring AIDS by transfusion.

Opposition to the designated donor approach

The three major blood banking organizations that provide the nation's supply of whole blood and its components—the American Association of Blood Banks, the American National Red Cross, and the Council of Com- munity Blood Centers—have stated their opposition to the designated donor approach, as have many public health officials and the agencies they represent, such as the New York City Department of Health.

There are two primary public health reasons for opposing designated, or directed, donations:

1. There is no evidence that a designated donation source would provide safer blood. In fact, concern exists as to whether it would be as safe as blood from a community supply.

2. There is concern that this approach would jeopardize the adequacy, availability, and efficiency of the nation's blood supply, therefore compromising the health and safety of blood recipients throughout the United States.

Evidence for higher risk from designated donations

As I noted earlier, the first defense against disease transmission by transfusion has been the application of medical and epidemiologic criteria for the exclusion of individuals at high risk of virus transmission. This is accomplished through medical history and the enlistment of donors' cooperation with exclusion criteria. Factors that influence this compliance, such as payment for blood donation, have been shown to select a donor base at higher risk of disease transmission than the all-volunteer donor base enlisted through the community blood service system (Aach et al. 1981). The designated or directed donation approach introduces an important pressure on the donor to give blood that compromises his or her privacy in exercising a decision not to give blood. For example, if a healthy person refuses to give blood for a specified recipient, he or she might be suspected of being in a high-risk group. This is considered to have a negative impact on the person's ability to comply with medical history criteria that are so important in donor screening.

Supportive evidence for this conclusion is derived from a national study carried out in the late 1970s to determine the incidence of post-transfusion hepatitis (Aach et al.). This study revealed that patient-recruited donors had a risk of transmitting post-transfusion hepatitis that was almost three times higher than that of community donors. Recent data from blood-collecting institutions which have implemented a directed donation program confirm that directed donations do not have less evidence of transmissible diseases. These data fail to support the contention that designated or directed donations are a safer source of blood. Unfortunately, although the blood source is not safer, the impression of two classes of blood, one better than the other, is created.

Designated donation jeopardizes the nation's blood supply

Great concern also exists about both the logistics of carrying out a designated or directed donation program and the threat to the nation's blood supply of such an approach. An alarming aspect of a designated donation system is its negative impact on the volunteer community blood supply. As healthy, willing donors ceased to donate, holding themselves in reserve to meet family needs, the availability of blood to treat all patients in need would soon be compromised. This is especially true for the older population—and almost 50 percent of blood recipients are over 65 years of age (Friedman et al. 1980). These individuals are least able to marshall designated donors and would be seriously jeopardized by decreased community donor support. A similar problem would be experienced in the care of patients who require extensive blood component support. Patients with leukemia, for example, often need platelets from hundreds of donors. For these reasons, designated or directed donation has not been endorsed by the blood services and has been neither advocated nor implemented as a national policy.

However, the pressure for a response to the demand for designated or directed donations has been great in some areas and in some hospitals throughout the United States. As a result, a variety of local responses have emerged, ranging from refusal to permit directed donations to their full implementation within an area, and controversy continues to rage in regard to this issue. The pivotal question that has remained unanswered is how to appropriately respond to the demands of some recipients for the right to refuse blood from the community supply if they need to receive blood transfusions.

Autologous donation: An acceptable alternative

One responsible approach, which has been widely adopted by the blood service system, is to encourage donors who can donate their own blood for elective surgery to do so. This procedure, known as autologous donation, has long been advocated by blood services because it does provide the safest blood source for the individual. As a result of the concerns about disease transmission by transfusion, autologous donation has now gained increased support from the public and the medical community.

BALANCING RIGHTS AND ENSURING A SAFE SUPPLY

How should transfusion recipients' rights to self-determination be respected, when they cannot be reassured about the safety of the community blood supply and must receive blood for health reasons? One possible approach is to permit these individuals to receive blood from "designated donors," in specific medical situations, after issues of safety and availability are fully explained. Consent from the recipient would be obtained indicating that he or she accepts this kind of transfusion, releasing the providing organization from liabilities associated with the transfusion, and including the permission to use community blood sources if additional blood is needed. Donors could be given a special consent form indicating the risks to them of being designated donors, since these risks differ from those of community donors. However, the blood would not be released for others because of concerns about its safety in comparison to the community supply. This is the approach that has been adopted by the New York Blood Center in an effort to balance the rights of the public to the safest supply, the rights of seriously concerned recipients to determine the source of blood they receive, and donors' rights to privacy.

Recommendations for measures such as directed donations, which arise from fears in the mind of the public, need to be subjected to the same careful analysis that has been applied to the public health measures which have been implemented. As noted, satisfactory resolution of the problems that arise from public fear are difficult to achieve but must be addressed.

CONCLUSION

The blood service system has wrestled with a number of issues in implementing steps to protect the safety of the blood supply. The two policies which have been adopted nationally to protect the safety of the supply have been scientifically sound. They provide a history of early decision-making in prevention of the spread of AIDS by one recognized route, and may establish precedents for future decisions. Importantly, these policies evolved from extensive dialogue among public health officials, scientists, blood service staff, and the involved risk communities. Evidence has emerged supporting the hypothesis that educational efforts can be effective in changing behavior that leads to the spread of AIDS. The lessons we have learned in trying to achieve a balance between public health and safety priorities and individual rights and freedoms provide a model which may be helpful in achieving rational decision-making as efforts to prevent the spread of this disease expand.

REFERENCES

Aach, R. D., et al. 1981. Serum alanine aminotransferase of donors in relation to the risk of non-A, non-B hepatitis in recipients. *New England Journal of Medicine* 304:989–94.

Carroll, M. 1986. Revised bill would limit AIDS test use. *New York Times,* 24 February.

Centers for Disease Control. 1983. Prevention of acquired immune deficiency syndrome (AIDS). Report of Interagency Recommendations. *Morbidity and Mortality Weekly Report* 32:101–04.

_____. 1984. Declining rates of rectal and pharyngeal gonorrhea among males—New York City. *Morbidity and Mortality Weekly Report* 33:295–97.

_____. 1985a. *Acquired immunodeficiency syndrome (AIDS) weekly surveillance report*, 30 December.

_____. 1985b. Acquired immunodeficiency syndrome (AIDS). In 1985 STD Treatment Guidelines Supplement. *Morbidity and Mortality Weekly Report* 34(4S): 75S.

_____. 1985c. Self-reported behavioral changes among homosexual and bisexual men—San Francisco. *Morbidity and Mortality Weekly Report* 34:613-15.

_____. 1985d. Update: Public health service workshop on human T-lymphotropic virus type III antibody testing—United States. *Morbidity and Mortality Weekly Report* 34:477-78.

_____. 1986. Additional recommendations to reduce sexual and drug abuse-related transmission of human T-lymphotropic virus type III/lymphadenopathy-associated virus. *Morbidity and Mortality Weekly Report* 35:152-55.

Council of Community Blood Centers. 1985. *Newsletter*, 27 September.

Dahlke, M. B. 1984. Designated blood donations. *New England Journal of Medicine* 310:1195.

Forstein, M., et al. 1985. Alternative sites for screening blood for antibodies to AIDS virus. Letter. *New England Journal of Medicine* 313:1158.

Friedman, B. A., T. L. Burns, and M. A. Schork. 1980. *A study of national trends in transfusion medicine*. Ann Arbor, Mich.: University of Michigan Medical School and School of Public Health.

Kristof, N. D. 1985. More insurers screen applicants for AIDS. *New York Times*, 26 December.

McKusick, L., W. Horstman, and T. J. Coates. 1985. AIDS and sexual behavior reported by gay men in San Francisco. *American Journal of Public Health* 75:493-96.

Office of Biologics, Food and Drug Administration. 1983. Recommendations to decrease the risk of transmitting acquired immune deficiency syndrome (AIDS) from blood donors. 24 March.

_____. 1984. Revised recommendations to decrease the risk of transmitting acquired immunodeficiency syndrome (AIDS) from blood and plasma donors. 14 December.

_____. 1985. Revised definition of high-risk groups with respect to acquired immunodeficiency syndrome (AIDS) transmission from blood and plasma donors. 3 September.

Osborn, J. E. 1986. The AIDS epidemic: An overview of the science. *Issues in Science and Technology* 2:40.

Pindyck, J., et al. 1985. Measures to decrease the risk of acquired immunodeficiency syndrome transmission by blood transfusion. Evidence of volunteer blood donor cooperation. *Transfusion* 25:3.

Pindyck, J. 1986. Unpublished observations.

CHAPTER 10

Blood Policy Dynamics: An Overview

NANCY R. HOLLAND

Early in 1986, there were numerous media reports on the results of a poll, taken by the American Association of Blood Banks, addressing the public's perceptions about blood donation and transfusion in the context of the AIDS epidemic. The poll was remarkable in its revelation that, despite all scientific evidence and everything written to the contrary in both the professional literature and the lay press, 34 percent of those surveyed believed that one could become infected with AIDS by donating blood (*New York Times* 1986).

Undoubtedly, this percentage of the misinformed or unjustifiably paranoid will diminish over time, as public education and information programs about AIDS and how it is—and is not—transmitted reduce the irrational fears and misconceptions. As Johanna Pindyck points out in Chapter 9, however, the AIDS epidemic clearly has posed a significant challenge to the blood supply system of the United States and has required a revision in some of the methods by which blood has been collected in the past. What we have seen, as a result of AIDS, is a revision in national blood policy. The American Blood Commission has played a significant role in that policy assessment and revision.

The American Blood Commission serves as a private sector, public policy forum for blood services. Its members are national organizations representing blood service operators, blood recipients and donors, third-party payers, and health care professionals. Since it was founded in 1975, the Commission has addressed numerous national issues concerning blood service delivery throughout the country. The United States is unique in that it has a national blood policy that calls for a safe, adequate blood supply available at a reasonable cost to everyone who needs it. This policy was announced by the federal government in 1973, shortly after President Richard M. Nixon declared blood a unique, precious national resource. The American Blood Commission was subsequently established in the private sector to implement the national blood policy.

Undoubtedly, the public's misperception that there is a risk of becoming infected with AIDS virus as a result of blood donation is a result of the widely publicized danger of infection through blood transfusion. There is, of course, a risk associated with transfusion, but, as Dr. Pindyck indicates, less than 3 percent of reported AIDS cases involve this transmission route. Furthermore, since the introduction of the HTLV-III/LAV* antibody test for screening donations, the blood supply is decidedly safer. We do not know yet just how much safer, but data are being collected to answer this question.

In addition, blood banks have had substantial experience in dealing with transmissible disease, beginning with post-transfusion hepatitis in the early 1970s, and with additional strains of hepatitis in the 1980s. This experience has effectively informed the various approaches the blood service system has implemented to protect the blood supply from HTLV-III/LAV contamination.

ISSUES IN FORMULATING PROTECTIVE POLICY

The problems associated with protecting the blood supply from contamination with disease-causing viral agents have both social and public policy implications. In the 1970s, the American Blood Commission addressed two major issues in this regard, which resulted in significant changes in collection and transfusion policy.

The switch to all-volunteer donors

The first issue dealt with developing an all-volunteer blood supply. The need to do this became apparent as a result of studies indicating that volunteer donors were safer sources than paid donors. In the early 1970s, approximately 25 percent of the blood available for transfusion in the United States came from paid donors. By 1980, as a result of revisions in collection policy, 99 percent of the blood available for transfusion came from volunteer donors—and this percentage has remained constant.

Changes in donor recruitment

The second issue dealt with how blood donors were recruited. There were two schools of thought: One viewed blood supply as a community and, ultimately, national responsibility; the other believed blood to be an individual responsibility to be borne by those who needed it.

The "community" concept maintained that the community was responsible for acquiring and providing the blood supply that was to be used in the community and that would also be available to other areas of the country, as needed. The "individual responsibility" school of thought believed that blood should be provided by the patient's family or friends. If it could not be provided by these groups, then the patient should be charged a nonreplacement fee in lieu of being able to replace the units

*Human T-lymphotropic virus type III/lymphadenopathy-associated virus.

used. This practice was viewed by some as imposing a penalty on the patient for not being able to cover his or her own blood needs. The "community" concept prevailed, however, and by 1980 the practice of imposing a fee for nonreplacement of transfused blood units was virtually nonexistent, as most of the country had embraced the idea of community responsibility for the blood supply.

The resurgence of interest in directed donations

With the interest that is being expressed today in directed donations, as a result of the AIDS epidemic, one might say that the idea of individual responsibility is undergoing a resurgence. In the context of the AIDS epidemic, however, the concept of directed, or designated, donations becomes a problematic one.

As Dr. Pindyck points out, one of the pitfalls of directed donations is the coercion of those who are asked to donate under these conditions. There are documented cases of sons being asked by their mothers to donate blood, which subsequently tested positive for antibody to HTLV-III/LAV. Through counseling of these donors, it was determined that the sons were members of a group at high risk for AIDS, unbeknownst to their mothers until this event.

In addition, there have been no controlled studies conducted to determine whether or not directed donations are an effective alternative, and some believe that they actually undermine a community's ability to provide adequate blood supplies. However, there are areas of the country that have large directed donation programs, some that have none, and some that manage directed donation requests on an individual, case-by-case basis.

CHANGES IN THE DONOR–BLOOD CENTER RELATIONSHIP

While post-transfusion hepatitis was a major health and blood supply safety issue in the 1970s, it was viewed as a chronic disease problem, not a fatal one. AIDS is considered uniformly fatal. This posed a multifold dilemma for the blood service system, which in the past had notified donors of positive test results for hepatitis B, but whose responsibility to the donor tended to end there.

With AIDS, blood centers were once again faced with the necessity of notifying donors about positive test results. There were grave concerns about the impact of this information on the donor, since the implications of the positive result for antibody to HTLV-III/LAV are unknown or ambiguous beyond an indication that the individual has been exposed to the AIDS virus. Ironically, and in spite of the unknowns and ambiguities, broad public health concerns were the primary basis for notifying blood donors of positive HTLV-III/LAV antibody test results.

These have been trying decision-making times, and they have resulted in the altering of the former relationship between blood centers and donors because for the first time it appears that the responsibility to the donor has to extend beyond simple notification of the possibility of exposure to a disease. In some parts of the country, blood centers have assumed responsibility for the important donor follow-up counseling phase. In other areas, referrals are made to local organizations with counseling experience.

In addition, donor-informed consent was not a common practice in blood centers before HTLV-III/LAV antibody screening and this, too, has changed dramatically. Donors are now informed that their blood will be tested for certain infectious agents and that they will be notified if the results are positive.

Donor rights in an environment of voluntarism

As was pointed out at a 1985 AIDS conference, "Ethics and the Blood Supply," sponsored by the American Blood Commission and The Hastings Center, the blood donor is a volunteer participant in a compact with the blood center. There are rights, responsibilities, and expectations on both sides. The best way for the donor to exercise the right to donate or not to donate is to have the information about what donation entails presented prior to donation through an informed consent process. This procedure provides for informed self-determination, and is covered by Dr. Pindyck in the preceding chapter.

Confidentiality has been practiced in blood centers at varying levels for years. As a result of the AIDS epidemic, additional measures to protect donors and medical records and to restrict access to this information have been instituted. There are several court cases pending now, however, in which donor confidentiality is at issue.

ADDITIONAL QUESTIONS RAISED BY THE AIDS EPIDEMIC

The blood service community is the first group to introduce anti-HTLV-III/LAV screening in a broad population. As a result, it is acquiring a substantial amount of experience and data to address—after a reasonable amount of time has elapsed—questions of both test efficacy and adequate blood supply.The experience to date has raised additional questions about the blood supply.

At the December 1985 meeting of the American Blood Commission board of directors, for example, there was a special session on voluntarism.

Questions addressed included: Is the volunteer donor the safest donor? The findings can be summarized as follows:

- The safest donor is one who donates for his or her own blood needs in advance of an anticipated surgical need, that is, the autologous donor.

- Directed donors or paid donors may be as safe, less safe, or safer than the community-based blood supply. There are not adequate data available to make a distinction. However, all donations are screened for the presence of infectious agents, regardless of the source.

- The patient least at risk is the one who does not receive any transfusion.

Other questions arise in pursuing the goal of a safe blood supply. For instance, persons belonging to groups considered at high risk for AIDS are being excluded as blood donors. Certain other groups, by virtue of their ethnic origin, their profession, or by being housed in a prison are known to be at higher risk for either being exposed to, carrying, or contracting infectious diseases. Should these groups also be excluded as blood donors? Should we have a blood supply derived mainly from female donors?

AIDS is not the only problem

There continues to be a substantial amount of effort devoted to reducing the transmission of AIDS through the blood supply. However, there are data emerging that show that great challenges are ahead. There is a marker for AIDS and there is a screening test to detect the HTLV-III/LAV antibody. Nevertheless, there are still strains of hepatitis for which there are no markers and no specific screening tests. If ways could be found to prevent the transmission of these hepatitis strains through blood transfusion, chronic liver disease and the risk of cancer of the liver could be reduced significantly.

CONCLUSION

Some observers contend that blood banking is behind the rest of the medical domain in terms of being subjected to legal and moral strictures and ethics of medical practice. I would suggest now that blood banking has responded both rapidly and well to the ethical and legal concerns raised by the AIDS epidemic. Blood centers find themselves interacting a great deal more with public interest groups. There is a great deal of listening done and a significant amount of weighing of the risks and benefits, as evidenced by the blood service system's actions regarding donor notification, informed consent, and confidentiality.

Implementing the anti-HTLV-III/LAV screening test in blood service facilities was not easy, but it was done in a very short period of time—about three months—and it was done effectively. Consensus to alter procedures, introduce new testing programs, change relationships, and accept new responsibilities can be slow to achieve. These were all accomplished in a short time, while recognizing that all the critical issues would not be resolved by the time screening for AIDS exposure began.

It is clear, however, that the blood service system, even with its considerable experience in managing transmissible disease, faces new challenges posed by AIDS and other infectious agents that threaten the safety and adequacy of the blood supply. Currently, the best solution for sustaining a safe, adequate blood supply is a combination of individual exclusion and preventive personal health measures, coupled with continued, universal donor screening. This can be accomplished only if the need to elicit direct cooperation in the chain from the donor to the patient is met. In blood banking, it is important to remember, that the public is both the provider and the consumer.

REFERENCE

New York Times. 1986. Blood banks cite false fears. 16 January.

CHAPTER 11

Is Honesty the Best Policy?

HARVEY M. SAPOLSKY

Blood banking is an AIDS success story. As Johanna Pindyck describes in Chapter 9, blood service organizations in the United States have attempted to cope with the challenge of AIDS in a generally sensitive and sensible manner. Unfortunately, blood banking stands nearly alone. Most societal institutions have thus far faltered terribly in their encounter with this new, fatal disease.

Blood banking's success is twofold: It has apparently blocked effectively the main pathway for AIDS quickly spreading from current high-risk groups to the general population, and it has also been effective in limiting the spread of the other "disease" about which we must be concerned, AIDS panic.

A survey released at the beginning of 1986 reported that one-third of the American public believes that AIDS can be contracted by donating blood, but the rest of the population knows the truth (New York Times 1986). Another poll indicated that over three-quarters of Americans favor making it a crime for "homosexuals and others in groups at high risk for AIDS to donate blood" (New York Times 1985a). Most Americans, however, believe the blood supply to be safe. More important, the medical profession believes transfusion services to be safe. Think of what our predicament would be if the profession came to the conclusion that the blood supply was contaminated—that a blood transfusion was not the gift of life, but the opposite.

Blood banking's success, however, may be fleeting. There is no certainty that the safety of the blood supply can be maintained. Public and professional faith in the competence of blood service organizations to provide safe products is likely to be tested continually. To consider these problems, I examine two sets of public policies. One concerns the presentation of information about AIDS by blood service organizations to the public and the medical professions. The other deals directly with protecting the blood supply from contamination.

INFORMATION POLICY OPTIONS

In personal behavior, honesty is the best policy. Hopefully, our parents teach us so. We trust one another when we believe we are speaking the

107

truth. But in presenting information to the public, it is at least an open question as to whether or not honesty really is the best policy.

The opposite of honesty is, of course, dishonesty, or lying. No one can advocate lying as a public policy. The memories of Vietnam and Watergate are too fresh in our collective political mind. But there are at least two other options:

- exaggeration

- underplaying

Exaggeration is the shading of the truth to excite or frighten people. For hypothetical example, we might read:

> "The number of air traffic near misses has gone up substantially since the air traffic controllers' strike. Worse yet, the Federal Aviation Administration (FAA) is not requiring all encounters be reported. There are disasters waiting to occur because of the way the FAA has been operating the air traffic system."

The second option, underplaying, involves minimizing, the shading of the truth to comfort or reassure people:

> "The air traffic incidents are up somewhat because air traffic has increased. Most, though, do not involve dangerous situations. The reporting regulations were recently revised to avoid unnecessary paperwork and do not in the least jeopardize air safety."

In politics, depending on which side of an issue you are on, the temptation is to either exaggerate or minimize.

Using exaggeration

I recently completed a study of the political dynamics of product risks in which I compared controversies involving six classes of products that are said to be health risks (Sapolsky 1986). For these hazards, like so many others that are part of modern life, we must depend upon intermediaries—scientists, public interest groups, the news media, government agencies, and others—to help us interpret the risks. What I found is that the intermediaries distort the risks. Most often, they exaggerate risks, making both big and small risks bigger, but not proportionately. The result is, I believe, that the public thinks product risks to be more alike than they actually are. There is more fear of small risks, and less of bigger ones, than there needs to be.

The distortion is not necessarily intentional. Rather, it usually is the result of competition for patronage, in this case the patronage of a public frightened by the recognition of its own mortality. There is exaggeration to attract attention, to gain a competitive advantage over rivals. Scientists, for example, are likely to overstate the importance of their own work. Recall that I have just mentioned prominently my recently completed book. Television news editors prefer the most shocking presentation, hoping to win the ratings war. Businesses emblazon their products with package bursts proclaiming that the item is "Salt Free" or "Caffeine Free," seeking no doubt to imply that rival offerings that retain these ingredients are dangerous.

This kind of competitive exaggeration is in large part the cause of AIDS panic. You know the headlines: "AIDS to Bankrupt Hospitals," "AIDS Stalks the Schools," "The AIDS Time Bomb."* Scientists contribute with their constant resort to straight-line extrapolations of current virus exposures and infections, demonstrating their political rather than their epidemiological sophistication (Norman 1985; *Harvard Medical Area Focus* 1985). Gay activists, in their determination to force what they perceived to be a homophobic administration to provide more resources to combat AIDS, seriously overstated the immediate threat to the general population (Altman 1986; Lieberson 1986; Randal 1984). Even business firms have found a way to exploitation: I recently received a direct mail advertisement for the first monthly newsletter devoted exclusively to AIDS (*AIDS Alert*, published by American Health Consultants, Inc., Atlanta, Georgia). Soon, I am sure, there will be AIDS-free vacations available, with beachfront hotels certifying that their rooms and lounge chairs were never occupied by a homosexual, a hemophiliac, a heroin addict, or a Haitian.

Opting for minimization

Blood service organizations, however, have followed the opposite strategy. If competition breeds exaggeration, cartelization breeds minimization. Since the early 1970s, blood banking in the United States has been controlled by a government-arranged and -sanctioned cartel, one dominated by the three largest whole-blood collection agencies—the American Red Cross, the American Association of Blood Banks, and the Council of Community Blood Centers—and managed by the American Blood Commission (Drake et al. 1982; Office of Technology Assessment 1985). Cartels prefer the quiet life, far from public scrutiny. The AIDS epidemic promises something else for blood banking. Not surprisingly, the blood service organizations have chosen not only to guard the blood pathway with care but also to reassure the public and the medical profession that the blood supply is as safe as ever.

---

*It is worrisome how irresponsibly even professionals can behave. The last headline is on the cover of the January 5, 1986, issue of *Hospitals*, the semimonthly magazine published by the American Hospital Association for the nation's hospital administrators.

Reassurance is the constant theme. When the first transfusion-related AIDS cases were identified, blood bankers denied the possibility. There must be some mistake, they argued (Eckert 1985, 59-61). After the evidence of the linkage could not be denied, they then claimed that interview screening of donors was enough to protect the blood supply. Those who were in high-risk groups for harboring the virus would be discreetly asked to step aside from the line of blood donors. But not everyone who is in these groups is identifiable or admits the risk. The effect on the blood supply of lost donations was downplayed. Johanna Pindyck (in Chapter 9) is the first to report that blood donations at her center declined significantly when agreements were reached with gay community organizations to dissuade donors. Note that she only reports the decline for the first two months following the new policy and says nothing about the difficulty in maintaining an adequate supply of blood for New York City since then. If there had not been an unexplained parallel drop in blood usage (Riffer 1986), would not the donation decline have been a major crisis?

DESPITE REASSURANCES, DOUBTS LINGER

In March 1985, blood banks across the nation began using the test for HTLV-III/LAV antibody to protect the blood supply. There is reassurance offered that, this time, the test prevents the transfusion of tainted blood (Altman 1985). The high rate of false positives produced by the test is admitted to be a problem, but not the certain existence of some false negatives. One study, for example, found 4 of 97 AIDS victims with false-negative test results (Cohen 1986; Baum 1985). We are told by Dr. Pindyck that the number of missed infected units is on the order of 1 in 250,000 (see Chapter 9). But how certain can we be that the test is effective (Lieberson 1986)? Is not the incubation period for AIDS upwards of five years? And what about reports that the blood of some AIDS victims tests negative for antibodies (Levine and Bayer 1985; Weiss et al. 1985)?

The blood service organizations and Dr. Pindyck are quick to reject the use of directed donations (donations of blood for specific individuals by friends and relatives) as a way to gain additional protection. The claim of Dr. Pindyck and other officials is that the pressure placed on individuals to donate for a friend or a relative is likely to lead to less safe, rather than more safe, blood being contributed. Yet directed donations are tested for HTLV-III/LAV antibodies, as Nancy Holland indicates in Chapter 10. Moreover, blood banks could find ways to avoid situations in which the sexual and drug-using behaviors of donors are revealed to recipients when blood is rejected. Privacy issues and administrative problems associated with directed donations can be overcome. The assertion that community blood is always safer than family or tribal blood is difficult to accept as correct.

We have to ask ourselves whether or not the minimizing approach of blood banks is in society's interest. Exaggeration leads to panic, but so too might reassurance constantly proved wrong. Shading the truth is a risky practice. The reputations of institutions doing the shading are in jeopardy, but so too is the health of the society that follows their advice. We need to avoid AIDS panic, for there is real danger that we will sacrifice the civil liberties of all in a mad rush from a hazard that has been exaggerated. We need also to avoid thinking that things are better than they are if readily available measures to protect us from a real hazard are at hand.

EXAMINING OTHER OPTIONS AND
THE BLOOD BANKS' DILEMMA

The ability of blood service organizations to choose wisely needs also to be questioned because their perception of measures that could enhance the safety of the blood supply may be clouded by very powerful organizational interests. The establishment of a national blood policy in the early 1970s laid the basis for the cartelization of blood banking by reducing inter- and intra-regional competition and by eliminating paid donations of whole blood. But competition and paid donations are among the possibilities that must be raised again if transfusion persists as a source of AIDS transmission. The dilemma of the blood banks becomes clearer when the options for further protecting transfusions are considered.

Autologous donations

The safest blood is one's own, predeposited in advance of need. Autologous donations eliminate the risks of both AIDS and hepatitis infections, the other killer stalking the blood supply. About half of blood transfusions are for emergencies or for those too ill to donate. The rest occur in elective surgery where blood need can be anticipated. Blood service organizations admit the medical advantages of autologous donations and yet have been slow to accommodate those who wish to avoid the community supply. The desire to retain familiar routines endangers patients able to protect themselves from exposure to unnecessary risks.

Directed donations

A second option is the increased use of directed donations. The blood service organizations prefer to consider their enterprise not as a true bank with individual accounts but rather as a community chest to which those who can donate do so for those in need. Directed donations threaten this community obligation ideology. Claims of administrative inconvenience and even the problem of providing for those without friends or family are secondary, for they can be met in a variety of ways. The true danger for the blood service organizations is that pressures for protection from AIDS will revive discarded views of the blood enterprise. And yet, as the fear of AIDS increases, the movement to directed donation grows, much to the consternation of the Red Cross and other large blood service organizations (McGrath 1985; Sherman 1985). If these organizations fail to respond by providing directed donations, it seems likely that enterprising patients and their physician advocates will make alternative arrangements, thus leading to increased competition, which is also an anathema to the established organizations (White 1985; *Medical World News* 1985a).

Paid donors

Another option is to return to the use of paid donors. Blood bankers are quick to cite the experience with hepatitis as evidence that financial incentives for donors increase the risk of contamination. To be sure, some collection agencies that relied upon paid donors had high rates of hepatitis infections, but so did some of those that relied only upon volunteer donors. Ignored is the experience of prominent medical institutions, such as Massachusetts General Hospital and the Mayo Clinic, both of which used cash payments in order to obtain a pool of "biologically clean" repeat donors and an enviably low rate of hepatitis transmission (Sapolsky and Finkelstein 1977). If AIDS remains a blood banking problem, there likely will be attempts to use money to encourage high levels of donations from those free of contact with the virus. The major blood service organizations are certain, however, to resist a return to payments, because their adherence to the national blood policy was intended in large part to protect themselves from the competition of agencies that paid donors (Drake et al. 1982, 129-34; Eckert 1985, 6-31).

Imported blood from safe locales

A third option is to import blood from safe locales. Finding such safe sources may be increasingly difficult, but one could imagine Alsatian peasants or Laplanders providing blood to contaminated Americans, having demonstrated to the Food and Drug Administration (FDA) their social purity and clean living habits. A distasteful notion? Perhaps, but since the 1960s, the New York Blood Center, under an FDA-approved arrangement, has imported approximately 250,000 units of blood each year from West Germany and Switzerland to overcome persistent shortages and hepatitis problems (Drake et al. 1982, 122-23). The foreign donors are not paid, but the New York Center does provide the German and Swiss Red Cross with equipment and supplies of appropriate value as compensation for the blood. AIDS may well enhance international trade in blood, as people come to believe the safety of the local or national supply has been compromised.

Technological solutions

Finally, there may be technological solutions, most especially the development of artificial blood or blood components. Blood bankers tend to dismiss the suggestion that viable substitutes for the real thing will be found soon, but just as the AIDS research budget can be increased, so too can the support for artificial blood research. Already there are claims of substantial progress being made (*Hospitals* 1985; *Medical World News* 1985b; *New York Times* 1985b; *Science* 1985). The blood service organizations, however, had institutional reasons to disparage attempts to find artificial substitutes for blood. They are, after all, essentially blood collection agencies. Transfusions are the province of hospitals, not blood centers. If blood substitutes do become available, it is likely to be DuPont, Genentech, or Baxter-Travenol that would then be the supplier to hospitals, rather than the Red Cross or any of the other existing whole-blood collection agencies.

CONCLUSION

I offer these comments not to make light of the significant efforts that blood service organizations have made to protect the nation's blood supply. I am impressed by their sensitive handling of the privacy issue for donors and their compassionate provision of counseling for those testing positive for exposure to the virus. Rather, I think it is necessary to add to the congratulations questions about what the future might bring. Shading the truth may not be a wise choice for blood banking. Moreover, I worry about the reasons that some in blood banking see this strategy as desirable. Do we not have to ask ourselves what it is that we are trying to protect? Is it blood banking as its professionals prefer it to be practiced, or is it the benefits of a safe blood supply?

REFERENCES

Altman, D. 1986. *AIDS in the mind of America.* New York: Anchor Press/Doubleday.

Altman, L. K. 1985. Blood supply called free of AIDS. *New York Times,* 1 August.

Baum, R. M. 1985. AIDS epidemic continues, moving beyond high-risk groups. *Chemical and Engineering News* 63 (1 April): 19-26.

Cohen, R. L. 1986. AIDS: The impending quarantine. *Health/PAC Bulletin* 16 (4):9-14.

Drake, A. W., S. N. Finkelstein, and H. M. Sapolsky. 1982. *The American blood supply.* Cambridge, MA: M.I.T. Press.

Eckert, R. D. 1985. Blood, money and monopoly. In *Securing a safer blood supply: Two views.* Washington, DC: American Enterprise Institute.

Harvard Medical Area Focus. 1985. Can AIDS be stopped? 10 October, 4.

Hospitals. 1985. Artificial red cells show promising results in studies. 59 (1 October): 46.

Levine, C., and R. Bayer. 1985. Screening blood: Public health and medical uncertainty. *Hastings Center Report* 15 (August): Special Supplement, 9.

Lieberson, J. 1986. The reality of AIDS. *New York Review of Books* 32 (16 January): 43-48.

McGrath, A. 1985. The bad blood between us. *Forbes* 136 (30 December): 107.

Medical World News. 1985a. Directed donation donnybrook? 26 (25 October): 52

_____. 1985b. Closing in on a red blood cell substitute? 26 (11 November): 10.

New York Times 1985a. Poll indicates majority favor quarantine for AIDS victims. 20 December.

_____. 1985b. Advances seen in search for blood substitute. 3 December.

_____. 1986. Blood banks cite false fears. 16 January.

Norman, C. 1985. AIDS trends: Projections from limited data. *Science* 230:1018-21.

Office of Technology Assessment, U.S. Congress. 1985. *Blood policy and technology,* OTA-H-260. Washington, DC: Government Printing Office.

Randal, J. 1984. Too little aid for AIDS. *Technology Review.* August/September, 10-13.

Riffer, J. 1986. Blood banks still cope with AIDS fears and myths. *Hospitals* 60 (5 January): 74.

Sapolsky, H. M. (ed.) 1986. *Consuming fears: The politics of product risks.* New York: Basic Books.

Sapolsky, H. M., and S. N. Finkelstein. 1977. Blood policy revisited—A new look at the 'gift relationship.' *Public Interest,* 46 (Winter): 15-27.

Science. 1985. Artificial red blood cells. 230:1091.

Sherman, B. 1985. Many patients due for surgery storing own blood in fear of AIDS. *New York Times,* 17 November.

Weiss, S. H., J. J. Goedert, M. G. Sarngadharan, A. J. Bodner, The AIDS Seroepidemiology Collaborative Working Group, R. C. Gallo, W. A. Blattner. 1985. Screening test for HTLV-III (AIDS agent) antibodies. *Journal of the American Medical Association* 253:221-25.

White, E. C. 1985. Blood banks pressured to change policies to allow 'direct' donations. *Modern Healthcare* 15 (25 October): 56.

PART FIVE

Acute
Medical Services:
Four
Case Studies

St. Luke's-Roosevelt Hospital Center
MICHAEL H. GRIECO

M. D. Anderson Hospital and Tumor Institute
PETER W. A. MANSELL

New York City Health and Hospitals Corporation
OMAR L. HENDRIX

San Francisco General Hospital
PAUL A. VOLBERDING

CHAPTER 12

St. Luke's-Roosevelt Hospital Center

MICHAEL H. GRIECO

I want to begin by imparting some sense of the dimensions of the acquired immune deficiency syndrome (AIDS) epidemic from the point of view of a voluntary hospital in New York City. St. Luke's-Roosevelt Hospital Center has a total of 1,350 beds at two sites in Manhattan: one at Amsterdam Avenue and 113th Street, and the other at Columbus Avenue and 59th Street. The site at 113th Street is closer to the Harlem area, and its AIDS patient population is characterized by a predominance of members from the intravenous (IV) drug-using risk group. Meanwhile, the site at 59th Street is on the West Side of Manhattan and is characterized by a higher percentage of patients who are middle-class male homosexuals.

At St. Luke's-Roosevelt, the annual AIDS patient caseload has grown from one case in 1979 to 227 in 1985, for a total of 522 diagnosed cases (see Table 12. 1), with an average daily census of 50-60 AIDS inpatients at the beginning of 1986. These patients occupy about 4 percent of the total beds at St. Luke's-Roosevelt. I believe the numbers are similar for other New York City hospitals, and it is extremely important, when discussing medical services for people with AIDS in New York, to understand the dimensions of the problem in the city—and the differences—as they relate to other cities and to the nation as a whole.

THE DIMENSIONS OF AIDS IN NEW YORK CITY

The number of AIDS cases diagnosed in adults annually in New York City has grown from 6 in 1979 to 1,902 in 1985 (see Table 12.1). With over 5,200 cases diagnosed to date, New York City accounts for almost one-third of all AIDS cases in the United States (New York City Department of Health 1985). It is an enormous number, even in relative terms. More than 2,800, or 54 percent, of those diagnosed with AIDS in the city since 1979 have died, which is similar to the national case fatality rate of approximately 51 percent (Centers for Disease Control 1986). In 1984, in fact, AIDS became the leading cause of death in New York City for men in the 30-39 age range, was the third and fourth leading cause of death, re-

Table 12.1
Adult AIDS Cases at St. Luke's-Roosevelt Hospital Center and in New York City
and the United States, by Year, 1979-1985

	YEAR						
	1979	1980	1981	1982	1983	1984	1985
St. Luke's-Roosevelt Hospital Center (N = 522)	1	4	5	30	85	170	227
New York City (N = 5,210)*	6	24	144	454	976	1,684	1,902
United States (N = 15,901)†	9	44	251	971	2,656	5,280	6,690
N.Y.C. percent of U.S. total‡	66.7	54.5	57.4	46.8	36.7	31.9	28.4

*Total includes 20 cases for which the year of diagnosis is unknown; New York City data are as of 20 December 1985.
†U.S. data are as of 7 January 1986.
‡The decrease in the New York City proportion of total U.S. AIDS cases over the period reflects the increase of cases elsewhere in the nation, not a decrease in the disease incidence in New York City. Total AIDS cases in New York City represent 32.8 percent of cumulative U.S. cases.
SOURCES: St. Luke's-Roosevelt Hospital Center, New York City Department of Health, and the Centers for Disease Control.

spectively, for men in the 20-29 and 40-49 age group, and the second leading cause of death for women aged 30-34 (New York City Department of Health 1986). It is important to note, of course, that the case fatality rate for AIDS, over time, is virtually 100 percent, and that thus far no one has recovered from AIDS.

The demographics of AIDS in New York City differ from the national profile, a fact which also influences the acute medical services picture. For example, although most AIDS patients in New York City are homosexual/bisexual men, as they are across the nation, in the city overall there is a significantly higher percentage (34 percent) of total AIDS cases among the IV drug-abuser group than is reflected in the national distribution (see Table 12.2). With more than 100 cases, New York City also accounts for nearly 44 percent of pediatric AIDS cases nationwide, another important factor in the scope of the epidemic and the problems associated with it here.

HOW RESPONSES DIFFER

In comparing how health care providers in different cities have responded to AIDS, I think we should examine the concepts of care rather than the procedural methods that have been used to execute and carry out those

Table 12.2
AIDS Cases by Patient Group, in New York City and the United States*

PATIENT GROUP	NEW YORK CITY		UNITED STATES	
	NUMBER	PERCENT	NUMBER	PERCENT
Adults				
Homosexual/bisexual men (not				
IV drug users)	3,027	58.1	10,600	65.3
Homosexual/bisexual IV drug				
users	305	5.9	1,310	8.1
IV drug users	1,462	28.1	2,766	17.0
Hemophilia patients	8	0.1	124	0.8
Heterosexual contacts	80	1.5	182	1.1
Transfusion recipients	38	0.7	261	1.6
None of the above/other				
Other	109	2.1	N.A.	N.A.
No identified risks	51	1.0	586	3.6
Born outside U.S. †	130	2.5	398	2.5
SUBTOTAL	5,210	100.0	16,227	100.0
Pediatric				
Parent with AIDS or at				
increased risk for AIDS	87	84.4	175	75.8
Hemophilia patients	—	—	11	4.8
Transfusion recipients	8	7.8	33	14.3
None of the above/other	8	7.8	12	5.2
SUBTOTAL	103	100.0	231	100.0
TOTAL	5,313	100.0	16,458	100.0

Note: Percents may not total due to rounding.
N.A., not available.
*New York City data as of 20 December 1985; U.S. data as of 13 January 1986.
†Includes persons born in countries in which most AIDS cases have not been associated with known risk factors.
SOURCES: New York City Health Department, monthly data; Centers for Disease Control, *Morbidity and Mortality Weekly Report* 35:20.

concepts. For example, if we compare the response of the health care system in New York with that in San Francisco, it is important to realize that there are two basic differences:

1. There is a significant difference between the health providers. At St. Luke's-Roosevelt, private physicians provide a significant amount of primary medical care for AIDS patients in a voluntary hospital setting.

A recent study of resource utilization by AIDS patients at St. Luke's-Roosevelt, which I will discuss in more detail later, found that private physicians provided primary care for 67 percent of all AIDS admissions and 61 percent of all AIDS patients—and at no time were patients transferred from private to staff physicians, even when insurance coverage changed. These private physicians provide a continuity from inpatient to outpatient, and are an extremely important part of the health care system in New York voluntary hospitals.

In contrast, in San Francisco, acute medical services for AIDS patients are largely based in a municipal hospital setting (see Chapter 15). In New York City, the majority of AIDS patients are cared for in two large systems—a municipal system and a voluntary system—and my estimate is that approximately two-thirds of all patients are cared for in the voluntary hospitals.

2. In dealing with the AIDS epidemic in San Francisco, there was significant leadership developed at the institutional level early on, but until recently there was little in the way of an organized approach among the health care institutions of New York City. However, that has changed dramatically in the last year with the recognition that the AIDS problem could no longer be effectively handled by merely reallocating existing resources.

CHANGES IN NEW YORK CITY'S RESPONSE

What changes have occurred in the response of New York City's health care delivery system to the AIDS epidemic? One is that the New York City Health and Hospitals Corporation, the city agency that operates the municipal system, has proposed and is in the process of implementing a significant program for confronting the AIDS epidemic within the municipal hospitals. However, that its planning was not done in conjunction with the voluntary hospital group, to develop an integrated approach in New York City, represents, I think, a failing that should have been recognized and avoided.

The second change is that the voluntary hospitals have become active in the last year with the Greater New York Hospital Association (GNYHA), have established a joint task force, and, again, have made significant strides in dealing with and understanding the impact of the AIDS epidemic on the voluntary system, and in developing guidelines for confronting the problems it has engendered. As a result, GNYHA (1986) has compiled and made available a package of information that deals with three elements of the AIDS epidemic that affect hospitals:

1. Infection control guidelines.

2. Hospital workers with AIDS.

3. Legal issues.

This package has begun to pull the voluntary system together and point the way to the development, with the municipal system, of an integrated health care plan for New York City.

The third change is that the AIDS Institute, a state agency, is helping guide the New York State Department of Health to recognize the needs of the voluntary hospital system. The way the health care system is organized, New York City assumes primary responsibility for the municipal hospitals, and New York State assumes primary responsibility for the voluntary hospitals. And the state government has begun to realize that one cannot care for AIDS patients through only the standard methods of reimbursment, especially as the Diagnosis Related Groups (DRGs) system becomes established in the state, which will make it much more difficult to cope financially with a disease that requires so much medical care.

Finally, as a result of the efforts of Cyril Brosnan, assistant to the chairman of Empire Blue Cross and Blue Shield, The Health Services Improvement Fund, Inc., a foundation sponsored by Empire Blue Cross and Blue Shield, has underwritten a study at St. Luke's-Roosevelt—and is planning other studies—to examine key issues regarding the medical care of AIDS patients and the resource utilization in acute care hospitals. The results of the study have been made available through the Empire Blue Cross and Blue Shield Health Services Improvement Fund Office (Belmont 1985).

In addition, I think I should emphasize that one of the advantages of a pluralistic society is that where the existing institutions fail to act, new institutions arise, and in New York City the Gay Men's Health Crisis (GMHC) has played an outstanding role in helping organize health care for people with AIDS and in providing the community support that the formal agencies were not able to offer. GMHC effectively bridges the care gap until these other institutions pull themselves together and mount an orderly and effective response.

DIFFERING DEMOGRAPHICS

Aside from the differences with respect to health care delivery systems in other cities, in New York we also have, as noted earlier, a different profile of AIDS patients. The difference is particularly apparent when we compare the New York City data with that for San Francisco (see Table 12.3).

Table 12.3
AIDS Cases in New York City and San Francisco through 1985

	NEW YORK*	SAN FRANCISCO†
Total number of adult cases	5,210	1,628
Percent AIDS cases by race/ethnic group		
White	46.6	87.7
Black	30.8	5.0
Hispanic	21.9	5.7
Other	0.7	1.5
Percent male	90.0	99.2
Percent homosexual/bisexual	58.1	84.5
Percent homosexual/bisexual and IV drug users	5.9	13.0
Percent IV drug users (not homosexual/bisexual)	28.1	0.7
All others	7.9	1.8
Number of AIDS cases in children aged 13 years and under	103	3

*New York City data as of 20 December 1985.
†San Francisco data as of 31 December 1985.
SOURCES: New York City Department of Health; Institute for Health Policy Studies, University of California, San Francisco.

While in San Francisco, for example, about 98 percent of AIDS patients are homosexual/bisexual men, in New York that category accounts for 64 percent. In New York, heterosexual IV drug abusers account for 28 percent of AIDS cases, but in San Francisco only about 1 percent of cases are from that risk group. We also have, in New York, over 100 children—a number that is increasing—who meet the narrow definition the Centers for Disease Control (CDC) has established for pediatric AIDS, while the number of afflicted children in San Francisco is very small.*

Furthermore, we must realize that AIDS, the disease syndrome per se, represents only the tip of the iceburg; it is the retroviral infection caused by human T-lymphotropic virus type III/lymphadenopathy-associated virus (HTLV-III/LAV), which causes AIDS, that is the real problem. AIDS itself, albeit ultimately fatal, represents only a serious set of symptomatic complications for some AIDS virus carriers. And while there are numer-

*The Centers for Disease Control defines a case of pediatric AIDS as a child who has had a reliably diagnosed disease at least moderately indicative of underlying cellular immunodeficiency and no known cause of underlying cellular immunodeficiency or any other reduced resistance reported to be associated with that disease.

ous cases of symptomatic infection with HTLV-III/LAV in both New York and San Francisco, as well as across the nation, as Philip Lee and Peter Arno point out in Chapter 1, there are even more cases of infection that are asymptomatic. Estimates of the number infected in the United States run to 1.5 million persons (Curran et al. 1985), and while some researchers believe that as many as 40 percent of these will eventually develop AIDS (Boffey 1986), I do not think we can make any reliable predictions at this time. We know, of course, that there will be many medical sequelae, but only time will reveal the true dimensions of this epidemic. Nevertheless, the health care problem that we have to address is clearly going to be an enormous one. I think that instead of guessing, we should concentrate on what we know, and we know enough; we do not have to provide specific numbers to prove that a lot has to be done to organize health care.

Thus, in New York we have a pluralistic health care system, we have a heterogeneous group of patients whose needs are not identical, and we need elasticity in the system because one simple format for providing service or meeting patient needs is not going to provide what is required by everyone to whom we must deliver care.

THE RESOURCE UTILIZATION STUDY

The results of the resource utilization study at St. Luke's-Roosevelt Hospital Center mentioned earlier (Belmont 1985) provide some indication of what these needs are, what has been done to meet them, and what needs to be done. The study had four essential purposes:

1. To describe the utilization of hospital-based medical, nursing, and social work resources.

2. To identify predictable patterns of patient needs at different stages of illness.

3. To identify barriers to discharging patients from the acute care hospital.

4. To suggest cost-effective alternatives to acute care hospitalization of AIDS patients.

The study involved an evaluation over 16 months, by chart review, of 152 AIDS patients hospitalized from January 1984 to April 1985. For those 152 patients, there were 273 admissions. Here is a summary of the findings:

• The average number of hospital admissions per AIDS patient over that period of time was two. The number varied, however, from one to eight.

- The length of stay was initially 26 days in the first four months of 1984, and it decreased to 18 days by the last four-month period in 1985. Again, the study was done for all of 1984 and the first four months of 1985, and was divided into four periods of four months each. So, there was a spontaneous change, not decided by any bureaucratic process but developing from the natural course of the illness, where there was a tendency toward reduced length of stay because the physicians and nurses involved ascertained that prolonged stays did not serve a useful purpose. The average number of hospital days per patient was 40.

- Almost all patients required a private room. It is almost impossible to provide AIDS care without facilities for private rooms. In New York City, this is an extremely difficult problem to deal with because our hospital system is in the pincer grip of the state and federal governments, and we are, from the point of view of facilities, relatively poor. Approximately 15 percent of our AIDS patients were admitted to intensive care units. That percentage appears to be declining as time passes.

- Private physicians were involved in 67 percent of the patient care. They represent a tremendous resource in the voluntary hospital system.

- Consultations were common. The majority of the consultations were with the infectious disease and pulmonary services.

- The most common invasive diagnostic procedure was bronchoscopy.

- Only 61 of the 152 patients were seen by a social worker. I think this reflects the fact that hospitals have been slow to develop social resources, and some of the other community services actually provide the needed care.

- The average amount of nursing care for these patients was 10.3 hours per day. One of the pupuses of the study was to establish and verify data from other sites that the nursing care required was much greater than that for the average non-AIDS patient at our institution. For a frame of reference, the general guideline at St. Luke's-Roosevelt is that each patient averages approximately 3.5 hours of nursing care. That 10.3 hours for AIDS patients was overall. In a general nursing unit, the average was 8.9 hours. In intensive care, it was 17.35 hours. It was estimated that in a general nursing unit up to 4.1 hours could be provided out of the total of 8.9 by a nurse's aide, and that approximately 5 hours had to be provided by a nurse. This is very important because the provision of nursing services is the foundation of in-hospital care for AIDS patients.

- On discharge from the initial hospitalization, one out of five AIDS patients did not need support services, and two out of five were cared for by significant others. One-third of the patients died during their first hospitalization, and of the two-thirds that survived, about one-third did not need support services and two-thirds had significant others who provided that support.

- There was proportionally less support for dietary, substance abuse, and discharge planning activities. It is in these areas that program development has to occur, especially when we deal with large numbers of patients.

- There was a neurological diagnosis in one-quarter of the patients, but a problem behavior in four out of five. Thirty-five patients received neurologic consultations, and 19 received psychiatric consultations.

It is worth emphasizing again, I think, that the study clearly underlines the need to identify and hire the additional support staff needed to provide the social, psychiatric, dietary, discharge planning, and other aspects of care that have received less attention than acute medical services and procedures.

OTHER AREAS OF CARE

What about the other areas of care outside the in-hospital focus of the Belmont report? In most of our acute care institutions there has been, basically, a lack of institutionally organized and integrated ambulatory care for AIDS patients. At the Roosevelt Hospital site at 59th Street, we have an AIDS ambulatory clinic that is open one a week. It has been a limited program, but one that we think has worked out quite well, and we have begun to examine the idea of expanding it to provide the sort of support required for the 33 percent of patients who do not receive integrated care from their voluntary private physician. What we need in our ambulatory systems is not only integrated care but also the ability to treat AIDS patients in a way similar to the ambulatory surgery system. Other areas that need further development to accommodate AIDS patients include the home care programs, long-term care facilities, and nursing homes.

Another important item that should be on the agenda for voluntary hospitals is the development of facilities in the outpatient department for dispensing difficult-to-administer drugs. For example, both the San Francisco General Hospital AIDS Activities Division and the M. D. Anderson

Hospital in Houston have developed oncology services with an organized system for the administration of toxic drugs to ambulatory patients. However, in New York City hospitals, it remains difficult to administer, on an ambulatory basis, some of the oncolytic and other powerful drugs utilized in the treatment of infections and the sequelae of AIDS.

In summarizing the unit developed at San Francisco General Hospital as a model for the care of AIDS patients, Paul Volberding, in an article in the *Annals of Internal Medicine* (1985; see also Chapter 15), indicated certain critical elements:

- multidisciplinary team medical care, including oncologists, infectious disease specialists, pulmonary physicians, neurologists, neurosurgeons, dermatologists, ophthalmolgists, radiation therapists, and others

- multidisciplinary psychosocial care—for health care providers as well as for patients and their significant others

- integration of inpatient and outpatient services

- community involvement to support these efforts and extend them into the community

Dr. Volberding also pointed out that the development and implementation of this sort of comprehensive care system requires a high degree of planning and commitment by the institution. This is a valid statement, except that the commitment, in New York at least, involves much more than that of hospitals alone. As I mentioned earlier, New York voluntary hospitals are state-regulated, and any planning and commitment has to be supported at the government level—both state and federal—because, especially in today's cost-containment atmosphere, government essentially controls the ability of hospitals to plan and function.

Much has been said about the importance of developing AIDS units in hospitals, usually meaning physical units, but to me this concept can just as well symbolize a *system* of integrated health care in the hospital center. The decision about whether or not there should be a physical unit specifically for AIDS patients is up to the individual institution, which alone can best determine how to allocate its resources and organize care.

Intensive care and informed consent

In discussions of acute medical services the question of admitting AIDS patients to intensive care units is also frequently raised and is another area of decision acute care providers must confront. At St. Luke's-Roosevelt, intensive care for AIDS patients is not ruled out. Even though the percentage of AIDS patients who come out of intensive care is very small, once they reach the stage of illness where intensive care is indicated, we feel there is a place for ventilatory support. For example, we have had four patients who survived their stay in the intensive care unit and left the hospital. Ventilation will sometimes tide over, for a period, a patient with acute *Pneumocystis carinii* pneumonia, particularly at the very acute onset of the first episode.

However, with slowly progressive cases, we discuss the use of intensive care and the likely outcome with the patient early on, so the issue of intensive care and the issue of informed consent regarding treatment are dealt with before the need arises, as is done in a transplant program. This assumes even greater importance because of the neurological sequelae of AIDS, which, although they can occur early, usually are progressive. In any event, we certainly do not administer experimental drugs to patients who are neurologically impaired and unable to provide informed consent.

RESOURCE REALLOCATION—AND ITS LIMITS

In regard to the future, I think it is absolutely clear that, with the massive numbers of AIDS patients such as we have in New York, we have reached the limits of dealing with an epidemic of this size through resource reallocation, which has largely characterized our approach to date at St. Luke's-Roosevelt. Because of the financial constraints imposed by current reimbursement systems, we have not hired a new full-time employee in any area to deal with AIDS. Instead, we have attempted to meet patient and program needs by reallocating existing resources. In some instances, individuals have raised their own funds to participate in special AIDS-related programs, but the system can no longer depend on these methods of providing or paying for the special sorts of care AIDS patients require.

Organizing care

Hospitals that have fewer than ten AIDS patients can provide that average 8.9 hours of nursing care needed by distributing patients throughout the institution, which is the way St. Luke's-Roosevelt has handled the problem. Without additional resources, we have been able to provide the necessary level of nursing by distributing patients on certain floors of the hospital. If, for example, we have 30 patients at one of our sites, we have five to seven floors that can handle up to five AIDS patients each. We try to limit the number to five patients on a floor so as not to overwhelm the available nursing care facilities, which are the major limiting factor in providing hospital care.

In this way, some of the nursing time that the average patient on a floor receives can be shifted to the AIDS patient without detriment, and the need for additional nursing can be met without hiring additional personnel. However, once there are more than ten patients, then greater structure around which to organize care is needed. My own view is that, at that point, it makes a tremendous amount of sense to consider dedicated facilities, or AIDS units, as were developed in San Francisco. At the same time, I do not think that the state should make that decision for the institution. The institution should bring its staff together, assess the needs for care and the resources available, and decide how to operate.

Of course, whether you have a separate physical AIDS unit or a system of care that constitutes a figurative unit is not the critical question. Personally, I like the idea of having AIDS patients physically in one unit, but I think it is more important that an institution have an organized system of care for its AIDS patients. Naturally, the system of care an institution decides upon should be based upon both the needs of its patients and its ability to identify and allocate or reallocate the resources necessary to meet those needs.

Assessing other needs

I think psychosocial program development is critical and needs explicit funding that, in large part, can probably be handled through existing reimbursement systems. There is also a vital need in New York City for a markedly improved system of ambulatory services to provide intravenous therapy on an outpatient basis, as previously mentioned. We also need a multidisciplinary program, so that the consultations that are required in dealing with the spectrum of AIDS illnesses are reasonably available.

A good internist, of course—and many now have experience with AIDS—can become expert in all aspects of AIDS diagnosis and treatment. This means that fewer consultations are needed than might otherwise be indicated. A well-trained internist can learn about the characteristic infectious diseases and oncology.

I think there are additional things that we can do in regard to inpatient education, improving recreational facilities, and generally enhancing the quality of life for AIDS patients within our institutions. And these, too, will vary depending on the individual institution, the resources it has available, and the profile of the AIDS patients in its care programs.

MEETING THE NEEDS: WHAT WILL IT COST?

At St. Luke's-Roosevelt, we have examined our AIDS program needs and tried to estimate what it will cost to try to meet them in our system. We considered, for example, setting up AIDS inpatient units at each of our two sites. We looked at the cost for units with 20 beds each, with the idea that we would have extended-care AIDS patients outside the unit, while the unit would provide the coordination of services. We found that merely to increase the nursing hours to eight per patient per day would cost $500,000 annually for a 20-bed unit. For two units, one at each site, we were looking at approximately $1 million in additional costs.

We have asked our psychiatrists to tell us what it would take for them to develop and operate a coordinated psychiatric program for the two sites, including psychiatrists, social worker, and occupational therapist. They tell us that it would take about $200,000.

Currently, we do not have enough private rooms to care for our daily average of 50-60 AIDS inpatients, and, if projections hold up, by 1990 or 1991 we can expect 100 AIDS patients a day. We will need construction funds to provide the private rooms and facilities that that many AIDS patients will require. Thus, the state of New York not only must reimburse us for the care we are already providing—and current reimbursement is inadequate and does not cover what we spend on AIDS care—but also must provide construction funds for unit development.

We also had a group examine costs and produce an estimate for the development of ambulatory care units at each of the St. Luke's-Roosevelt sites. According to the study, assuming a case-managed primary care model with a multidisciplinary team serving 75 patients a week in units operating for at least half of each day, the projected cost was close to $700,000 a year.

CONCLUSION

All of these things add up, so a tremendous amount of money will be required to pay for an adequate and effective system of care for the number of AIDS patients we are and will be seeing. And even if the caseload growth slows, if doubling takes three years instead of one or two, the absolute numbers—and the implications—are still enormous.

The evidence indicates that the mean incubation period for the development of CDC-defined AIDS is about five years. As time goes by, the incubation period will probably become even longer, simply because it takes time to identify cases that have a longer incubation period. It would seem obvious that health care providers must plan for a very large number of patients who will have to be hospitalized. Above all, one thing is certain: although we can probably shorten the hospitalization period AIDS patients require, even from the current 16- or 18-day average length of stay, and even with a good ambulatory care system further reducing the need for expensive hospitalization, caring for AIDS patients is not going to be cheap.

REFERENCES

Belmont, M. F. 1985. *Resource utilization by AIDS patients in the acute care hospital.* St. Luke's-Roosevelt Hospital Center. New York: Empire Blue Cross and Blue Shield, Health Services Improvement Fund, Inc.; December.

Boffey, P. M. 1986. AIDS in the future: Experts say deaths will climb sharply. *New York Times,* 14 January.

Curran, J. W., W. M. Morgan, A. M. Hardy, H. W. Jaffe, and W. W. Darrow. 1985. The epidemiology of AIDS: Current status and future prospects. *Science* 229:1362-67.

Centers for Disease Control. 1985. Revision of the case definition of acquired immunodeficiency syndrome for national reporting—United States. *Morbidity and Mortality Weekly Report.* 34:373-75.

_____. 1986. Update: Acquired immunodeficiency syndrome — United States. *Morbidity and Mortality Weekly Report* 35:17-21.

Greater New York Hospital Association. 1986. *AIDS: Infection control guidelines for hospitals, recommendations for personnel diagnosed with AIDS, legal issues for hospitals.* Report of the Task Force on Hospital Services for AIDS Patients. New York, January.

New York City Department of Health. 1985. *AIDS—Surveillance update.* 26 December.

New York City Department of Health. 1986. Office of Epidemiological Surveillance and Statistics. Unpublished data.

Volberding, P. A. 1985. The clinical spectrum of the acquired immunodeficiency syndrome: Implications for comprehensive care. *Annals of Internal Medicine* 103:729-33.

CHAPTER 13

M. D. Anderson Hospital and Tumor Institute

PETER W. A. MANSELL

In early 1982, in the Department of Cancer Prevention at M. D. Anderson Hospital and Tumor Institute, a state cancer facility in Houston, Texas, we became aware of the fact that individuals with AIDS are among the group of people in our society at the very highest risk for getting malignant diseases. As a result, the Department of Cancer Prevention set up a program with the Department of Immunology and opened a special clinic, with the thought that we would be able to do some very quick epidemiological surveillance, find the answer to the problem of AIDS, and probably close down the clinic within nine to ten months.

Since January 1982, we have seen over 825 AIDS patients in our clinic and, in the intervening four years, it has become quite clear that the problem of AIDS is not going to be an easy one to solve and that its effect reaches into all branches of medicine. At M. D. Anderson, we now have a multidisciplinary team for dealing with AIDS; it is also an inter-institutional team, with the participation of Baylor College of Medicine, the University of Texas Medical School, and other local institutions in Houston.

EMPHASIS ON OUTPATIENT CARE

The basic care plan for AIDS patients at M. D. Anderson emphasizes outpatient care. The reason for this is twofold: First, M. D. Anderson is a relatively small hospital; we have only about 500 beds and an occupancy rate of 98 percent. Second, our charter mandates that we look after people in Texas who have malignant diseases. As a result, it is often very difficult to defend having a young man or a young woman with toxoplasmosis or *Pneumocystis carinii* pneumonia in a bed that might otherwise be occupied by someone with breast cancer, leukemia, or cancer of the lung. That priority for cancer patients is one of the problems we have had to face in treating people with AIDS, who may or may not be suffering from some form of malignant disease.

An additional factor affecting our ability to care for AIDS patients is that M. D. Anderson, as a state institution, has a responsibility to look

131

after the medically indigent. It makes no difference in our care system whether an individual has funds or not, and, except for one other hospital, located in Galveston, M. D. Anderson is the only state institution serving the medically indigent in southern and southeastern Texas, a very large area geographically with a population of about 10 million people. This increases the demand on our care services and contributes to our high occupancy rate.

Furthermore, because of M. D. Anderson's widespread reputation as a cancer treatment center, we find it difficult to refuse cancer patients, who come to us from all over the world. However, we have had to refuse AIDS patients from outside Texas simply because we do not have the facilities to look after everyone.

Two-tier care system for AIDS patients

What we have in Houston—and I think it is important to realize that this is probably the case elsewhere—is a kind of two-tier care system for AIDS patients. In many cases, the patient initially is seen by a private physician and treated in the private hospital care system. At that early point in the disease trajectory, the patient is likely to have funding from either insurance or private sources. Depending on the location, however, the average lifetime hospital care costs for an individual with AIDS have been estimated to be as much as $150,000. As a result, many AIDS patients quickly exhaust their insurance coverage and other sources of private funding. Once that happens, the patient becomes dependent on city, county, or state facilities. In the Houston area, this means one of two county hospitals that have relatively small units for AIDS patients, or the Veterans Administration hospital—if that is appropriate—or M. D. Anderson.

Reduced length of stay

At M. D. Anderson, therefore, our approach to treating AIDS has been to concentrate our energies on outpatient, or ambulatory, care, providing extended and long-term care for patients in their homes, and relatively short inpatient stays at the hospital.

Since M. D. Anderson is a cancer hospital, we already have the facilities to deliver drugs to patients on an outpatient basis, and the great majority of our patients on treatment protocols that require intravenous drug therapy go about their lives for months with a subclavian catheter in place. They come into the hospital once or twice a day—or three times a week, or whatever is appropriate—receive treatment and ongoing ambulatory care, and then go home.

This emphasis on ambulatory care treatment has allowed us to significantly reduce the average length of hospital stay for AIDS patients.

In the early days of our unit, the average length of stay was about 30 days; by January 1986, it was down to between 15 and 20 days. Obviously there are exceptions to this rate, but we attempt, with discharge planning, to get people out of the hospital as soon as possible, and to get them home.

Discharge planning is complicated, however, by the fact that no nursing home in the state of Texas will accept an AIDS patient. This has made it extremely difficult to discharge some patients and, simultaneously, has made community care programs extremely important. Consequently, programs for providing community care and support urgently need to be developed and expanded in Houston.

Other patient services and resources

All of our AIDS patients at M. D. Anderson are seen by a medical social worker, a majority receive neuropsychiatric consultation, and some 45 percent are also counseled by a dietician. We are fortunate in that we have state-funded positions for all of these staff people, as a part of our cancer treatment program, and to that extent, we may be better off than a lot of private institutions. In many parts of the country, for instance, these sorts of services for AIDS patients are in short supply and in desperate need of development.

We have also been fortunate in Houston to have available group therapy for AIDS patients, much of it through the Montrose Counseling Center, a well-developed counseling service for the gay community. A number of therapists both at the facility and in private practice have set up therapy groups. These efforts have been very successful as support groups, and this is something of which I think we, in Houston, can be justifiably proud. Another source of local pride is the KS/AIDS Foundation, which has developed AIDS educational systems and materials in Houston that are now internationally famous.

ISSUES IN AIDS PATIENT CARE

Obviously, the traditional objective of acute medical care has been to try to cure the patient's illness. Sadly, as we know, in the case of AIDS this has not yet proved to be possible. In view of this unhappy reality, there are a number of sociopolitical, ethical, and psychosocial issues that I think need to be addressed in considering the care of people with AIDS.

Why treat AIDS patients at all?

One of the issues—as banal as it may seem—is whether, in fact, to give care at all, in view of the thus far invariably negative outcome of AIDS treatment. This is a question that has been raised—and is still being raised—in places that are perhaps less enlightened than New York and San Francisco. There are, for example, those who ask why one should care for a group of people who might be regarded—as some AIDS patients some-times are—as being, to some extent at least, responsible for what has hap-pened to them. One has to have an answer for that question, and it is not simply good enough, I think, to say that, well, of course one must look after people. My response is to ask, "Why should we look after the in-dividual who smokes and gets lung cancer, or the one who eats too much and gets a coronary infarction?"

Intensive care

The same question has been asked about the usefulness of admitting AIDS patients to intensive care units (ICUs). Studies indicate that the majority of AIDS patients admitted to ICUs seldom, if ever, get out of them (Murray et al. 1984). Our findings at M. D. Anderson confirm these observations. And, although we did admit large numbers of AIDS patients to intensive care in 1982 and 1983, we have subsequently taken the view that it should be possible to care for them on the general ward and avoid the majority of admissions to ICUs. As a result, in 1985 we did not admit a single AIDS patient to intensive care.

Informed consent

Caregivers are also facing ethical issues. How, for example, does one cope with the facts of the increasing effects of AIDS on the central nervous sys-tem? As we have learned more about this retroviral infection, it has become quite clear that the virus that causes AIDS is a neurotropic as well as lymphotropic virus. Dr. Grieco points out (in Chapter 12), for example, that as many as four out of five AIDS patients admitted to the St. Luke's-Roosevelt Hospital Center sites in New York exhibit behavioral problems resulting from the AIDS virus infection.

Faced with patients whose mental capacities may be impaired, how does one deal with questions of informed consent, of people being aware of how to dispose of their lives and their affairs, of how to refuse care, and so forth? Questions about how we will cope with these sorts of problems are still not completely resolved, but at M. D. Anderson we believe that it basically depends on having effective communication with the patient from the very first contact. As doctors who have been trained to believe that we can cure disease, and who are now confronted with a situation where—at present, at least—it is quite obvious that we cannot, we tend to ignore the importance of explaining to the individual, at the outset, the whole spectrum of future events. Although it may seem callous and cruel to say to someone whom you are seeing for the first time, "This is what I think may happen to you in the future," I think it is very important that this be said.

In the clinic at M. D. Anderson, we spend a great deal of time with each new patient. A resident ethicist attends patient interviews, and, as mentioned earlier, every patient sees a medical social worker, and more than 50 percent are also seen by the staff of the hospital's neuropsychiatric consultation service, which shares our clinic area. In this way, we try to deal with the informed consent problem at the very beginning of a patient's treatment.

Obviously, the use of experimental drugs in people with diminished ability to give consent requires that decisions in many cases be made as situations arise. However, we certainly would not exhibit a drug to anyone who did not understand what was happening to him. Ethically speaking, I agree with Dr. Grieco that there should not even be a question about that.

Financial problems

One cannot discuss acute medical services for AIDS patients without considering the financial problems for facilities providing care. The cost of caring for patients with AIDS is very high by any account, and caregivers are constantly confronted with the need to make decisions about how to allocate resources.

At M. D. Anderson, we have no state or city funds for our AIDS patients, other than those that are provided for the hospital in general. We have none of the munificence from the state of Texas that the states of California and New York have shown, or are beginning to show, in providing for the treatment of AIDS in their hospitals, nor do we receive any funding from the city of Houston. In addition, we have not been very successful in obtaining federal funding to any great extent; therefore, the financial problem with which we must contend in operating our AIDS treatment program is a considerable one. The question we must continually address is how does one allocate resources that are necessarily very limited?

Experimental drugs

There are two additional problems at M. D. Anderson—and they are not ours alone—to which attention should be paid. One of these problems, especially pressing from the acute medical care provider's viewpoint, relates to the availability of special or experimental drugs for the treatment of AIDS.

For those of us who look after patients in the acute care system, one of the most distressing things is trying to explain to the individual suffering—indeed, dying—from AIDS why some purportedly effective therapeutic drug that he or she has heard about on television news or read about in a magazine is not available. We also must deal with the problem of explaining to the patient that reports about the drug may not be true, and why M. D. Anderson, a prestigious cancer center in South Texas, does not have access to that drug.

Although I think the Food and Drug Administration and the federal government have done a good job in many respects, their failure to make certain drugs available in areas where there are people who desperately need treatment—whether or not these drugs have received all of the multitude of bureaucratic approvals that are necessary these days—is indeed distressing and difficult for many people to understand. Certainly, when one is faced with a lethal illness, or a life-threatening, dire situation, it should sometimes be permissible to allow the use of agents that show at least some hint of promise, without severe toxicity, more rapidly than has been the case thus far.

Caregiver burnout

The other problem facing providers of acute medical care for AIDS patients is that we tend to concentrate—and rightly so—almost exclusively on our patients, often to the detriment of the nurses, technicians, social workers, maintenance staff, chaplaincy, and even ourselves, the physicians, who are trying to look after these people.

Caring for AIDS patients, for example, obviously puts an enormous strain on the nursing staff. At M. D. Anderson, we are fortunate, on the one hand, that all of our beds are in private rooms, which obviates the problem of not having enough of the private rooms that many AIDS patients require. But, on the other hand, having all your patients in private rooms means that nursing intensity is very high, and so is the resultant potential for burnout. This is particularly true when all the other beds are occupied by cancer patients.

Personally, confronting the AIDS epidemic has been the most distressing, most frustrating, and most saddening experience that I have gone through in my 25 years of professional life. I think attention needs to be paid to the situation of all of those who are engaged in acute caregiving, and to the stresses with which they must live and work on a day-to-day basis. It is not good enough simply to say, "You're a nurse, you're a doctor; look after yourself." That may be possible in some situations, but very often, and especially in the one with which we are currently confronted, it can be a disastrous attitude.

CONCLUSION

Finally, I am also distressed at how long it has taken for the medical community and health care policy-makers to recognize and address such problems as organizing and funding efficient and humane systems of care, involving the community, coping with the sociopolitical issues, obtaining access to experimental drugs, and caring for the AIDS caregivers. There are now well over 16,000 cases of AIDS, and many scores of thousands of cases of AIDS-related complex and asymptomatic retroviral infection. It is clear that we should have been discussing these issues—and others—at least three years ago.

REFERENCE

Murray, J. F., C. P. Felton, S. M. Garay, M. S. Gottlieb, P. C. Hopewell, D. E. Stover, and A. S. Teirstein. 1984. Pulmonary complications of the acquired immunodeficiency syndrome: Report of a National Heart, Lung, and Blood Institute Workshop. *New England Journal of Medicine* 310: 1682–88.

CHAPTER 14

New York City Health and Hospitals Corporation

OMAR L. HENDRIX

The New York City Health and Hospitals Corporation (HHC) is the largest municipal hospital system in the United States. It operates eleven acute care facilities, five neighborhood family care centers, five long-term care facilities, and the city's Emergency Medical Services. The mission of the Corporation is to guarantee to all New York City residents the right to high quality, compassionate health care, regardless of their ability to pay.

The AIDS epidemic has placed a tremendous burden on the human, medical, financial, and technological resources of New York City's municipal hospital system. The best delineator of this is that, in the last quarter of 1985, the municipal hospital system had a daily census of approximately 250 AIDS patients. The HHC's institutions were among the first in the nation to care for AIDS patients, and to meet their needs the HHC has developed a philosophy of care and a wide range of programs for persons with AIDS.

THE MUNICIPAL APPROACH

As early as 1983, the HHC began a concerted, ongoing AIDS program. As developed, the program involves

- providing corporate-wide employee training and education, including the use of print and film materials and group conferences for specific personnel, such as education for house staff about the social problems of AIDS patients

- convening interdisciplinary groups of health care professionals to review AIDS-related issues and assist in the development of AIDS programs and policies

- conducting studies of resource utilization to determine the resource needs for AIDS patient care

- monitoring AIDS patient census and demographics, including illness histories, lengths of stay, and other variables

138

The Corporation has also evolved a philosophy of service provision for AIDS patients. This philosophy involves a system-wide commitment to the following policy:

• AIDS patients must have access to services within their own communities and neighborhoods, rather than at some distant, centralized location.

• AIDS patients should not be segregated or isolated, except when medically necessary.

• All health care workers much have an awareness of AIDS. While a core team of care givers will have particular expertise, the provision of care must be shared throughout the health care setting.

• Factual, responsible education of staff, patients, their families, and all who use HHC facilities for their health care is a critical component of the response to AIDS.

• The HHC is committed to case management of AIDS patients across all levels of care and to close collaboration with other New York City agencies, the voluntary sector, and private groups involved in caring for people with AIDS.

PROGRAMS KEYED TO PATIENT DEMOGRAPHICS

To a large extent, the shape of an AIDS treatment system and the demands made upon it are determined by the demographic profile of the patients served by that system. While the vast majority of AIDS patients fall into discrete risk groups, the distribution of patients by risk group varies from city to city and even from facility to facility. A comparison of the demographics of AIDS patients in HHC facilities, in New York City as a whole, and in the city of San Francisco indicates significant differences (see Figure 14.1).

AIDS patients profiles: San Francisco and New York City

San Francisco has a homogeneous AIDS patient population composed almost entirely of homosexual/bisexual males, as Michael Grieco has indicated (in Chapter 12). They constitute about 98 percent of the total caseload, with homosexual/bisexual intravenous (IV) drug users accounting for about 15 percent of that group. Heterosexual IV drug users account for only about 1 percent of AIDS patients in San Francisco and the remaining 1 percent comprises heterosexual sex partners of AIDS virus carriers, children born to infected mothers, and persons infected by receiving contaminated blood products or in other unusual ways.

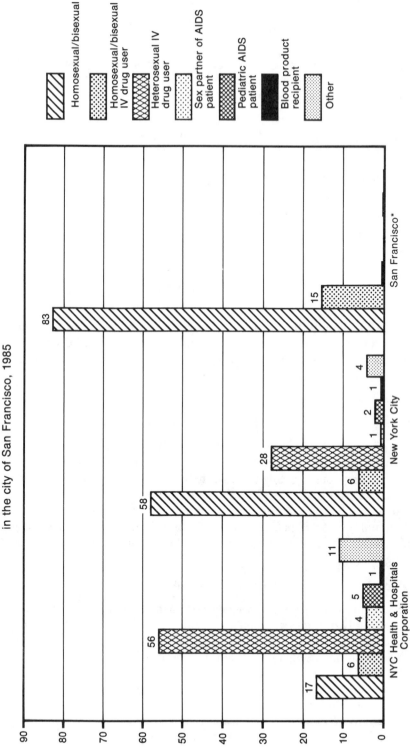

Fig. 14.1. Demographics of AIDS patients by risk group in New York City Health and Hospitals Corporation facilities, in New York City as a whole, and in the city of San Francisco, 1985

Legend:
- Homosexual/bisexual
- Homosexual/bisexual IV drug user
- Heterosexual IV drug user
- Sex partner of AIDS patient
- Pediatric AIDS patient
- Blood product recipient
- Other

Risk group (percentage of patients)

San Francisco*   83   15
New York City   58   28   6   1   2   1   4
NYC Health & Hospitals Corporation   56   17   6   4   5   1   11

*Remaining risk groups account for only 2 percent of AIDS patients in San Francisco.

SOURCES: New York City Health and Hospitals Corporation, New York City Department of Health, San Francisco Department of Public Health.

New York City as a whole shows a larger percentage of heterosexual IV drug users (28 percent) among its AIDS patients than San Francisco, but overall gay men (64 percent) still are predominant. In contrast, HHC facilities have an overwhelming majority of IV drug users (62 percent) as AIDS patients and a significantly larger number of children (5 percent) and heterosexual sex partners (11 percent) of persons infected with the AIDS virus than either San Francisco or New York City as a whole.

In addition, San Francisco's AIDS patients are predominantly white (88 percent), while the majority of AIDS patients in New York City (51 percent) are black or Hispanic. The HHC's AIDS patient population comes almost entirely from minority groups, black or Hispanic, which account for 89 percent of the caseload in HHC institutions (see Figure 14.2).

Different patterns of illness and needs

The AIDS patient census has climbed steadily in HHC facilities since the first cases were identified in 1981. In March 1985, HHC had an average daily census of 140 AIDS inpatients; by the last quarter of 1985, the average was 250 patients per day. The unadjusted mean length of stay of AIDS patients across all HHC facilities is 26 days, while the median length of stay is 17 days. This discrepancy is caused largely by a relatively small group of patients with exceptionally long lengths of stay, the result of overwhelming discharge problems. When outliers with exceptionally long or short lengths of stay are excluded from the calculations, the adjusted mean length of stay drops to 22 days.

The vast majority of the HHC's AIDS patients—about 85 percent— are appropriately placed in the acute care setting at any given time. The remaining 15 percent are on alternative-level-of-care status, awaiting discharge to lower levels of care: 7 percent to home with services; 4 percent to home without services; 3 percent to a skilled nursing facility; and 1 percent to a health-related facility (see Figure 14.3).

The HHC's experience with AIDS-related illnesses also differs from that of San Francisco and that of New York City as a whole. The HHC's AIDS patients present with a greater number and different variety of opportunistic infections. For example, although 24 percent of all AIDS patients have been diagnosed with Kaposi's sarcoma, only 2 percent of IV drug users with AIDS have that otherwise rare form of cancer. However, 15 percent of IV drug users with AIDS have common tuberculosis (TB), a significantly higher rate than among AIDS patients as whole. The New York City Department of Health and several independent researchers have documented a parallel rise in the incidence of TB and AIDS among IV drug users and believe that the rise in TB incidence represents a more subtle manifestation of immune suppression resulting from infection with the AIDS-causing virus.

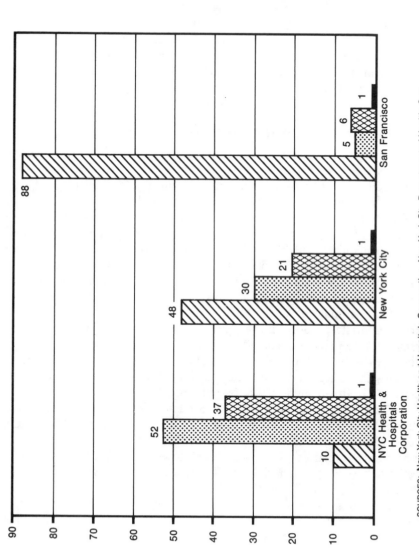

Fig. 14.2. Demographics of AIDS patients by race/ethnicity in New York City Health and Hospitals Corporation facilities, in New York City as a whole, and in the city of San Francisco, 1985

SOURCES: New York City Health and Hospitals Corporation, New York City Department of Health, San Francisco Department of Public Health.

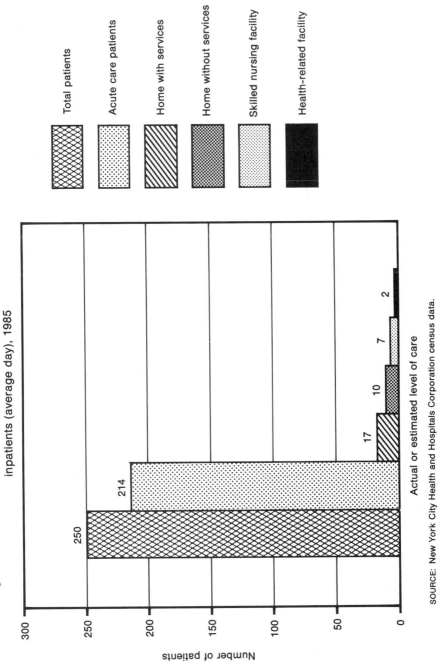

Fig. 14.3. Status of New York City Health and Hospitals Corporation AIDS inpatients (average day), 1985

SOURCE: New York City Health and Hospitals Corporation census data.

Intravenous drug users have lengthy histories of illness and poor nutrition, and, because of a variety of social problems, present later and sicker than AIDS patients in other risk group categories. They often avoid ambulatory care clinics, presenting, instead, to emergency facilities and with relatively advanced illness. In addition, the relative lack of social supports for IV drug users creates difficulties in securing post-acute services for patients in this risk group. All of these factors contribute to more frequent and lengthier hospitalizations for HHC's AIDS patient population.

The HHC has implemented, or is in the process of implementing, a number of programs to address the problems arising from its particular mix of AIDS patients.

HEALTH AND HOSPITALS CORPORATION STRATEGY

At the heart of HHC's strategy for treating AIDS patients is the provision of interdisciplinary teams for all HHC hospitals with a significant AIDS patient population. These teams consist of infectious disease specialists, nurse clinicians, and social workers with particular expertise in the needs of AIDS patients. Their primary role is consultative. They work with existing hospital staff to ensure appropriate case-managed care for AIDS patients in both inpatient and outpatient settings. It is their responsibility to educate and inform other staff and patients and their families about AIDS issues. Each facility has also been provided with increased levels of nursing staff and additional supplies to meet the increased needs of AIDS patients.

Institutional flexibility to meet particular needs

The individual municipal hospitals in the HHC system have been allowed the flexibility to tailor the team concept to meet their own particular needs. They have also developed particular programs to meet the distinctive needs of their respective AIDS patient populations. For example, Bellevue Hospital, which has consistently had the highest census of any HHC facility, created a dedicated AIDS unit that serves as a triage base for its AIDS team. It is not, however, an isolation unit to segregate AIDS patients; rather, new admissions and patients with special needs receive intensified assessment and attention. Bellevue has also implemented an ambulatory AIDS assessment clinic as a joint effort with the Community Health Project. There, persons at risk for AIDS can receive thorough physical assessment, as well as counseling on psychosocial issues related to AIDS.

The number of pediatric AIDS patients is a growing problem in New York City. Pediatric patients constitute 5 percent of the HHC's AIDS in-patient caseload. The experience of Bronx Municipal Hospital Center (BMHC) is indicative of the future: It has an average daily AIDS pediatric census of five patients, of whom as many as half, having been abandoned by their parents, live in the hospital. The nurses and volunteers at BMHC are devoted to these children, providing extra attention, clothes, games, and outings. However, the children's greatest need is for foster care. Although the New York City Human Resources Administration provides enhanced foster care funds to encourage their placement, many of these children with AIDS remain abandoned.

To address at least part of the deprivation experienced by children with AIDS, the HHC has opened an AIDS pediatric day-care center at BMHC. The center serves as many as 25 children, providing needed socialization for them, respite for their families, and on-site medical evaluation and follow-up to facilitate early intervention and reduce the need for acute hospitalization.

Post-acute care for AIDS patients

Because of the intensity of need in the wake of AIDS, the AIDS epidemic exacerbates existing weaknesses in the provision of services outside the acute care setting. The provision of post-acute care for AIDS patients who are also IV drug users is further complicated by the already existing poverty, homelessness, and lack of social supports that, in general, charac-terize this population subgroup. The result is unnecessarily lengthy—and costly—acute hospitalizations.

The majority of HHC's AIDS inpatients on alternate-level-of-care status could be discharged to home, with or without services, but this is stymied by their lack of either housing or appropriate home settings in which to receive services. The HHC has relied on other municipal and voluntary agencies, such as the Human Resources Administration and the AIDS Resource Center, to address the difficult task of providing housing and home-based services.

For some patients, however, a non-acute institutional setting is the most appropriate care environment. The HHC responded to this particular need by establishing an AIDS long-term care program. Begun at Coler Memorial Hospital in August 1985, this specialized program was later ex-panded to Goldwater Memorial Hospital. Coler was the first long-term care facility in New York City and one of the first in the nation to provide a long-term level of care for persons with AIDS. Protocols and policies that were developed at Coler for the long-term care of AIDS patients are being studied by other facilities and other agencies for their potential application in non-HHC settings.

Dedicated long-term care

The goal of the HHC's AIDS long-term care program is to provide skilled medical, nursing, and psychosocial care to those AIDS patients whose needs exceed the level that could be met with services in the home but who, nevertheless, do not need the level of care provided in the acute hospital setting. Freed from the demands of acute care, the AIDS long-term care program environment is dedicated to achieving the maximum degree of long-term comfort and well-being for each AIDS patient. Interdisciplinary teams, similar to those employed in the acute hospitals, direct the care of up to 16 patients. The teams provide medical services and early intervention on-site to reduce, as much as possible, transfers between levels of care. The teams also travel to acute care facilities throughout the city to assess potential candidates for admission to the long-term care program. Because of the demand for long-term care beds for AIDS patients, there are plans to double the program's capacity in the near future. And not to be overlooked, of course, is the cost-effectiveness of this alternative to care in the acute hospital setting.

Staff education to allay fears

AIDS patients at Coler and Goldwater hospitals are neither isolated nor segregated, but are integrated with the other patients. As patients with AIDS were introduced into the Coler and Goldwater facilities, fears about the communicability of AIDS and concerns about the extraordinary needs of the AIDS patients themselves developed as obstacles that had to be overcome in order for the program to be implemented as planned. AIDS patients had never been in residence at either hospital, and the time frame of their appearance was much more compressed than in the acute care facilities where their numbers had grown gradually, giving staffs and other patients time to adjust. At Coler and Goldwater, the value of AIDS education programs for both staff and residents and their families has been convincingly demonstrated. Initial concerns and fears have been overcome, and the AIDS patients participate in the facilities' activities to the limit of their abilities, accepted by staff and other patients alike. Staff members are particularly proud of their success in rehabilitating some of the AIDS patients to the point that they could be discharged to the community.

Planning for the future

The HHC programs described here are the major components of the HHC's effort to date to address the needs of persons with AIDS in the municipal hospitals of New York City. The major tasks before us in the AIDS epidemic are related to decreasing the use of inpatient services, both by encouraging a somewhat resistant AIDS patient population to use outpatient services appropriately and by working together with other agencies and health care providers to expand the range of available post-acute and community services.

To plan for the future, the HHC regularly convenes an advisory group, composed of representatives from all of its facilities, to monitor the performance of existing programs and to plan future projects. Infectious disease specialists from HHC facilities also meet regularly to discuss a wide array of clinical and policy issues related to AIDS. A central management team includes a project coordinator and a consulting physician to provide day-to-day supervision of the full range of the HHC's AIDS activities.

CONCLUSION

The AIDS epidemic presents health care providers everywhere with an enormous challenge. The problems resulting from AIDS not only have placed extraordinary fiscal and physical burdens upon health care systems but have also imposed a heavy emotional toll on providers and patients alike. Solving these problems will require the full measure of our ingenuity. The New York City Health and Hospitals Corporation has accepted the challenge and is confronting the problems of the AIDS epidemic with programs designed to be accessible, appropriate, cost-effective, and humane—for all persons with AIDS.

CHAPTER 15

San Francisco General Hospital

PAUL A. VOLBERDING

The system of caring for people with AIDS in San Francisco is one of which any of us who are involved are probably too proud. For the clinicians among us, I hasten to note that the following comments are not meant to reflect, in any way, less favorably on the work that other people in this country have done, and are doing, because everybody has struggled with this epidemic and done the best they can with whatever options they have had in their own facilities.

Indeed, one of the comments that we in San Francisco have made in the past is that we cannot brag too much about our care system because the job we have is a lot easier than that of some of the others involved in caring for AIDS patients elsewhere. This stems from the fact that the AIDS patient population in San Francisco is very homogeneous, as noted by Michael Grieco (in Chapter 12) and Omar Hendrix (in Chapter 14), and is largely composed of middle-class gay men who are very motivated, very compliant, and very educated about most aspects of the disease.

However, I do not think we can rest either on our laurels or on assumptions about care delivery that are based on that statistical profile because, as we see the epidemic affecting more and more people, increasingly we expect to see a more heterogeneous patient population in San Francisco. And I acknowledge that providing care to the intravenous drug-using AIDS patients in San Francisco is more difficult than taking care of our gay patient population.

I want to elaborate upon a few points that Michael Grieco makes about the program at San Francisco General Hospital (SFGH), a public hospital owned by the City and County of San Francisco, because it does serve, I think, both as a contrast, in some senses, to the work that is going on in other places, and as a model that other hospitals can and, in my opinion, should look at closely.

THE AIDS ACTIVITIES DIVISION

Early on, we realized at SFGH that AIDS is, of course, a disease requiring a multidisciplinary approach; all of us with academic medical backgrounds and with our subspecialty blinders on, so to speak, had to enlarge on our fields of vision to some degree. We realized, for example, that an infectious disease specialist had to be at least aware of the treatments for the various malignancies that we were seeing, and that the reverse was true for an oncologist. As a result, what we did at SFGH was create a separate Division of AIDS Activities, integrating several medical subspecialties with general internal medicine. As a result, we have infectious disease, oncology, and general medicine as part of the same multidisciplinary division of the Department of Medicine.

We also recognized immediately that the psychosocial aspects of the disease were often much more important for the patient than the medical aspects, and we did more than pay simple lip service to that awareness. We integrated psychiatry, psychiatric social work, and medical social work into our AIDS care system from the very beginning.

The outpatient clinic

Our goal was to have a clinic that focused on outpatient care. We also have an inpatient unit of which we are very proud at SFGH. However, with the outpatient clinic, the idea was to create a system where patients would not have to go from one specialist to another but where the vast bulk of care could be delivered at one site. This allowed us to develop a group of physicians and nurses who were more sensitive to the AIDS patients' social and medical needs and to eliminate some of the problems of compliance and miscommunication that can result when more than one subspecialist takes care of a patient.

The inpatient unit

In the middle of 1983, we decided that we needed to reorganize the way in which we were handling the care of AIDS inpatients. At that time—and over many people's fears and objections—we started the first AIDS inpatient unit in the country. We were careful to avoid an atmosphere of isolation or of a "leper colony," which many people were afraid would be associated with this unit, and we did that, in part, by involving the gay community in the unit's development. We invited members of the gay community to provide input at the early stages of planning, to increase communication and foster a sense of mutual trust.

With the tremendous support of Mervyn Silverman, who was then the director of the San Francisco Department of Public Health, and Merle Sande, who is the chief of medicine at SFGH, we put together an inpatient unit for AIDS patients that still serves as a very useful model of integrated of care. This approach has allowed us to create a nursing staff that is devoted to the care of these patients and can provide immense amounts of education. This is important because it reduces hospital stays and limits the burden that the care of these patients places on the house staff.

The AIDS inpatient unit at SFGH was created in an existing 12-room unit. Most of the rooms were originally constructed as double, semiprivate rooms; however, we decided early on, when there was still some question about cross-infection with opportunistic infections, and because of social problems with dying patients and so forth, that we would have all private rooms. So the previously semiprivate rooms were made into private ones. For a lot of reasons, I favor AIDS patients' being in private rooms, and I feel the same way about cancer patients. In general, I think it simply works better.

Our AIDS unit patients are cared for by one of seven general medical teams; we do not have a team of doctors assigned specifically to the AIDS unit. This makes rounds time in the morning a little more difficult, but it decreases the burden on any one team. Because it is such stressful work, I think it would be very difficult, for many interns especially, to take care of AIDS patients only.

We do not always admit AIDS patients directly to the AIDS unit because, since it is only a 12-bed unit, it is always full. Thus, we usually admit patients to other wards in the hospital and then move them into the AIDS unit, depending on need. If patients have been in the AIDS unit before, we try to get them there again, because usually the contrast between that unit and a general medical unit is too dramatic and they feel more comfortable on the AIDS unit. Also, if they are having behavioral problems, or are on experimental drugs, or having a lot of stress reactions, we can take care of them better on the AIDS unit. So we tend to move people from other units to the AIDS unit, rather than bringing them there first and then moving them out. We are also expanding the unit to 20 beds, so we should be able to admit more patients to it directly.

Reduced utilization of ICUs

One result of the creation of the special AIDS unit has been a dramatic decrease in the utilization of the intensive care unit (ICU) by AIDS patients in the hospital. We found that the use of the ICU was a result of AIDS patients not being eduated about the outcome of ICU admissions. We do not have a policy that limits ICU availability for AIDS patients; all we have done is explain to the patient, before he becomes critically ill, the likely outcome of mechanical ventilation. We then encourage the patient and family, friends, or lovers to make a decision about the kind of care they feel is appropriate. And we support their decision, whatever it is. We find, however, that more people are declining that type of care, and, as a result, our own use of the ICU for AIDS patients has become negligible.

In addition, because there are many ethical problems surrounding the treatment of AIDS, particularly in terms of informed consent for people with central nervous system problems, we have an ethics consultation service with a major focus on AIDS. When issues such as informed consent come up, we can quickly bring ethicists onto the health care team to provide assistance.

INVOLVING THE COMMUNITY

There are two other important points to be made about our service. One, to which I have already alluded, is that we realized in San Francisco that we were dealing with a community problem, not just an isolated medical one, and that community resources could play a vital role in our program. With this awareness, we very aggressively went to the gay community, which is where our patients come from, and looked at existing resources and organizations. We encouraged the development of needed community resources that did not exist and participated in the development process. We also brought in representatives from some of the groups as active staff members in our care program. Thus, when patients are admitted, or when patients are observed to have problems in the outpatient setting, we can quickly refer them to appropriate community resources, limiting the impact on the hospital system.

This use of community resources also has involved the private medical and hospital system in San Francisco. At SFGH, where we have a medical service of about 110 beds, we found that at least 30 of them were filled by patients with AIDS on a regular basis. We were afraid that at some point, if that continued, we would begin compromising the other missions of the hospital, including the training of house staff—that is, giving them a good, balanced experience in treating a variety of medical problems. To remedy the situation, we began an aggressive program of meetings with community physicians. As a first step, we drafted a list of physicians who were willing to take AIDS referrals from us. That was an interesting switch, because usually the referrals have come in the other direction, but it has worked out very well.

Now, when we see a new patient at SFGH, we encourage him to maintain a relationship with any private physician that he may know already, so that as the illness progresses, he will have the option of going back to the private sector. When we have as many AIDS patients hospitalized as we can comfortably care for, we encourage that new ones be admitted to a private hospital. And we have not had any problems with that at all. Private hospitals in San Francisco have been willing, from the start, I think, to accept AIDS patients. I have not heard, at least, about any private hospital that categorically refuses to take care of AIDS patients.

PARTICIPATING IN CLINICAL RESEARCH

The last point I want to emphasize is that, as Peter Mansell says (in Chapter 13), the care of AIDS patients is incredibly stressful. There is no way to deny that it is very stressful for me and my staff to see people our own age dying of this disease and to realize that, in reality, we cannot do very much to reverse the process. However, one of the things that I think gives us the most support is our own involvement in clinical research, and what we have done is take a very aggressive stance in using whatever experimental drugs we find available for our patients. In that process, we increase our own knowledge of AIDS, and we can offer patients more than simple palliation of an otherwise fatal disease. Even if our experimental drugs do not change the outcome, the patient participates in an active program that tries to reverse the disease process. I personally think our AIDS program would not be as successful if we were not so involved in clinical research. Therefore, I agree that there is a need to keep encouraging the expansion of clinical research programs on a nationwide basis.

CONCLUSION

As a result of our efforts, the AIDS treatment program at San Francisco General Hospital is one that I think people should look at and of which we are very proud. I think we have a system that can very efficiently take care of large numbers of AIDS patients—we care for about the same number as St. Luke's-Roosevelt Hospital Center in New York—that can deliver both cost-effective and very sensitive care, and that can involve the patient and the providers in current state-of-the-art clinical research.

PART SIX

Community
Care
Services

CHAPTER 16

New York City:
Gay Men's Health Crisis

RICHARD DUNNE

In July 1981, the *New York Times* printed its first story about an unnamed and, at that point, mysterious disease that was affecting previously healthy homosexual men (Altman 1981). It was only a month later that a group of about 40 gay men, who were very concerned about what was happening to them and to their friends, got together in New York to see what they could do.

The Gay Men's Health Crisis (GMHC) was formed initially to raise money to fund medical research on what has since become known as acquired immune deficiency syndrome (AIDS). In fact, in early 1982, GMHC gave a grant to St. Luke's-Roosevelt Hospital Center in New York to conduct a prospective epidemiologic study of gay men. That GMHC grant for AIDS research preceded any research funding from the National Institutes of Health. It quickly became apparent to GMHC, however, that the amount of money that would be required to fund medical research on this new disease would be extraordinary and well beyond the resources of a community-based organization. Although GMHC's focus has shifted since that time, the organization still remains very interested and involved in the issue of medical research, and funds a lobbying effort in Washington that, thus far, has been very successful in getting federal funds allocated.

The next mission that GMHC undertook was in the area of AIDS education. Again, initially there was very little being done by local government, so GMHC created and distributed the first AIDS information literature in New York City; it still puts out the majority of what is available. In conjunction with its focus on education and information, GMHC also decided to open a telephone hotline service, with the intention, at the time, of referring callers to other services and agencies dealing with AIDS and the problems of people with AIDS or at risk of getting it. What GMHC soon discovered was that there were no such services or agencies. At that point, the oranization took on its third mission: providing services to people with AIDS.

Although only five years old, GMHC today is the largest AIDS service and education foundation in the world. To date, it has provided counseling, financial, legal, and home-care services to more than 2,500 people. GMHC currently has about 1,000 clients, and gains approximately 100 to 150 new ones each month (see Figure 16.1). GMHC has also developed educational programs and has done psychosocial research into behavior modification that may well represent models for the future. Most of the work that all of this activity entails is done through the extraordinary efforts and the devotion of over 1,000 volunteers, and, until recently, much of it has been done without government support.

GMHC's early funding was provided by private contributions raised primarily within New York's gay community by a variety of methods, including direct appeals, sidewalk solicitations in Greenwich Village and at community events, and special benefits. In the spring of 1983, for example, more than 18,000 people purchased tickets for a GMHC benefit performance of Ringling Brothers, Barnum and Bailey Circus at New York's Madison Square Garden, an event which proved successful at both fund-and consciousness-raising. Although GMHC now receives a significant amount of government support, private donations still accounted for more than 50 percent of its $3.6 million budget in 1986 (see Figure 16.2).

CONFRONTING THE EPIDEMIC OF FEAR

In the five years since GMHC was formed, the number of known AIDS cases in the United States has grown from a relative handful in New York and Los Angeles to include nearly 17,000 men, women, and children across the nation—over half of whom have died from the disease—and the incidence continues to climb every year. As Michael Grieco has pointed out (in Chapter 12) AIDS is now the leading cause of death in New York City for men between the ages of 30 and 39, and the second leading cause of death for women between the ages of 30 and 34. In addition, it is predicted that by the end of 1986 AIDS will be the leading cause of death for all men in New York City between the ages of 25 and 44 (New York City Department of Health 1986).

Science has discovered the virus that causes AIDS and its principal routes of transmission, but we are years away from a vaccine and cure, and research into antiviral agents and immune response modulators seems to move at a glacial pace. Badly needed funding and coordination of research efforts seem to be lacking. Meanwhile, a poll conducted by the *Los Angeles Times* in November 1985 indicated that half of all Americans believe that one can get AIDS from casual contact, and a small but still significant percentage thinks, like conservative columnist William Buckley, that persons with AIDS should be tattooed (Balzar 1985; Buckley 1986).

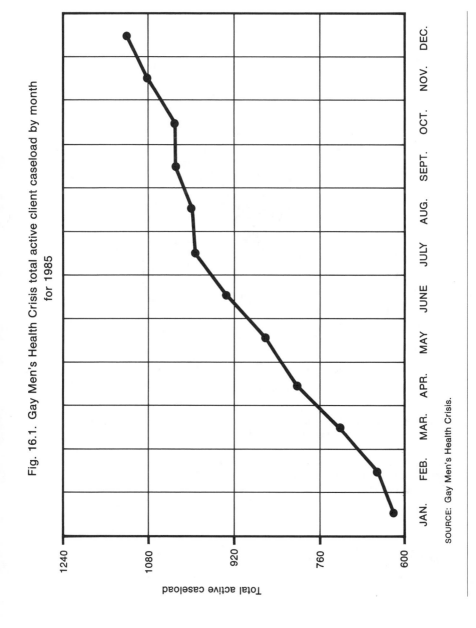

Fig. 16.1. Gay Men's Health Crisis total active client caseload by month for 1985

SOURCE: Gay Men's Health Crisis.

Fig. 16.2. Gay Men's Health Crisis funding for fiscal year 1986

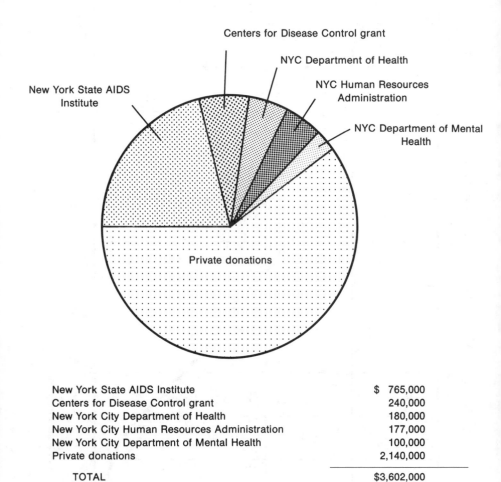

New York State AIDS Institute	$ 765,000
Centers for Disease Control grant	240,000
New York City Department of Health	180,000
New York City Human Resources Administration	177,000
New York City Department of Mental Health	100,000
Private donations	2,140,000
TOTAL	$3,602,000

SOURCE: Gay Men's Health Crisis.

According to the Centers for Disease Control, somewhere between 500,000 and 1 million Americans have already been infected with the AIDS virus, and, according to one government authority, that number could climb to 2 or 3 million within five to ten years, with 40 percent of those eventually dying of the infection (Boffey 1986). Millions of others are not infected, or at least do not know that they are, but are members of what we call "the worried well," worried that a slight cough may be the first sign of *Pneumocystis carinii* pneumonia, or that a never-before-noticed spot on an ankle is surely the first Kaposi's sarcoma lesion. As recently as the fall of 1985, 11,000 children were kept out of school in the New York City borough of Queens because of irrational fears that one student, who may or may not have had AIDS, somehow represented a threat to the public's health. During the community meetings held in Queens to discuss this issue, there were no representatives present from the New York City Department of Health to attempt to allay the panic.

Hysteria hampers care

In the fall of 1985, New York City announced a plan to open the first city nursing home to AIDS patients, then dropped it almost immediately because of opposition from community members and existing residents of the facility, who feared exposure to AIDS victims. In early 1986, there were over 3,000 AIDS patients in New York City and a total of just six nursing home beds available for those who needed long-term care.

Also during 1985, the Catholic Archdiocese of New York announced and then, because of the irrational fears and protests of parishioners and neighbors, immediately cancelled plans to open a hospice for AIDS patients on Manhattan's Upper West Side. Following that debacle, Mother Teresa succeeded in opening an AIDS hospice in Greenwich Village, where, although some neighbors expressed concern, there was no panic and the facility was accepted. However, GMHC's attempts to assist the Archdiocese in setting up appropriate and sensitive programs have been rebuffed, and we have not been allowed to see GMHC clients who have been placed—and subsequently died—in Mother Teresa's facility. Following the opening of the hospice, Mother Teresa next announced a preposterous scheme to open farms in the countryside for persons with AIDS from New York City, a plan of which nothing more has been heard (Friedman 1986).

In addition to requests for assistance and information, GMHC also receives many reports of discrimination against people with AIDS. Every single day, we receive reports of meals not being delivered in hospitals, or of persons who have been fired from their jobs, of patients who are neurologically damaged walking out of hospitals and wandering the streets, and of funeral homes demanding exorbitant fees to handle the body of someone who has died of AIDS.

A woman whose son had been a GMHC client before he died became a volunteer. The first client to whom she was assigned was a young woman, an intravenous (IV) drug user, who died about a week later. The volunteer was with her at the very end and stayed to make sure that appropriate arrangements were made for the body. Appropriate arrangements in this case consisted of someone coming in with a body bag, throwing chemicals inside the bag with the body, and closing it—and that is how that person with AIDS left this world.

AIMING FOR A DURABLE COMMITMENT

Until AIDS, many of the people involved at GMHC had avoided gay and lesbian politics and all of the baggage that frequently goes with those politics. GMHC's founders foresaw the need for a foundation that would be durable and so full of promise that it would endure beyond the rise and fall of individual charismatic leaders. This durability has been built into GMHC in a number of ways: by relying on organizational development rather than on individuals; by a creative mix of private and public funding; and by fiscal caution. GMHC, it is hoped, will outlast AIDS, so that generations of gay men and women can enjoy a healthier future.

Meanwhile, many at GMHC are frightened more than they ever thought possible. Some of its organizers have been diagnosed with AIDS. The founder and president of GMHC, for example, has a triple diagnosis of Kaposi's sarcoma, *Pneumocystis carinii* pneumonia, and tuberculosis. The irony that the founder, five years ago, of the first AIDS service and education foundation should now himself be a client of that organization is simply too sad for words. Others, although they have not yet been diagnosed as suffering from AIDS, know or suspect that they are infected with a virus that has several names but one grim meaning. Many GMHC members have lost a lover and/or friends, and they have grieved for so long that sometimes it seems the pain cannot be borne any longer. Many are also angry and outraged because they have not seen our official institutions doing enough to ameliorate the pain and suffering.

The truth, as I comprehend it, is that gay men and women and people with AIDS have fallen into a terribly complicated medical situation and, as a result, their political situation is even more complicated. AIDS is not, as all of us know, just another infectious disease, and it has shaken the world of medical science as badly as it has shaken the wider community and the world of gay men and women. Still, GMHC and its members have been fortunate to witness, every day, countless examples of compassion and sacrifice by people, from every walk of life, who have simply shown up at its offices to help in whatever way they can. Whatever happens in the years ahead, their heroism is a permanent and indelible monument to GMHC's mission, not to mention to their own nobility.

Doing simply what had to be done

The success, if one can call it that, of GMHC and the growth of organizations like it around the country, are more than a testament to the selflessness of those men and women who have created and who operate these organizations; it is also an indictment of the existing social welfare and health institutions that failed to respond to the AIDS epidemic. When its members began to establish programs at GMHC, it was without any awareness that they were creating models. GMHC simply did what had to be done, and what ought to have been done—but was not—by others.

PROVIDING SERVICES

The following is a brief outline of some of the services GMHC provides:

Crisis intervention

GMHC has crisis intervention workers who establish a one-to-one friendship with each client. When they come to us, typically, the clients have been referred by their physician, by a hospital, or by a social worker; sometimes, they are self-referred. Usually they come because they have just recently been diagnosed with AIDS or, if they have been diagnosed earlier, have just had their first major opportunistic infection. Crisis intervention workers provide emotional and psychological support and also act as case managers in referring clients to other GMHC services.

Buddies

Crisis intervention workers are assisted by "buddies," who also provide emotional support but basically take care of routine daily-living chores such as shopping, cooking, cleaning, paying bills, and accompanying clients to the doctor or hospital. It would be difficult to list all of the things that buddies do, but let me cite one example from when I was a team leader:

The volunteer assigned to one of the team's homebound clients reported a problem with walking the client's dog. Beyond the basic problem of walking the dog once or twice or three times a day, which the client was unable to do, was the additional problem that the dog, a 15-year-old dachshund with arthritis, had to be carried up and down several flights of stairs to the client's walk-up apartment. And since the dog frequently had been waiting 10 or 12 hours to be walked, as soon he was picked up, he typically would urinate on the volunteer. Fortunately, another volunteer on the same team was a veterinarian who specialized in acupuncture for animals. Hearing of the problem, he took it upon himself to visit the other volunteer's client, and did so over a period of two months, to give acupuncture to the arthritic dachshund. It worked, and, with his arthritis relieved, the dachshund was able to go up and down the stairs by himself for a period of several more months, until he finally died, resolving the problem altogether.

Group support services

GMHC provides a wide range of group services, including group therapy led by professionals, and open support groups, so people can come and go as they please. Just before Christmas 1985, a new person appeared in one of the open support groups: a white, 60-year-old grandmother. Members of the group assumed that she was the mother of a person with AIDS and that that was why she was there. Over the course of the discussion, however, it became clear that she herself had AIDS. And the other clients in the group, primarily gay men and IV drug users, felt bad for her, and said, "Oh, isn't that terrible. You must have gotten it from a blood transfusion."

"No," she replied, "I didn't get it from a blood transfusion, and I don't use intravenous drugs. I presume I got it by sexual transmission."

I think that the people in that support group realized for the first time in their lives that AIDS is really just a viral disease and that it is not a punishment of some kind from God, for sin. And that 60-year-old grandmother brought that message home to them.

"Care-partners" groups

In addition to therapy and support groups for clients, GMHC also has "care-partners" groups for lovers, friends, and family members who are frequently unable to share their own pain and anger with others. Several of the care-partners groups consist entirely of women.

Recreational therapy

GMHC also provides recreational therapy to reduce the isolation and loneliness that often accompanies a stigmatizing and debilitating disease. Programs include trips to Broadway shows, brunches, a Friday night movie series with a meal and time for socialization, workshops, exercise classes, and day trips to nearby resorts, such as Atlantic City and New Hope, Pennsylvania.

Financial advocacy

Because people, particularly when they are ill, often need help in finding their way through the incredible bureaucratic mazes of entitlement programs—that frequently seem designed to make sure that no one finds his or her way through them—GMHC provides financial advocacy and assistance. When necessary, the organization can make direct financial grants to clients who do not qualify for entitlement programs, often because they are undocumented aliens, or to tide them over until they get their first check.

Legal assistance

GMHC provides legal assistance, especially for wills and powers of attorney, and, more and more frequently, in cases of discrimination against people with AIDS. These discrimination cases are by no means restricted to gay men. One of them, for example, involves a heterosexual Hispanic male who does not have AIDS but who, like many young Hispanic—and non-Hispanic—males in New York, wears an earring in his left ear. When he went for dental care, his dentist assumed, based on the earring, that the man was gay. He accused him of being homosexual, which is a slanderous offense in New York State, and refused to treat him. So GMHC is in the rather peculiar position of taking on the case of a heterosexual male who has been slandered in being accused of being gay. It should make an interesting legal study.

Meanwhile, GMHC has been informed of many instances of discrimination without regard to sexual orientation but because of AIDS. In New York, if someone discriminates against a person because he or she has AIDS, or because they think that he or she has or may develop AIDS, there are some legal protections. If someone fires a person merely because he or she is gay, however, there is no case.*

Information services

GMHC has created and supports a variety of educational and information programs designed not only for people with AIDS and in AIDS risk groups but also for health care workers and the general public. These programs include the development and publication of pamphlets and other materials about AIDS, and the operation of a telephone counseling service that receives over 7,000 calls each month, an increasing proportion of which are from heterosexuals concerned about AIDS.

*In New York City, discrimination in employment because of actual or perceived sexual orientation has been prohibited by an act of the City Council, passed on March 20, 1986, subsequent to this conference.—ED.]

ORGANIZING TO MEET UNMET NEEDS

All of the services that GMHC provides, especially those directed at clients, could be organized in different ways. There is no one *right* way to do these things, and organizations responding to AIDS around the country will find their own ways to provide services for which they identify a need in their communities. I think, however, that the common link between all of these services, and between all of these groups and their volunteers as well, is that they bear constant witness to the lives and deaths of the people they serve.

Whatever differences there are in the structures and services of the growing number of AIDS organizations scattered about the United States, I believe one of the principal motivations for their establishment has been the sense that the problem of AIDS was being ignored—until recently, at least—both by society at large and by society's traditional institutions. Although the AIDS groups that have sprung up are almost entirely new entities, one must acknowledge the preceding 15 years of organization-building in the gay community that resulted in the formation of groups such as the National Gay Task Force and the Lambda Legal Defense Fund and the development of a variety of political clubs and political action committees, as well as social, religious, cultural, and even bowling organizations. All of them have been important in establishing the cultural medium in which organizations such as GMHC can take root and grow.

New York City, for example, has a large and very visible gay population, but it has not had the sort of strong gay political movement that exists in San Francisco. In New York, it was in the context of a reasonably secure, successful, and financially well-off middle-class gay population—but one without much in the way of a political structure—that GMHC was created. In some other cities, there already existed a medically oriented organizational basis for confronting the AIDS epidemic. Examples of these groups include the Whitman-Walker Clinic in Washington, the Howard Brown Clinic in Chicago, and the Fenway Clinic in Boston. And what we are now beginning to see is that the AIDS programs have grown far larger than the original institutions of which they are a part.

In San Francisco, and in Los Angeles to a lesser extent, an AIDS care model has been developed for the provision of community-based services with government funding and support, and with a professional, salaried staff supervising a corps of volunteers. The New York City model did not begin that way, but it is clearly moving in that direction. Government support now accounts for approximately 50 percent of GMHC's funding (see Figure 16.2), and there is a paid staff of 40 people who recruit, train, and supervise—but largely are there to support—over 1,000 volunteers.

Difficulties in other cities

Outside of New York, San Francisco, and Los Angeles, AIDS organizations have had a much more difficult task. In Houston, in Dallas, and in Atlanta, for example, there has been an almost complete lack of government support, funding, or even recognition. This problem is particularly acute in cities such as Newark and Miami, where a large proportion or even majority of AIDS cases are among IV drug users and heterosexuals. In these places, educational and support services are only beginning to be developed, and there are, not surprisingly, deep suspicions among IV drug users and Haitians about gay, typically white, middle-class organizations. Nevertheless, after five years, GMHC is still providing services in New Jersey, in the absence of any viable local organizations or effort to take on the task.

ADJUSTING TO A CHANGING EPIDEMIC

GMHC has had to adjust to a very different and changing epidemiology of AIDS in New York City, where, unlike in cities such as San Francisco, an increasingly large proportion of AIDS cases are IV drug users and/or heterosexuals (see Figure 16.3). GMHC also provides services to an increasing number of infants and children, with a special volunteer team just for pediatric cases. And as the AIDS epidemic spreads, so does GMHC's geographic service area (see Figure 16.4). The typical volunteer on one of our Brooklyn teams is a gay white male; the typical client of that volunteer is a heterosexual black female.

A new volunteer described an experience he had at his first meeting with a new client, a black, male, IV drug user who lived in Queens. During that first encounter, the client felt it was important to assure the volunteer that he, the client, was not a "homo," as he put it, and he told the volunteer that three times, just to be absolutely clear about it. On another level, it is not infrequent for people to ask us to send them information but to make sure that the organization's name does not appear on the envelope. I think the irony of an essentially gay organization providing services on a volunteer basis to people anxious not to be perceived as gay should not be overlooked.

Neither should the contribution of gay women to the growth and development of these community-based organizations. If the situation had been reversed, if AIDS had primarily affected lesbians, would gay men have responded in a similar fashion? In our male-dominated society, I think the answer is clear: They would not have. In addition, the very real

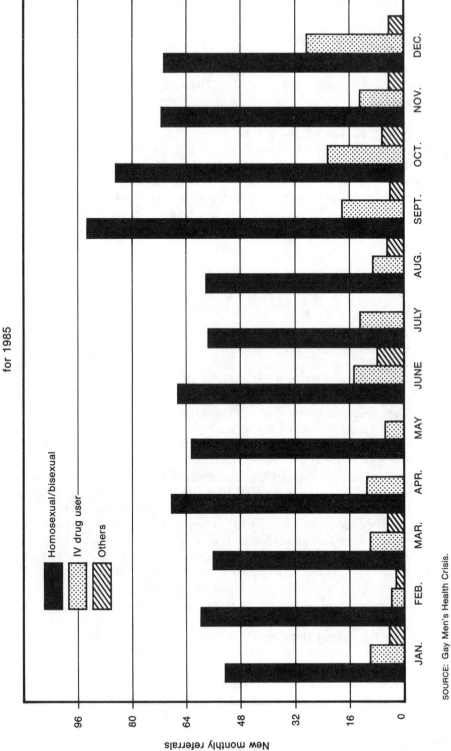

Fig. 16.3. Gay Men's Health Crisis new monthly referrals by risk group for 1985

Homosexual/bisexual

IV drug user

Others

New monthly referrals

96   80   64   48   32   16   0

JAN. FEB. MAR. APR. MAY JUNE JULY AUG. SEPT. OCT. NOV. DEC.

SOURCE: Gay Men's Health Crisis.

Fig. 16.4. Gay Men's Health Crisis new monthly referrals by place of residence for 1985

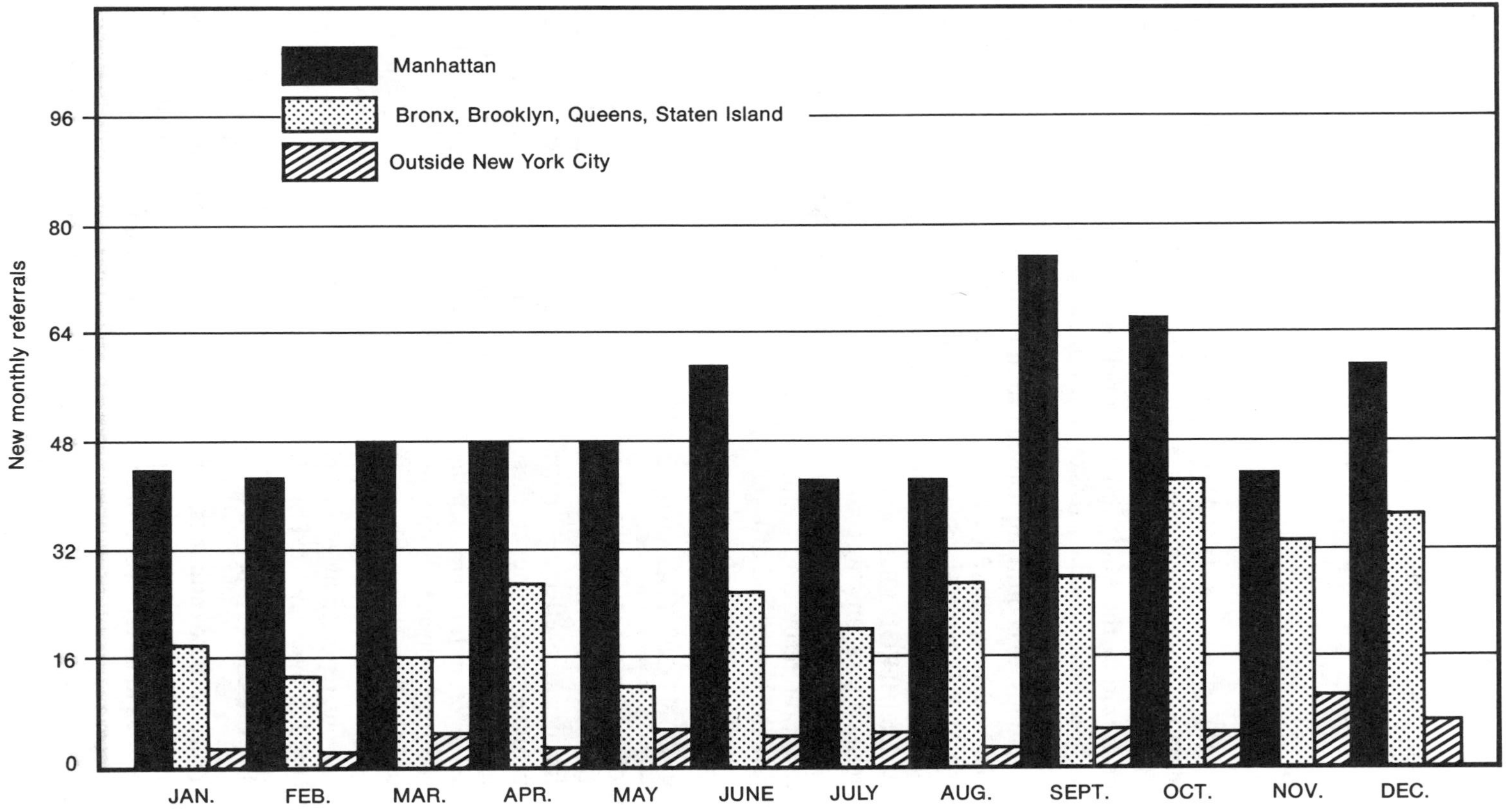

New monthly referrals

Legend:
- Manhattan
- Bronx, Brooklyn, Queens, Staten Island
- Outside New York City

SOURCE: Gay Men's Health Crisis.

contributions of persons with AIDS also need to be acknowledged. Their courage and dignity in the face of this terrible scourge inspire all of us to go on.

ORGANIZING ON A NATIONAL LEVEL

One of the current needs of AIDS-related organizations is for contact and coordination among themselves on a regular basis. Although these groups have been remarkably successful in creating, in 1982, an effective lobbying organization, the AIDS Action Council, in Washington, there is a desperate need for a national AIDS organization to act as a clearinghouse for information, to provide technical assistance, especially to newly emerging organizations, to coordinate national fund-raising efforts, and to sponsor psychosocial research. As a result, the executive directors of a group of leading AIDS organizations, including GMHC, AIDS Project/Los Angeles, the San Franscisco AIDS Foundation, Health Education Resources Organization (HERO) in Baltimore, and the AIDS Action Committee in Boston, formed an organizing committee and have established an office with a small start-up staff in Washington for a new National AIDS Network. However, the resources for this project are very limited, especially considering the task ahead of us.

CONFRONTING THE AIDS COST PANIC

One of the issues which all of us involved with AIDS must confront is the reported high cost of hospital care for persons with AIDS, and the potential for negative effects—especially on the already panicky insurance companies—from some of these reports. Admittedly there is a wide variance in the lifetime hospital costs of treating AIDS patients; a widely quoted report in the *Journal of the American Medical Association* (Hardy et al. 1986), based on a study conducted under the auspices of the Centers for Disease Control, cites a figure of "approximately $147,000 . . . being expended for the hospital care of each patient with AIDS." Other studies, including one reported by Anne Scitovsky, Mary Cline, and Philip Lee (see Chapter 21), have reported much lower numbers.

Putting the costs in perspective

The range of these estimates may be due to faults in the different studies, differences in the patient samples, or other factors. We should, however, be cautious in interpreting these data and be on guard for an overreaction to the costliness of caring for people with AIDS. One is struck by the social and psychological reactions to the sums being quoted just for hospital treatment. In considering the cost to the health care system, and, hence, to all of society, I think we should be mindful of the expense of treating patients with other disorders that are also costly and which have an even higher incidence than AIDS. Head and spinal injuries due to automobile accidents, not to mention lung cancer, are also expensive and high in incidence. Although we know that many patients treated for these problems also die, we do not talk a lot about how terrible the expense of taking care of them is; we simply do it.

CONCLUSION

The burden of AIDS is not just the burden of death and dying. For many it is also the burden of contending with fear and hatred and prejudice, and it is the burden of caring for the dying. By and large, it has been the gay community that has borne that burden, and it is the gay community, with help from our friends, that by and large has reached out to those who are suffering and to those who are alone, and the gay community has done it without regard to age, gender, race, religion, or sexual orientation. It has been the gay community that has provided the muscle, the resources, and the dollars to educate the public and those most at risk. The gay community has done its part, and it will do far more in the years ahead. But it cannot do it alone; it needs the help of the health care community.

We are not "The Other"; we are not "them." We are your children, your nephews and your nieces, your brothers and your sisters, your neighbors and your co-workers. We are persons with AIDS, we are persons with AIDS-associated virus infection, we are caregivers to those with AIDS, and we are the lovers and friends of persons with AIDS and of those who have already died. AIDS is not only our problem; AIDS is a community problem. It requires a community solution.

REFERENCES

Altman, L. K. 1981. Rare cancer seen in 41 homosexuals. *New York Times*, 3 July.

Balzar, J. 1985. Tough new government action on AIDS backed. *Los Angeles Times*, 19 December.

Boffey, P. 1986. AIDS in the future: Experts say deaths will climb sharply. *New York Times*, 14 January.

Buckley, W. F., Jr. 1986. Combating the AIDS epidemic: Identify all the carriers. *New York Times*, 18 March.

Friedman, S. 1986. Cardinal open to AIDS farm idea. *Newsday*, 8 January.

Hardy, A. M., K. Rauch, D. Echenberg, W. M. Morgan, and J. W. Curran. 1986. The economic impact of the first 10,000 cases of acquired immunodeficiency syndrome in the United States. *Journal of the American Medical Association* 255:209-11.

New York City Department of Health. 1986. AIDS Surveillance Office. unpublished data.

CHAPTER 17

San Francisco: Coordinated Community Response

MERVYN F. SILVERMAN

The response to AIDS in San Francisco, the city with the second highest caseload in the United States, is remarkable and, I think, instructive, because it indicates how a coordinated community response can be effective not only in the delivery of vitally needed services but also in reducing costs—and not just dollar costs, but the toll of human suffering as well.

It is, by now, a cliche to observe that a community's response to the AIDS epidemic will need to vary according to the local caseload and demographics of the disease, but the point remains valid. Whether what has been done in San Francisco to provide care and community services to persons with AIDS is applicable to other communities depends, of course, upon the situation with which each of those other communities is confronted, and upon the resources available to it.

Michael Grieco and Omar Hendrix have drawn some demographic comparisons between the AIDS case mix in San Francisco and New York (in Chapters 12 and 14 respectively). Therefore, I will not reiterate the details here, beyond observing that, as of January 10, 1986, in San Francisco, there had been 1,647 cases of AIDS and 879 deaths. Of these AIDS cases, 98 percent were in homosexual/bisexual men; 88 percent of the victims were white, 5 percent were black, another 5 percent were Hispanic, and 2 percent belonged to other ethnic groups. Ninety percent of the victims were in the age group of 20 to 49 years, with males accounting for 99 percent of the total. The survival time for AIDS patients in San Francisco, from diagnosis to death, has ranged from zero to 60 months, with 13 months as the median. Of all cases, 50 percent survived less than 12 months. For 50 percent of the survival time, people with AIDS are in fairly good health; 40 percent of the time, they are chronically ill and in a debilitated condition; and 10 percent of the time, they are in the terminal stages of the disease (San Francisco Department of Public Health 1986.)

THE BASIC CONCEPT—A NEW APPROACH

The basic concept underlying our approach to the AIDS epidemic in San Francisco when I was Director of the Department of Public Health, way back when the epidemic began—and it seems more like 30 years ago than five—was that government cannot do everything. Rather than expect the community alone to plan, initiate, and implement all AIDS programs, however, we began, in San Francisco, with the idea of a cooperative and collaborative arrangement—in essence, a partnership—between government and community groups. We looked at the situation as a new type of health crisis that needed a new approach.

A network of care

One of the things that emerged from that collaborative concept, and which Paul Volberding discusses (in Chapter 15), was the inpatient team for acute care services, a multidisciplinary hospital team that, although previously seen in some intensive care units and trauma centers, was both without parallel in treating a disease such as AIDS and unique in the way in which its members work together. In addition, this team approach was applied in an outpatient clinic that was combined with an inpatient program to create, in effect, a network of care.

The result of this coordinated approach to services has been to reduce, as mentioned at the outset, both the financial and human costs of the AIDS epidemic. If anything positive can come of dealing with this disease, it is the possibility that this kind of model for a health care delivery system—that is really not AIDS-specific—can be applied to other types of chronic illness. In doing so, the services and care we provide will be much more humane, and considerably less costly.

Groundwork for a collaborative response

Prior to 1981, when we started seeing the first AIDS cases in San Francisco, I had established a lesbian-gay coordinating committee in the Health Department, so that we would be more responsive to the needs of the lesbian-gay community and could make sure that we were aware of what their problems were and that our staff understood the various cultural aspects of the lesbian and gay community.

In retrospect, it was fortunate that this committee was in place because, when the cases started to increase—and the numbers were very few at that time—the committee saw a pattern and started reporting it to us. Then, working with the rest of the department, they created a resource document—probably the first in the country—for health care professionals and anyone referring somebody with AIDS, so that people would know where to go and what services were available, and have some information about this strange new disease.

In July 1981, I established, within the San Francisco Department of Public Health, a reporting system and registry for AIDS cases. We tried to investigate and interview all persons with AIDS, when it was possible. We established liaisons between the department, the hospitals, private physicians, and the Centers for Disease Control, and tried to keep these lines of communication open.

In October 1982, a multidisciplinary outpatient clinic, which Dr. Volberding also describes, was established in Ward 86 at San Francisco General Hospital (SFGH). It is an outstanding clinic, providing screening, diagnosis, follow-up, education, and counseling. As the number of AIDS cases increased, screening clinics were added at two city health centers; at these clinics, people are frequently referred to the outpatient unit at SFGH.

AIDS ACTIVITY OFFICE

In 1983, I established an AIDS Activity Office in San Francisco to

• coordinate and link the continuum of services

• identify service gaps and develop plans to address them

• oversee, monitor, and support AIDS-related contract services

• anticipate funding requirements and make the necessary requests

• maintain and expand the department's liaisons in the community

In 1983, we also opened the country's first dedicated inpatient ward for AIDS, with 12 beds, at SFGH. Initially, I was among those who doubted the wisdom of this approach, fearing, as Dr. Volberding reports, the possibility that a "leper colony" analogy might develop around a special AIDS unit. I was very reluctant to support its creation. Fortunately, I was persuaded, because it is now an absolutely incredible facility. Every staff person on the unit volunteered to work there. In fact, there have been more people who want to work on the unit than slots available, and there has been almost no attrition from that ward. I think that is indeed remarkable when you think of the psychological problems that are faced by the health care workers who are involved in AIDS care and daily see young people, in the prime of their lives, wasting away and dying. It gets very depressing for them to realize how many friends, made in that setting, have died. However, the team approach, the emotional support that is provided, and the one-on-one support from the community has been superb.

We also funded, through the Department of Public Health, counseling services, involving both professional and lay practitioners, to work with people with AIDS, the worried well, their loved ones, family members, and others.

Education and information

In cooperation with gay organizations in San Francisco, especially the San Francisco AIDS Foundation, which grew out of the Kaposi's Sarcoma Research and Education Foundation, and also working with businesses in the city, we distributed, in the first year, over a half-million pieces of literature to the gay and the general populations. In the 1982-1984 period, we conducted over 500 training sessions, education programs, and forums about AIDS. We established an AIDS hotline which very quickly began receiving tens of thousands of calls a year. We posted signs in city buses and in gay bars. We even put messages on some billboards. We also put public service announcements on radio and television, and, in the summer of 1983, though we were providing a great deal of information, we still had the highest level of anxiety that I had ever seen in a city. (In fact, the hysteria around the country during the latter half of 1985 was like deja vu for us in San Francisco.) My phone was ringing constantly with questions like, "Can I sit on a bus?" "I work in a court, can I accept a piece of paper from someone who is gay?" "Will I get AIDS?" "I have a swimming pool. A gay man's going to swim in it. Will I get AIDS from that?"

I could not understand how we were constantly saying what we thought, what we believed about AIDS and its transmission—of course, the virus had not been identified at that time—and nobody was listening. Instead, people were getting more upset. And then I realized very quickly the reason for this level of anxiety. First of all, it was the government— local, state, and federal—telling people not to worry. The same government that says not to worry about Love Canal, not to worry about Three Mile Island, and so forth. The point is that the government does not tell us to worry about much of anything in these areas and, here it was again, saying not to worry, not to worry about a disease for which there was no known agent, no cure, no vaccine, and which was known to be universally fatal. So the ingredients for anxiety were certainly there, and so was the anxiety.

Reducing anxiety

In an attempt to reduce this AIDS anxiety, we reconcentrated our efforts on the entire community. Information was directed not just to the gay community through gay-related newspapers, but to the general community and through the general community to bisexuals, for example, who live in and out of the city, with families, and who cannot simply walk into the house with a copy of the *Advocate*, or any of the other gay-oriented magazines or newspapers. We had to provide information that could be disseminated and received through the general media, as well as through selected media. As a result, I think that the anxiety level has come down considerably.

Establishing advisory committees

In addition, we established, very early, both a general AIDS advisory committee, with people from the community and the providers, and also an AIDS medical advisory committee. And this, I felt, was very important, because with all the aspects of a disease that can cause anxiety, such as its being sexually transmitted, a disease primarily of homosexuals—and a lot of people cannot deal with that—with no cure or vaccine, with a long incubation period, and a high fatality rate, one thing we did not need was to have the medical community giving conflicting information. And today, this is probably causing a bigger problem than all of the other six anxiety-producing factors: that is, when physicians and health care workers make statements based on lack of knowledge, confused information, or just plain bigotry. And just as an example, in Houston, Texas, during a discussion of AIDS, three physicians, wearing their white lab coats, with stethoscopes suitably draped, walked into the City Council meeting and made the statement to the Council that they should advise their citizens not to shake hands with strangers because perspiration could spread the AIDS virus.

One cannot imagine—or perhaps one can—what impact that has on anything that anybody else says, because everyone always assumes all physicians have the same degree of knowledge. And they do not look beyond that to see that the person is not speaking as a physician but as a bigot.

The AIDS Medical Advisory Committee included the medical society, hospital representatives, physicians—gay and straight physicians from the community—and the blood bank, and we met on a regular basis to make sure we all heard the same thing, received the same information, evaluated it, and all agreed. We were not trying to march in lockstep; however, one of the things I have been pleased with in San Francisco is that, for the most part, when it comes to giving out information, the city's physicians do so intelligently and consistently. So we were able to present a unified approach, and not have one part of the medical community saying one thing, and another part saying something else.

San Francisco's financial commitment

For fiscal year 1985-86, the City and County of San Francisco (CCSF) is spending about $9 million on AIDS (San Francisco Department of Public Health 1985.) In regard to these expenditures, I want to underscore something Richard Dunne mentions (in Chapter 16) about the cost of treating people with AIDS. AIDS costs are significant, especially in certain areas, but a science writer in San Francisco, reporting on the study of AIDS costs by Ann Hardy et al. (1986) in the *Journal of the American Medical Association*, estimated that the cost of AIDS today represents a nickel out of every ten dollars spent on health care. That is somewhat sobering. It does not mean there is no impact, but it puts the cost of AIDS care in proper perspective.

AIDS SERVICES IN SAN FRANCISCO

I want to describe briefly the services provided in regard to AIDS in San Francisco:

Screening and referral

We screen for AIDS at two health department district health centers and in the Haight Asbury Free Medical Clinic, seeing about 480 patients in about 940 visits per year. A person diagnosed with AIDS is often referred to Ward 86, the outpatient clinic at San Francisco General Hospital, or to a private physician in the community. In fiscal year 1984-85, outpatient registrations at the SFGH clinic averaged 891 per month; for fiscal year 1985-86, it is expected that the average will increase to over 1,200 registrations per month.

Emotional support at SFGH

The emotional support services made available by the Shanti Project are also very important at SFGH, where a team of counselors provides emotional support, advocacy, and education for AIDS inpatients and outpatients. Founded in 1974 to provide emotional support for the terminally ill, Shanti predates AIDS but has now focused its attention on the epidemic and those who suffer from it. Its rigorously trained volunteers offer a variety of services and support for AIDS victims. At SFGH, 81 percent of Shanti's counseling costs is funded by the CCSF Department of Public Health, and the remainder is covered by private donations.

Mental health services at SFGH

The Department of Psychiatry of the University of California, San Francisco (UCSF), oversees the AIDS Health Project, which provides crisis intervention, psychological assessments, short-term therapy for those on waiting lists for psychotherapy, and educational support groups to promote healthiness in people with AIDS. The mental health services component sees about 230 clients and provides over 2,600 hours of consultation and conference services annually at SFGH.

Physicians registry

Private physicians are also involved in San Francisco's community approach to dealing with AIDS. Working with the San Francisco Medical Society, which has been very supportive, and more recently with the California Medical Society, the Department of Public Health has been able to compile a registry of physicians throughout the state for patients with AIDS. This reduces the demand on services at SFGH. Although other hospitals in San Francisco do not want to put up big neon signs reading "AIDS Treatment—Everybody Welcome," the empty bed rate at many has been on the order of 50 percent, and they do not mind physicians' bringing AIDS patients in to fill the beds. However, they do not want to advertise it, and the registry has helped to get care for AIDS patients in these facilities without causing public relations problems.

Hospital services and extended care

In San Francisco overall, there are 14 hospitals providing inpatient services to people with AIDS and AIDS-related complex (ARC). Still, 35 percent of the AIDS/ARC patients in San Francisco are being cared for at SFGH, receiving both acute medical care and mental health services. Garden Sullivan Hospital, a subsidiary of Pacific Medical Center, officially provides about four beds for extended care of AIDS patients, although it has provided care for as many as seven at one time. As in the acute care setting, these are in single-bed rooms. About 75 percent of the extended care patients are covered by Medi-Cal (California's Medicaid program) or private insurance; CCSF reimburses Garden Sullivan for the uninsured or those ineligible for Medi-Cal.

Home health assessments and services

Public health nurses provide health assessments and referrals for people with AIDS in their patients' homes. They see about 150 clients and make approximately 450 home visits each year. The Department of Public Health has also contracted with Hospice of San Francisco to provide registered nurses, licensed vocational nurses, medical social workers, and home health aides and attendants to provide health monitoring, skilled nursing, and other home health care. The daily caseload is about 50 patients. About 63 percent of the costs is covered by CCSF subsidization, and the remainder is covered by Medi-Cal, private insurance, and private donations.

As I speak to various corporations about AIDS and the ways in which our institutions should be responding to it, I am urging them more and more to start looking at these types of in-home services when they review their benefits packages. They are certainly more humane, in many ways, and certainly a lot less costly than alternatives.

Telephone information and referral

The hotline operated by the San Francisco AIDS Foundation, with the support of the Department of Public Health, receives about 2,500 calls per month, and provides information about AIDS and referral to services. New York City has about three times the AIDS cases and its local hotline receives about three times as many calls as San Francisco's hotline handles, indicating, I think, a relative consistency in the relationship between AIDS incidence and not only inquiries but also the utilization of hotline services.

Case management and social services advocacy

In addition, the San Francisco AIDS Foundation provides case management and social services advocacy, including assistance in applying for financial aid for those people with AIDS or ARC who qualify but may have difficulty obtaining aid. This service deals with about 845 clients per year.

Emergency and long-term housing

Under contract to the Department of Public Health (DPH), the San Francisco AIDS Foundation leases a single residence in which it provides emergency shelter for from four to six people, with an average stay of two weeks, although some people with AIDS have stayed for up to two months. About 84 persons per year are housed in this way. Meanwhile, the Shanti Project, also under contract to DPH, provides low-cost, long-term housing for displaced people with AIDS. The aim is to provide a home rather than just a shelter; home health care services are also provided as needed. There are about 34 rooms available in three- and four-bedroom houses. The residents are assessed 25 percent of their current income, and the remainder of the cost is covered by the CCSF and private donations.

Emotional support services

The Shanti Project provides one-on-one emotional support, hospice counseling and information to AIDS patients, their families, and loved ones, helping them to deal with death and grieving. Currently, more than 220 trained volunteers are providing 70,000 hours of service—and these are counseling and/or conference hours—annually. CCSF funds 77 percent of the costs; 23 percent is covered through private donations.

Practical support for daily living

Another Shanti Project program assists persons with AIDS with activities of daily living, including transportation to a clinic or to other places they have to go. Trained volunteers also provide assistance with shopping, cooking, cleaning, laundry, and so forth. There are currently about 120 volunteers providing 30,000 hours of service annually to some 450 clients. The DPH pays for 84 percent of the costs, with 16 percent met by private donations.

Substance abuse services

Obviously San Francisco's problem with IV drug users and AIDS is not as great as New York's, but the incidence of AIDS in our IV drug-abusing community is growing, and 12 percent of the total San Francisco AIDS population consists of IV drug-abusing homosexual/bisexual men. The AIDS Health Project at UCSF operates a program that provides assessment and referral services for individuals with AIDS or ARC who are also substance abusers. Initially, the aim of the program was to train providers and others who deal with this group of patients, but it was expanded and now devotes about 25 percent of its time directly to people with the combined problems. The AIDS Health Project also is involved in AIDS preventive education for substance abuse groups.

Youth outreach

Another important AIDS prevention and education program is aimed at runaway youths—and many of them are young boys—who are hustling on the streets of San Francisco. There is an outreach program to try to reach them, literally, on the streets, and provide individual counseling and health education. Training is also offered for staff of other youth programs. In addition, the AIDS Health Project provides psychological and general health assessments, with special emphasis on dealing with situations that reduce the immune function—such as depression and stress—and on the promotion of safe sexual practices.

Education programs

In San Francisco, some $2.5 million is being spent on education and preventive information programs which include media advertising, news, and feature stories. Under contract to the DPH, the San Francisco AIDS Foundation manages an advertising campaign promoting AIDS prevention, and also provides pamphlets and collateral educational materials, as well as the above-mentioned telephone and information referral services. Educational events, such as forums, workshops, seminars, and other programs, some of which are televised or broadcast on radio, reinforce the AIDS information and education campaigns.

An important point of our education and information campaign has been to emphasize to everyone, especially to those members of the general public who are not particularly at risk for AIDS, that the only thing in this epidemic that can be transmitted by casual contact is AIDS hysteria. Through effective education and information, through the media, through whatever means possible, I believe that we must make sure that the American public knows and understands the facts.

THE RESPONSE OF THE MEDIA

The response of the media to AIDS and to our efforts to deal with the epidemic in San Francisco has, in general, been supportive and very good, although there have been exceptions. Two examples demonstrate two different types of response:

A motel in San Francisco was being used as an emergency shelter for some persons with AIDS, each in an individual room, with individual entrance and private bath. The accommodations sufficed, even if they did not have all the amenities. A number of people in the local media were aware of this arrangement and did nothing about it, but one newspaper decided they wanted to report this story. In my 20 years of public health work, I have never tried to kill a news story, but I tried on this one. Even the mayor got involved. We were up until one or two in the morning over several nights with the newspaper's editors, but they kept insisting, "It's the right of the people to know," which is obviously a very easy thing to say and which covers a multitude of sins.

I responded by asking, "Why should the people need to know? The people of San Francisco have no reason for being in that motel and, therefore, they don't need to know. And the person from Des Moines is not on the newspaper's mailing list, and very likely won't see the article anyway. And even if they saw it, whether they went to that motel or not would have nothing to do with the risk of getting AIDS. Whom are we trying to protect?"

Despite our arguments, we lost. When the paper came out with the story, the motel had to make the people with AIDS who were being sheltered there leave—people who had already been thrown out by either lovers or landlords or families, and some of whom were feeling that they had been thrown out by God, too. They were thrown out onto the street. The motel lost business—and it was not making a killing on this arrangement anyway—and we had to find another facility for these unfortunate people. But the public got to know.

On the other hand, KPIX-TV, a television station in San Francisco, has done a superb job of providing media support. They have a staff dedicated to the AIDS program and to public education rather than fearmongering. Among other things, KPIX-TV has shown two documentaries on AIDS, and shown them in prime time and with no commercials. The first one was seen by 28 percent of the people watching television in the Bay Area on the night it was telecast. Through the San Francisco AIDS Foundation, KPIX-TV has funded the production and dissemination of AIDS information literature, so people also will have access to the printed word. Overall, KPIX-TV and its staff have served as a good example of the positive support that the media can provide in a public health crisis.

THERE WILL ALWAYS BE PROBLEMS

Despite the general effectiveness of many of the programs we have developed in San Francisco to deal with the AIDS epidemic, there have been, and will undoubtedly continue to be, some problems.

Although the rate of increase of AIDS diagnoses in San Francisco is flattening out, it is flattening out, unfortunately, at the rate of two cases and one death per day. We are still seeing a great many AIDS cases. We still see a great many people with ARC who have debilitating conditions and need all the services that we can provide, yet some of them may not qualify for services because they do not have the strict AIDS clinical diagnosis, as defined by the Centers for Disease Control. We also have people with either AIDS or ARC who have mental problems as a result, or who may have had them before, and who come out of acute care also physically debilitated, making it very difficult to find daily living situations for them.

The question of continued funding

In San Francisco, we have been able to implement all of these programs to meet the challenge of the AIDS epidemic because the local government had a budget surplus from which funds could be made available to support them. Now that surplus is gone, and it will be interesting to see, especially with the advent of federal cutbacks mandated by the Gramm-Rudman-Hollings deficit reduction legislation, how San Francisco will continue to meet this challenge. However, I am firmly convinced that it will be met, and I say this as someone who left the city government over a year ago. I feel strongly that the commitment is there, from the top to the bottom, and that it will continue.

All of what has been accomplished in San Francisco could only have been accomplished with a responsive legislative body, a responsive executive branch of government, and a very supportive community. Without that kind of support, we could not be doing in San Francisco what we are doing today.

CONCLUSION

Recently, I was asked what I would do if I were the director of the health department in a community in which AIDS was just beginning to be observed. Jokingly, I said my first response would be, of course, to resign. However, I really would not say that. Actually, I think that being involved in this crisis and the response to it for the last four years has been all at once the most fascinating, the most frustrating, the most challenging, the most difficult, and one of the saddest experiences I have ever had. My recommendation to anyone who is in a position of public health responsibility—or any kind of responsibility, for that matter—in that unlucky community, and who is beginning to see a rise in AIDS cases such as we saw in San Francisco three and four years ago, can be summarized in three words:

- cooperation

- coordination

- education

We have to cooperate with everyone in the community at all levels, we have to coordinate our activities with everyone at all levels, and, by all means, we have to educate. The cost of the AIDS epidemic may be great, but the cost of ignorance is even greater.

REFERENCES

Hardy, A. M., K. Rauch, D. Echenberg, W. M. Morgan, and J. W. Curran. The economic impact of the first 10,000 cases of acquired immunodeficiency syndrome in the United States. *Journal of the American Medical Association* 255:209-11

Harris, R. 1986. AIDS cost: $6.2 billion in hospital bills, wages. *San Francisco Examiner,* 9 January.

San Francisco Department of Public Health. 1985. *San Francisco's response to AIDS: Status update.* October.

San Francisco Department of Public Health. 1986. AIDS Activity Office. Unpublished data.

CHAPTER 18

Community Care:
How Can Hospitals
Participate More Effectively?

LAMBERT N. KING

Richard Dunne gives us (in Chapter 16) an eloquent and moving descrip-
tion of the implications of the AIDS crisis, which has already killed or
painfully affected so many people. Mr. Dunne further describes how the
gay community and others have courageously responded to help those
touched by the epidemic.

Mervyn Silverman shows (in Chapter 17) how important it is to build
an organized community response to a disease which, now and for the
next few years, is unlikely to be cured by even the most advanced medical
techniques. Despite this fact, the great majority of resources directed at
AIDS have supported acute hospital services. There are, however, ways in
which hospitals can participate more effectively with community care
networks to help AIDS victims, whose genuine needs are often far more
extensive than acute hospital care.

It was in the hospitals of New York City, Los Angeles, and San Francisco that AIDS, in its diverse clinical manifestations, first emerged in the
United States. Faced with growing numbers of young people dying of this
implacable disease, physicians and hospitals responded by stressing the
necessity of understanding and confronting AIDS, by assembling the
resources to diagnose the opportunistic infections and malignancies
associated with it, and by applying every therapeutic means available to
help AIDS patients survive at least their current disease complication.

THE LIMITATIONS OF ACUTE HOSPITAL CARE

It has now been five years since we became aware of AIDS, and there has
been remarkable progress in understanding the etiology, pathogenesis,
and epidemiology of HTLV-III/LAV-related disease. Our understanding of
the mechanisms of retroviral infection and its effects upon the immune
system offer hope for the development of new preventive and therapeutic
modalities. Yet, at the same time, we have become more aware of the

182

limitations of acute hospital care in coping with the crisis we face. While almost 20,000 people in the United States have been diagnosed as having AIDS, and over half of them have died, we now know that far greater numbers of people are likely to be affected in a more chronic way. The necessity of a broader treatment concept—emphasizing community-based long-term care—has become obvious. One of the imperatives for hospitals, therefore, is to educate their medical, nursing, and social service workers about why and how we must move from an acute disease paradigm to a community strategy.

Financial squeeze for providers

In order for hospitals, expecially New York City voluntary hospitals, to participate more effectively in community care of AIDS patients, changes in the financing mechanisms for the hospital care of AIDS patients are undoubtedly necessary. The situation at many New York City voluntary hospitals is analogous to that of the man who, when asked by a friend how he had gone bankrupt, replied, "In two ways: gradually, and suddenly."

New York voluntary hospitals caring for AIDS patients continue to be severely limited in their capability to extend services into the community because of the New York State Prospective Hospital Reimbursement Methodology (NYPHRM), implemented in 1983. Under the NYPHRM system, the amount that hospitals receive for inpatient care depends upon their inpatient service activity in the base year of 1981, with costs trended forward each year to adjust for general, but not health care, inflation rates. The 1981 base year costs for New York hospitals did not include the substantial demands now being made upon hospitals for the professional staff, equipment, and supplies necessary to provide care for AIDS patients.* Because the per diem costs of treating AIDS patients in the hospital are, on the average, higher than those for most other acute illnesses, hospitals have absorbed the costs of AIDS by shifting resources from other programs and from previous priorities.

Not only have New York hospitals experienced a shortfall due to per diem rates that do not take into account the needs of AIDS patients, but they also may be financially penalized if their occupancy rates are significantly greater in years after 1981. Thus, at St. Vincent's Hospital and Medical Center, a financial volume penalty was imposed in 1984, even though the increased census in 1984, compared to 1981, was partly attributable to the care of AIDS patients. As a result, in 1984, St. Vincent's suffered a $3 million loss on the NYPHRM volume adjustment alone.

*In 1981, only 148 cases of AIDS were diagnosed in all of New York City, but, by the end of 1985, the number of annual diagnoses had increased by over 1,300 percent, with, it is reasonable to assume, a relative increase in hospital expenses in treating AIDs patients.—ED.

Risks in overestimating AIDS costs

However, it is important not to overestimate the hospital costs associated with caring for AIDS patients. In 1985, the average length of stay (ALOS) for AIDS and AIDS-related complex (ARC) patients at St. Vincent's was slightly more than 21 days. While this ALOS is almost twice that for AIDS patients at San Francisco General Hospital, it is also less than half the ALOS of 50 days that was used in a recent article to extrapolate the New York City hospital costs for AIDS patients (Hardy et al. 1986). Such projections, which overestimate the hospital costs attributable to AIDS, may have the unwarranted—and undesirable—effect of limiting the funds available for supporting community-based services. Faulty overestimation of actual AIDS hospital costs may also impede making funds available for those community services which would actually reduce hospital costs by reducing ALOS.

ALTERNATIVE CARE: A CRITICAL NEED

Another important aspect of hospitals' participating more effectively in community-based services for AIDS patients is the critical need for skilled nursing facility (SNF) services. On any given day at St. Vincent's, about 10 percent of our 35 to 40 AIDS patients are hospitalized on an alternate-level-of-care (ALC) basis. In reviewing 18 of our most recent ALC patients with AIDS, we found that 15 were male and three were female. Eight of the patients had Blue Cross coverage, of whom four had Medicaid applications pending for home care services. Six patients were covered by Medicaid, and four were uninsured, with applications pending for Medicaid coverage. Five of the patients accounted for 196 ALC days while awaiting care in a SNF. Eleven patients, with 255 ALC days, needed 12- to 24-hour home care services.

While resources for home care services are increasing, there are virtually no vacancies available in New York City for AIDS patients requiring SNF care. Our experience at St. Vincent's—similar to that at other hospitals in New York City—indicates that there should be an urgent emphasis on development of more SNF beds and facilities for AIDS patients. Rather than simply decertifying acute hospital beds in facilities with low occupancy, conversion of those acute beds to SNF beds should be aggressively supported by state and federal agencies.

An additional consideration for hospitals endeavoring to move from a narrow emphasis on acute hospital care to a continuum of community services resides in the willingness of many volunteers to respond to the AIDS epidemic.

The Supportive Care program

Beginning in 1983, St. Vincent's began to integrate AIDS patients into its Supportive Care program, which provides hospital- and home-based hospice care. Since that time, along with other patients that we have cared for in the hospice program, we have treated over 70 patients with AIDS, of whom 56 have died. At St. Vincent's, hospital- and home-based supportive care services are provided by registered nurses, social workers, pastoral counselors of various denominations, and, most importantly, by well-trained and experienced volunteers.

The Supportive Care program at St. Vincent's also includes a bereavement service for families, lovers, and friends of patients who have died. All of this has been accomplished without direct public financial support. A grant from the United Hospital Fund of New York was instrumental in expanding the Supportive Care program to include AIDS patients in 1984, and the Gay Men's Health Crisis (GMHC) also has been crucial in sustaining this program in many ways, particularly through good advice and the provision of volunteers.

HOSPITALS AND VOLUNTEERS

The remarkable effectiveness of GMHC in responding to all aspects of the AIDS crisis has demonstrated how important the work of volunteers can be in the AIDS epidemic. Mobilization of other community volunteers in meeting the complex needs of intravenous (IV) drug-using patients with AIDS will certainly be more difficult than within the more cohesive gay community. However, hospitals, many of which already have established volunteer programs for assisting patients of all types, can be important in stimulating broader community and voluntary support to help AIDS patients.

A final perspective from the hospital point of view relates to the inherent capabilities of hospital workers to identify those persons with AIDS who are likely to require coordinated medical and social care. Hospital social service departments can intensify their efforts to secure timely and full eligibility for Medicaid and other services. The development of multidisciplinary AIDS treatment teams, as well as discrete hospital units for AIDS patients, will undoubtedly be important steps in enhancing the effectivenesss of the hospital's role in the continuum of care.

AIDS IN THE CORRECTIONAL SYSTEMS

Before concluding, I would like to draw attention briefly to another important community concern about AIDS, which, although it does not relate directly to the hospitals, nevertheless should be addressed.

An important part of my professional career has been spent in caring for and trying to improve health care for people in prisons and jails around the country. I would, therefore, like to mention the effect of AIDS within correctional institutions. Because of its association with IV drug use, AIDS-related disease is, on the whole, more common among prisoners than among the general population (Centers for Disease Control 1986). From an epidemiological perspective, however, prison and jail populations account for only a small percentage—approximately 4.6 percent—of total AIDS patients.*

There is little or no evidence of significant intramural transmission of AIDS within prisons and jails; however, there has been intensive media attention directed at this question, as well as to other medical, legal, and correctional management issues in the context of the AIDS epidemic. There also has been an uninformed and sometimes hysterical response to AIDS among correctional officers in certain locations, including states in which there are no diagnosed AIDS patients in prison.

Wherever there are walls, there are likely to be abuses behind them, and it is important, I believe, to monitor carefully social and public policy initiatives for AIDS that might be tested first in prison and jail environments. At present, for example, there is serious consideration being given to policies mandating that all prisoners have mandatory blood tests for HTLV-III/LAV antibodies before being released. The value of such an approach to combating AIDS is extremely dubious. Instead, the focus should be placed upon gains that can be made in health education and risk reduction in prisons and jails, and upon the provision of adequate medical, health, and social services to AIDS patients in prison before, and after, their release.

CONCLUSION

Finally, I would like to emphasize how important it is to understand the AIDS crisis in a larger social context. We must build a national response to the AIDS epidemic similar to that which we have made to atherosclerotic heart disease, hypertension, and cancer. With increased federal and private support for AIDS research, we not only will help people directly affected but also will achieve a quantum leap in our understanding of the biological mechanisms of oncogenesis and of the intricacies of the im-

---

*As of early January, 1986, 766 cases of AIDS were reported in the correctional systems of the United States, an incidence rate of 151.2 cases per 100,000 population, while the rate for the general population, based on 16,458 cases diagnosed, was about 6.9 cases per 100,000 population (Centers for Disease Control).—ED.

mune response and aging, and perhaps also of chronic neurologic diseases, including the dementias. At a cost that is modest in comparison, for example, to that of just one Trident submarine, AIDS research will benefit not just AIDS victims but all of us and future generations.

It is likely that we will only begin to respond adequately to AIDS when we establish a new national agenda that will also care more for the needs of the homeless, the frail elderly, and the 13 million children in this nation who live in poverty. Either we will change the nature of the official policies that now limit the quality of our national response, or the AIDS epidemic will continue upon its tragic course. As Dr. Oliver Sacks observed in his book, *Awakenings* (1979): "Diseases have a character of their own, but they also partake of our character; we have a character of our own, but we also partake of the world's character."

REFERENCES

Centers for Disease Control. 1986. Acquired immunodeficiency syndrome in correctional facilities: A report of the National Institute of Justice and the American Correctional Association. *Morbidity and Mortality Weekly Report* 35:195-99.

Hardy, A. M., K. Rauch, D. Echenberg, W. M. Morgan, and J. W. Curran. 1986. The economic impact of the first 10,000 cases of acquired immunodeficiency syndrome in the United States. *Journal of the American Medical Association* 255:209-11.

Sacks, O. 1976. *Awakenings.* New York: Random House.

CHAPTER 19

The Contributions and Limitations of Voluntarism

PETER S. ARNO

Community-based organizations have played a key role in the nation's response to the AIDS epidemic. They have provided an important and otherwise missing dimension in patient care and social support services, and have been instrumental in developing and disseminating public health information and preventive strategies.

In the third quarter of 1984, the United States Conference of Mayors conducted a survey to determine what actions were being taken at the local level in regard to the AIDS epidemic. The survey revealed that 60 percent of local health departments had working relationships with community-based groups providing a range of AIDS-related services (U.S. Conference of Mayors 1984). By 1986, that number has surely grown.

COMMUNITY GROUPS: FILLING THE RESOURCE GAPS

The AIDS epidemic has generated a large and unanticipated need for a variety of medical, public health, social, and educational resources. Many of the community-based organizations were initially formed to close the gaps in government provision of these resources. The services they provide fall largely into two categories:

1. Public health education.

2. Social support and counseling activities.

Education and information

Public health education includes information for groups at risk, regarding safe sexual practices and hypodermic needle sharing, to limit exposure to the AIDS virus. Accurate information about AIDS is provided to persons outside the main risk groups in order to reduce unwarranted fears in the community, promote support for effective programs, and prevent further spread of the epidemic. Educational services are provided in a variety of ways, including telephone hotlines, forums, workshops, distribution of pamphlets and other literature, and documentaries and advertisements in the electronic and print media.

188

Social support

Social support and counseling activities are particularly important because the psychosocial needs of AIDS patients are extensive, complex, and unique (Dilley et al. 1985; Holland and Tross 1985; Morin, Charles, and Maylon 1984). An AIDS diagnosis is a terrifying experience that raises a number of difficult issues that an AIDS patient must immediately face. These include the reactions of employers and families and friends, treatment options, sexual behavior modification, community fear and ostracism, financial hardship, physical deterioration, depression, and the fear of death itself.

OFFERING A RANGE OF COST-EFFECTIVE SERVICES

Traditional health care systems have been unable or unwilling to develop an integrated approach to these areas of concern. As a result, community-based groups have sought to fill the void by offering a range of services that, while varying from one region of the country to another, generally include the following elements:

- psychosocial counseling

- practical support that includes help with day-to-day activities, such as cooking, cleaning, laundry, shopping, and transportation

- home health care services

- housing

- entitlements advocacy, such as helping those eligible to receive state and federal government benefits

- legal protection, such as fighting discrimination by landlords and employers

In addition to providing an important part of the care received by persons with AIDS, these services have a financial impact on local health care systems and the municipal governments that subsidize them. It has been argued that local government support for community-based services not only allows for a higher quality of care for AIDS patients but also is a rational and cost-effective fiscal policy.

The economic argument rests on two premises:

1. A link exists between the availability of community-based services and reductions in the length and expense of hospitalization of AIDS patients.

2. A hidden subsidy of large quantities of unpaid, or volunteer, labor exists that allows for a greater production of services per dollar expended than would be possible if local government supplied the services itself.

The largest component of direct economic costs imposed by the AIDS epidemic is the hospitalization of AIDS patients. Inpatient costs directly affect local government financing, particularly in cities, such as New York and San Francisco, that treat a large number of AIDS patients within the public hospital system. In New York City, municipal government already bears a heavy financial burden for its contribution to the Medicaid program, and, like San Francisco and other municipalities, for subsidizing those patients who have inadequate or no third-party health insurance coverage, public or private. An integrated system of outpatient clinical facilities and community-based services, such as exists in San Francisco, allows many AIDS patients to remain outside the hospital setting for longer periods of time and, once admitted to the hospital, to be discharged earlier, thereby reducing the overall level and expense of hospitalization.

GAUGING THE CONTRIBUTION OF DONATED LABOR

Unpaid labor provides the backbone of most community-based AIDS organizations in the United States. According to one national survey, nearly 80 percent of services provided by these groups was performed by volunteers (U.S. Conference of Mayors 1984). In New York City and San Francisco, the magnitude of donated labor is enormous, conservatively estimated to be between 100,000 and 150,000 hours per year in each city. Although the number of hours of donated labor at the Gay Men's Health Crisis (GMHC) in New York City and the combined total at the Shanti Project and the AIDS Foundation in San Francisco are comparable, the ratio of unpaid to paid staff hours is twice as large in New York City. Rather than reflecting any basic differences in local voluntarism in the two cities, however, the difference in ratios can be attributed to the pattern of funding of their respective organizations. During fiscal year 1984-85, the major community-based groups in San Francisco received 62 percent of their revenue from local government (Arno 1986). This compares with 3 percent of the total revenues received by GMHC in 1984 from the city of New York (Arno and Hughes 1985).

Looking out for limits

The role of unpaid labor raises some important questions for both high and low AIDS incidence areas around the country. For example, can the supply of volunteers continue to match the expected growth of the epidemic? In concentrated areas such as New York City and San Francisco, large gay communities exist from which the pool of volunteers has primarily been drawn. However, it is logical to assume that the level of volunteer support will at some point reach its limit. Furthermore, there are indications that the number of new AIDS cases among gay and bisexual men has begun to level off, at least in New York City and San Francisco. At the same time, the proportion of intravenous drug-related AIDS cases continues to rise. This reveals a potential flaw in a system so heavily dependent upon volunteer labor. While the gay community has done an extraordinary job thus far in supporting its afflicted members, in addition to caring for those of other risk groups, it is unclear whether this level of voluntarism will be maintained if the proportion of AIDS cases among gay men declines significantly. In low-incidence regions, there may not be a significant, identified at-risk population from which to draw volunteers. Thus, the gaps in service which many of these communities are already experiencing may become more severe as the epidemic continues to spread geographically.

Those who donate their labor clearly provide compassionate care for those afflicted with AIDS. There are, however, many health care services that cannot be provided by volunteers, including major aspects of hospital care, mental health care, and social services. Certainly, AIDS patients are entitled to treatment from trained professionals.

CONCLUSION

It is important to remember that community-based AIDS organizations are not viable without a steady stream of unpaid labor. In addition, these groups require a certain level of funding for administrative structures and paid staff who can recruit, train, supervise, and support their volunteers. There are, however, intrinsic limits to the current dependence on unpaid labor and the contributions from private charity and local government. As the epidemic continues to grow, the service needs will overwhelm even the most integrated of existing delivery systems. The pressures are quickly mounting for increased support and intervention at the state and federal levels.

REFERENCES

Arno, P. S. 1986. The non-profit sector's response to the AIDS epidemic: Community-based services in San Francisco. *American Journal of Public Health* 76:1325–30.

Arno, P. S., and R. G. Hughes. 1985. Local policy response to the AIDS epidemic: New York and San Francisco. Paper presented at the annual meeting of the American Public Health Association, 18 November, Washington, D.C.

Dilley, J. W., H. N. Ochitill, M. Perl, and P. A. Volberding. 1985. Findings in psychiatric consultations with patients with acquired immune deficiency syndrome. *American Journal of Psychiatry* 142:82-86.

Holland, J. C., and S. Tross. 1985. The psychosocial and neuropsychiatric sequelae of the acquired immunodeficiency syndrome and related disorders. *Annals of Internal Medicine* 103:760-64.

Morin, S. F., K. A. Charles, and A. K. Maylon. 1984. The psychological impact of AIDS on gay men. *American Psychology* 39:1288-93.

U. S. Conference of Mayors. 1984. *Local responses to acquired immune deficiency syndrome (AIDS): A report of 55 cities.* Washington, DC: United States Conference of Mayors, November.

CHAPTER 20

Integrated Services for AIDS Patients: Comments and Cautions

JOSEPH A. CIMINO

Governments at all levels are finally reacting to the crises posed by the AIDS epidemic to public health, in general, and to the communities most heavily affected by AIDS, in particular. Undeniably in some cases, governments are reacting somewhat later than they should have, but they are reacting. The news is both good and not-so-good.

THE GOOD NEWS

The basically good news for New York is that the state government is finally going to make funds available to support integrated services for people with AIDS. The New York State Department of Health has drafted a proposal for a comprehensive AIDS program and has issued regulations defining the criteria hospitals must meet in order to participate in the program. Facilities that qualify will be designated as AIDS centers and will be entitled to discrete reimbursement rates for providing coordinated and comprehensive services—including inpatient, outpatient, and post-hospital non-acute services—to AIDS patients. Since the average daily cost of acute care for the AIDS patient population in New York has historically been higher than the average cost for the non-AIDS patient population, this reimbursement plan should be good news for the facilities—largely clustered in New York City—that have been treating large numbers of AIDS patients. Hospitals designated as AIDS centers will be required to provide care to all AIDS patients, regardless of the patient's source of payment.

THE AIDS CENTERS PROGRAM

The overall goal of the New York State AIDS centers program for hospitals is to increase AIDS patients' access to essential services, through a case management approach organized around a continuum-of-care concept that emphasizes home care and community-based support services. Properly coordinated, such a program should enable AIDS patients to maintain the quality of their lives in a home environment for as long as possible

193

and should simultaneously reduce their need for hospitalization by addressing those patient needs that are currently not being met through existing health care and support systems.

Of course, the lack of available community support services has been identified as one of the factors in the longer average length of stay (ALOS) of AIDS patients in New York hospitals, compared with that of AIDS patients in San Francisco. Although the ALOS for AIDS patients in New York has been decreasing—from about 26 days in 1982 to about 21 days by the end of 1985—it is still far above the ALOS of about 12 days in San Francisco. The higher percentage of AIDS patients in New York who are intravenous drug abusers (IVDAs), who frequently present with more complicated clinical needs than AIDS patients who are non-IVDAs, is a significant factor in the longer ALOS of AIDS patients in New York. The AIDS centers program has at least the potential for narrowing the ALOS disparity. Since the average per diem cost of caring for AIDS inpatients is higher than that for non-AIDS patients, shortening the length of stay should reduce the overall costs of the epidemic, not only for individual institutions but also for the state, its affected communities, and all payers.

The services that New York hospitals designated as AIDS centers will be expected to provide for AIDS patients include

- ambulatory care

- inpatient services

- home health and personal care services

- psychosocial and psychiatric services

- housing

- legal and financial assistance

- residential health care services

- hospice care

AIDS centers requirements

In its qualification requirements for AIDS centers, the New York State Department of Health has formulated a set of program standards that facilities must meet. These standards call for

- designated units for AIDS inpatients. The requirement for a discrete AIDS unit may be waived for facilities demonstrating space or structural limitations that preclude such a physical unit or presenting valid reasons why such a unit is not preferable or practical.

- ambulatory/outpatient services for screening, diagnosis, and treatment of AIDS patients. Outpatient services may be provided both through the hospital's own clinics and by private physicians in their own offices.

- emergency services for AIDS patients, 24 hours a day. The emergency room service should be able to integrate new AIDS patients into the comprehensive care program and provide continuity of care for patients whose cases are already being managed.

- home health and/or personal care provided either by the center directly or by a licensed or certified home health care agency and including nursing; nutrition; home health aide services; occupational, physical, and speech therapy; and social services, as necessary. Home health and personal care providers must be able to address the special needs of different types of AIDS patients.

- provision or arrangements for residential health care, hospice services, and residential living programs appropriate to the needs of AIDS patients. Where sufficient housing facilities, hospice programs or residential health care services are not available, case managers are expected to make reasonable efforts to locate additional community resources.

- specialized diagnostic and therapeutic radiology and other services, as AIDS patients may require, either in the AIDS center facility or in a cooperating hospital.

- inservice AIDS-related education programs for all personnel caring for AIDS patients. These education programs should address both the special medical, psychological, and social needs of AIDS patients and the stress-management needs of staff caring for them.

- AIDS-specific infection control policies and procedures, based on the recommendations of the Centers for Disease Control, implemented and integrated into the hospital's existing infection control program.

- integration of protocols specific to AIDS patients and their comprehensive care plan into the hospital's existing quality assurance program.

- participation in approved AIDS clinical research programs.

- resource information and education programs for the public, especially targeting risk group populations in the AIDS center's service area with AIDS prevention and treatment information.

- crisis intervention and counseling services, provided through the center directly or through arrangements with community-based AIDS service agencies.

• individual patient care management plans specific to the patients' particular post-hospital care needs. Elements of such a program include a multidisciplinary professional team appropriate to the patient's needs for medical, nursing, nutritional, mental health, and social service support; a designated case manager; periodic reviews and updates of each patient management plan in conjunction with other service agencies involved in the patient's care; a comprehensive case management plan developed with input from the multidisciplinary team, the patient, and the appropriate representatives of other agencies involved in the patient's care. Oriented to post-hospital care and community support services, the case management plan should reflect the individual patient's ongoing needs and choices; include transfer, discharge, and follow-up planning; evaluate the patient's personal support system; be reviewed and updated to reflect the patient's current status; and be forwarded with the patient on transfer or discharge.

THE NOT-SO-GOOD NEWS

There is much that is laudable in this proposal for a comprehensive case-management approach to caring for people with AIDS. Certainly, as outlined, it offers the prospect of both better care for AIDS patients and, by providing alternatives to maintaining patients in expensive acute care settings, reduced costs for care of these patients. Using hospitals as the focus of the AIDS centers program, however, poses some dangers worth noting.

By making hospitals the coordinators of care for AIDS patients, the state is, in effect, creating a medical model for the management of the problems raised by the AIDS epidemic, whether people with AIDS are in the hospital or in the community, functioning relatively well. The program establishes a medical model for financial and reimbursement purposes as much as for care. One danger in this approach is that the acute care facilities may wind up getting the bulk of the funding that will be made available for the care of AIDS patients and the community-based health and support services that already provide services to AIDS patients may receive less than they deserve.

As the program requirements enumerated here indicate, the AIDS centers will integrate not only hospital inpatient and ambulatory services but also skilled nursing and home health services, which may be provided by the centers or by other contracted providers. This is likely to increase the problems of the voluntary home health industry in New York, which has played a critical role in the care of AIDS patients. There is already tremendous competition among home health agencies, most of which are struggling to make ends meet and are not prepared to compete with the for-profit home health agencies that are coming into the community. Thus, one result of the AIDS centers program may be to increase the financial pressures that the voluntary agencies already face.

In addition, when government comes in to provide funding for new programs, it often brings with it a host of rules and regulations for certification and licensure and other operational aspects. This happened with the Medicare and Medicaid programs in 1965, with the result that voluntarism in the hospitals was virtually destroyed. Now, the same thing is happening with the licensure of home health agencies and all of the community-based groups that are going to be providing services to AIDS patients. Even though the rules and regulations are absolutely necessary, there is a danger of making them so stringent, so systematized, that the unintended result may be the destruction of much of the voluntary effort that heretofore has been so important in helping people with AIDS.

Inevitably, as government becomes more involved, we must be increasingly careful that we do not lose the individuals with AIDS through the proverbial cracks in the system. We must be aware of the unfortunate tendency of government simply to allocate large sums of money, overregulate, and then assume that they have taken care of a problem. There are myriad problems for AIDS patients in the community that will not be entirely solved by current or projected efforts on the part of government—state or city. These problems include appropriate housing, adequate nutrition, simple socialization, and routine transportation for other than mere trips to and from medical facilities. For example, debilitated and weakened AIDS patients cannot be housed in apartments buildings that are three- or four-floor "walk-ups," because the pulmonary insufficiency that is often a complication of AIDS will make them virtual prisoners in their own homes. The need for delivery or provision of meals to homebound AIDS patients is another critical problem, as is the need for providing some sort of communication with friends and service agencies, on a 24-hour basis, both to relieve the patients' sense of isolation and to meet their emergency service needs as they arise. We have, in fact, the technology for two-way closed-circuit television systems that would be useful in these sorts of situations, but the provision of funding for such systems is very unlikely.

CONCLUSION

There is no question that the AIDS epidemic poses a wide range of problems, not only for people with AIDS but also for the medical systems that serve them and their communities and for the communities as a whole. And there are undoubtedly many things that could and might be done to improve both the quality of care and quality of life for AIDS patients, whether they are being cared for in our acute care medical institutions or living in the community. The voluntary sector has been very important in addressing some of the problems caused by the AIDS epidemic, and it should continue to be an important element in the overall service picture. However, if the focus of our—and our various governments'—efforts is too rigidly fixed on the acute care system, and if our models for dealing with AIDS become exclusively medical ones, some of our health care problems may be unintentionally exacerbated, and many things that could be done for AIDS patients either may be done less effectively than they might be or may not be done at all.

PART SEVEN

Financial Perspectives on AIDS: Footing the Bill

CHAPTER 21

Medical Care Costs of AIDS Patients in San Francisco

ANNE A. SCITOVSKY
MARY W. CLINE
PHILIP R. LEE

Acquired immune deficiency syndrome (AIDS) is a virulent disease, caus- ing its victims—mainly young persons in their twenties to forties—to come down with a variety of opportunistic infections and other diseases, such as *Pneumocystis carinii* pneumonia and Kaposi's sarcoma. AIDS ap- parently made its first appearance in the United States in 1979. Initially a rare occurrence, the incidence of AIDS has developed to alarming propor- tions and has been increasing at a near exponential rate. By January 13, 1986, according to the data from the Centers of Disease Control (1986), 16,458 cases had been reported nationwide, and a recent estimate places the number of new cases in the next two years at 40,000 (Quinn 1985).

AIDS is not only virulent, requiring frequent hospitalization, but also deadly. Of the 16,458 people with AIDS reported so far, 8,361—51 percent—have died. It has been reported that hospitalized patients with AIDS have an average life span of 224 days after being hospitalized for their first opportunistic infection (Landesman, Ginzburg, and Weiss 1985.) The average life expectancy of an AIDS patient from diagnosis to death has been estimated at 21 months for patients with Kaposi's sarcoma and nine months for those with *Pneumocystis carinii* pneumonia (Moss et al. 1984).

CONCERN OVER THE FINANCIAL BURDEN

Not surprisingly, the epidemic has caused widespread public anxiety. There is grave concern over both the deadliness of the disease and the fact that neither cure nor preventive treatment has been found to date, nor is

Participating institutions: The Palo Alto Medical Foundation/Research Institute and the In- stitute for Health Policy Studies, University of California at San Francisco.

This study was supported by a grant from the University-Wide Task Force on AIDS of the University of California. An earlier verison of the paper was presented at the Annual Meet- ing of the American Public Health Association in Washington, D.C., 19 November 1985.

likely to be found in the near future. There is also fear, based largely upon ignorance, that the disease may spread through casual contact to the population at large. Last but not least, there is concern over the financial burden AIDS imposes on its victims, on society in general, and, in particular, on the metropolitan centers—including most notably, New York, San Francisco, Los Angeles, Miami, Houston, and Newark—where the disease is concentrated.

Questions about cost data

Despite the seriousness of the situation, data on the use of and the expenditures for medical services for AIDS patients are fragmentary, generally based on small samples, and often little more than informed guesses. According to an estimate by researchers at the University of California at Los Angeles (UCLA) Medical Center, cited in an editorial some time ago, the average AIDS patient required two to three months of hospitalization, "with 1 to 2 weeks in the intensive care unit, at a total cost of between $50,000 and $100,000 per patient" (Groopman and Detsky 1983). The data on which this estimate was based were not given. Another estimate states that "the average direct lifetime hospital cost for the care of such patients is calculated to be $42,000. If there are at least 8,000 new cases of AIDS in 1985, then the estimated cost of inpatient care for patients with newly diagnosed disease will be approximately $336 million. This is an underestimate of the total medical care costs, since it does not include the costs of outpatient care or medication" (Landesman, Ginzburg, and Weiss 1985). No documentation of these estimates was given, nor were the figures broken out in more detail.

The most frequently cited estimate of the costs of treating persons with AIDS is one made by Ann Hardy of the Centers for Disease Control (Hardy 1985; Hardy et al. 1986). She estimated the direct costs of hospitalization of the first 10,000 AIDS patients in the United States at $1.473 billion over their lifetime, or an average of $147,000 per patient. This estimate is based on the assumption of an average length of initial hospital stay of 31 days (the average of some data from New York, San Francisco, and Philadelphia), an estimated lifetime use of 167 hospital days, an average survival time of 56 weeks, and an average charge (including inpatient professional charges) of $878 per hospital day (based on charges of 35 AIDS patients at one acute care hospital in Atlanta). However, Hardy concedes that, "The data available to make the necessary calculations were limited and often based on small samples of patients but represent the best and sometimes the only data that could be obtained."

A study undertaken in San Francisco

In order to obtain better and more detailed data on the costs of treating patients with AIDS, we undertook a retrospective study of the costs for patients treated at San Francisco General Hospital (SFGH), the city and county hospital, in 1984. We collected data on inpatient hospital and professional charges, as well as on charges for outpatient medical care provided by SFGH. Not included were charges for nursing home and home health care, hospice care, counseling and similar services, and outpatient drugs. It should be noted that our data refer to charges, not costs. While it is possible to convert hospital charges into costs, this cannot be done for other services, such as those of physicians; therefore, it seemed best to show the data only in terms of charges.

COSTS FOR AIDS PATIENTS TREATED AT SFGH IN 1984

Our study generated three sets of cost data:

1. Data on all AIDS admissions to SFHG in 1984 (Tables 21.1 through 21.3).

2. Data on all AIDS patients who received their inpatient hospital and inpatient and outpatient professional services at SFGH in 1984 (Tables 21.4 through 21.8).*

3. Data on lifetime inpatient costs for AIDS patients who died in 1984 and received all their inpatient hospital and professional care from diagnosis to death at SFGH (Tables 21.9 and 21.10).

AIDS admissions to SFGH in 1984

The mean charge per admission, including inpatient professional charges, was $9,024; the mean charge per day was $773, and the average length of hospital stay was 11.7 days (Table 21.1). The median charge per admission was considerably lower, amounting to $6,248. Charges varied substantially, depending on principal diagnosis and whether the patient spent one or more days in an intensive care unit (ICU). Mean costs by diagnosis ranged from $2,440, for admissions for diseases of the blood, to $14,120, for admissions for *Pneumocystis carinii* pneumonia. The relatively low cost of hospitalizations for diseases of the blood is explained by a high per-

---

*Outpatient professional services include physician services, laboratory tests, x-rays, and similar ancillary services performed at SFGH.

Table 21.1

Admissions, Charges, and Lengths of Stay, by Diagnosis, at San Francisco General Hospital in 1984

DIAGNOSIS*	ADMISSIONS	MEAN HOSPITAL AND INPATIENT PROFESSIONAL CHARGES PER ADMISSION	MEAN CHARGE PER DAY	MEAN LENGTH OF STAY (DAYS)
Total	445	$ 9,024	$ 773	11.7
Kaposi's sarcoma	59	5,695	747	7.6
Pneumocystis carinii pneumonia	136	14,120	782	18.1
Other infectious diseases	73	10,682	784	13.6
Other neoplasms	9	9,665	674	14.3
Diseases of blood	37	2,440	836	2.9
All other	131	6,125	759	8.1
All admissions having only regular room use	398	7,331	662	11.1
All admissions having at least one day in intensive care	47	23,360	1,399	16.7

*Diagnoses based on ICD-9 codes for discharge diagnosis as follows: Kaposi's sarcoma (173.8); *Pneumocystis carinii* pneumonia (136.3); other infectious diseases (001–139, excluding 136.3); other neoplasms (140–239, excluding 173.8); diseases of the blood (280–289).

Table 21.2
Distribution of Admissions, Hospital Days, Intensive Care Days, and Total Charges, by Diagnosis, at San Francisco General Hospital in 1984

DIAGNOSIS*	ADMISSIONS	DAYS	INTENSIVE CARE DAYS	TOTAL CHARGES
	(N = 445)	(N = 5,195)	(N = 240)	(N = $4,015,612)
Total	100.0%	100.0%	100.0%	100.0%
Kaposi's sarcoma	13.3	8.7	0.0	8.4
Pneumocystis carinii pneumonia	30.6	47.3	66.7	47.8
Other infectious diseases	16.4	19.2	14.6	19.4
Other neoplasms	2.0	2.5	0.4	2.2
Diseases of blood	8.3	2.1	0.4	2.2
All other	29.4	20.3	17.9	20.0

*Diagnoses based on ICD-9 codes for discharge diagnosis as follows: Kaposi's sarcoma (173.8); *Pneumocystis carinii* pneumonia (136.3); other infectious diseases (001–139, excluding 136.3); other neoplasms (140–239, excluding 173.8); diseases of the blood (280–289).

centage of one-night hospitalizations for blood transfusions. We understand that, beginning in 1985, such transfusions generally have been performed on an outpatient basis, which will raise the mean and median
charges per hospital admission for these conditions. The mean length of
hospital stay paralleled mean charges per admission, ranging from 2.9 days
for hospitalizations for diseases of the blood to 18.1 days for admissions
for *Pneumocystis carinii* pneumonia. The range of mean charges per hospital day by diagnosis was much more narrow than either mean total charges
or mean length of stay, ranging from $674 for neoplasms other then
Kaposi's sarcoma to $836 for diseases of the blood, but with charges for the
other diagnoses being very similar, ranging from $747 for Kaposi's sar-
coma to $782 for *Pneumocystis carinii* pneumonia. Patients who required
care in an ICU had very much higher charges than those not receiving
such care, averaging $23,360 per admission, compared with $7,331 for the
others. They also had considerably longer hospital stays: 16.7 days, compared with 11.1 days.

Another way of looking at differences in the costs of treatment for
different diseases which afflict AIDS patients is to compare the percentage
distribution of admissions by diagnosis with the distribution of all hospital days, all ICU days, and total charges (Table 21.2). This too shows that
Pneumocystis carinii pneumonia not only was the most frequent diagnosis
but also required a disproportionate share of hospital resources. It accounted for 30.6 percent of all admissions, but for 47.3 percent of all hospital days, 66.7 percent of all ICU days, and 47.8 percent of total costs of all
admissions. By contrast, diseases of the blood, which accounted for 8.3
percent of all admissions, accounted for 2.1 percent of all hospital days,
less than one-half of 1 percent of all ICU days, and 2.2 percent of total
charges.

Of the mean charge of $9,024 for all AIDS admissions, $8,380, or 92.9
percent, was for hospital services and only $643, or 7.1 percent, for in-
patient professional services (Table 21.3). Charges for the hospital room accounted for almost half of all charges, and laboratory tests for about one-
quarter. Despite the wide differences in mean charges per admission for
the different diagnoses, the distribution of charges by type of service was
found to be remarkably similar for all diagnoses.

Costs for patients receiving all their services at SFGH in 1984

Our next set of cost data relates to AIDS patients who received all their inpatient hospital and inpatient and outpatient professional services at
SFGH in 1984. These patients fell into three groups:

Table 21.3
Inpatient Charges and Number of Services per Admission, by Type of Service,
for All Diagnoses, at San Francisco General Hospital in 1984
(N = 445)

SERVICE	MEAN CHARGES		MEAN NUMBER
Total	$9,024	100.0%	—
Hospital total	8,380	92.9	—
Room	4,419	49.0	11.7
Regular room	3,665	(40.6)	11.1
Intensive care	754	(8.4)	0.5
Laboratory tests	2,211	24.5	—
X-rays	349	3.9	—
Prescriptions/materials	337	3.7	—
All other*	1,064	11.8	—
Inpatient professional services**	643	7.1	11.2
Medical	623	(6.9)	11.2
Surgical	20	(0.2)	†

*Includes: Emergency Room services prior to admission, EKGs, blood supplies, respiratory therapy, CT scans, surgery/recovery room charges, anesthesia, ambulance, EEGs, and miscellaneous clinic charges.
**Includes: Hospital visits, hospital surgeries and visits associated with respiratory function testing, EKGs, and EEGs.
†Less than 0.05.

1. Those who lived all 12 months of 1984.

2. Those who died in 1984.

3. Those who were newly diagnosed in 1984 and did not die in 1984.

Of the 201 patients who received all their inpatient and outpatient care at SFGH, 14.9 percent were in the first group, 41.3 percent were in the second, and 43.8 percent were in the third (Table 21.4).

Mean inpatient and outpatient charges for the entire group of 201 patients amounted to $15,993 (Table 21.5). Of this, 79.8 percent was for hospital inpatient services and 20.2 percent for professional services; one-third of the latter amount was for inpatient professional services, and two-thirds was for outpatient professional services. On average, these patients spent 18.0 days in the hospital. However, 25.4 percent of them had no hospital stays during the year. Those who had one or more hospitalizations spent an average of 24.1 days in the hospital and incurred mean total charges of $20,668.

Table 21.4
Percent Distribution of AIDS Patients, by Patient Status, at San Francisco General
Hospital in 1984

STATUS	DISTRIBUTION
	(N = 201)
Total	100.0%
Alive all 12 months	14.9
Died in 1984	41.3
Newly diagnosed in 1984 and did not die in 1984	43.8

Group 1.   Patients who lived all 12 months of 1984 had mean charges of $7,026, of which 44.4 percent was for hospital services, 4.1 percent for inpatient professional services, and 51.5 percent for outpatient services (Table 21.6). Only 43.3 percent of this group had hospital stays. Patients in this latter group spent an average of 11.1 days in the hospital and incurred mean total charges of $12,407. The majority of the patients who lived all 12 months of 1984 suffered from Kaposi's sarcoma, a condition which is treatable to a large extent on an outpatient basis.

Group 2.   Patients who died in 1984 had considerably higher costs, although on the average they had expenses for only 6.4 months of 1984 (Table 21.7). Mean charges amounted to $23,425, of which 84.1 percent was for hospital charges, 6.8 percent for inpatient professional charges, and 9.1 percent for outpatient professional charges. Patients in this group averaged 25.8 days in the hospital. All but three of the 83 patients in this group had one or more hospital stays.

Group 3.   Patients who were newly diagnosed in 1984 and did not die in 1984 averaged charges of $12,040 in the 4.6 months of 1984 during which, on average, they incurred expenses (Table 21.8). Of these charges, 78.9 percent was for hospital services, 5.7 percent for inpatient professional services, and 15.4 percent for outpatient professional services. Patients in this group spent an average of 15.2 days in the hospital. The two-thirds of this group who were hospitalized averaged 23.4 days in the hospital and had mean total charges of $17,453.

We have reason to believe that our cost data for outpatient professional services may be on the low side. Some of these services were provided at no charge, and some were provided at a fee lower than the

Table 21.5
Charges and Number of Services per Patient, by Type of Service, for All AIDS
Patients at San Francisco General Hospital in 1984
(N = 201)

SERVICE	MEAN CHARGES		MEAN NUMBER
Total	$15,993	100.0%	—
Inpatient total	13,759	86.1	—
Hospital total	12,755	79.8	—
Room	6,809	42.6	18.0
Regular room	5,649	(35.3)	17.2
Intensive care	1,160	(7.3)	0.8
Laboratory tests	3,338	20.9	—
X-rays	521	3.3	—
Prescriptions/materials	532	3.3	—
All other*	1,554	9.7	—
Inpatient professional services**	1,004	6.3	17.5
Medical	966	(6.0)	17.4
Surgical	38	(0.3)	0.1
Outpatient total	2,234	13.9	—
Physician	463	2.9	14.4
Medical	441	(2.8)	14.3
Surgical	22	(0.1)	0.1
Laboratory tests	1,186	7.4	56.9
X-rays	148	0.9	2.1
Prescriptions/materials	183	1.1	—
All other†	253	1.6	—

*Includes: Emergency Room services prior to admission, EKGs, blood supplies, respiratory therapy, CT scans, surgery/recovery room charges, anesthesia, ambulance, EEGs, and miscellaneous clinic charges.
**Includes: Hospital visits, hospital surgeries and visits associated with respiratory function testing, EKGs, and EEGs.
†Includes: CT scans, EEGs, EKGs, blood administration, anesthesia, and physical therapy.

scheduled fee when patients either had no insurance or had insufficient funds. At most, however, we estimate that they should be increased by 15 to 20 percent.

Lifetime costs for patients who received all their care at SFGH

Our final data set relates to AIDS patients who died in 1984 and had received all their inpatient hospital and professional services, from diag-

Table 21.6
Charges and Number of Services per Patient, by Type of Service, for AIDS Patients
Alive All of 1984 at San Francisco General Hospital
(N = 30)

SERVICE	MEAN CHARGES		MEAN NUMBER
Total	$7,026	100.0%	—
Inpatient total	3,405	48.5	—
Hospital total	3,117	44.4	—
Room	1,580	22.5	4.8
Regular room	1,580	(22.5)	4.8
Intensive care	0	(0)	0
Laboratory tests	855	12.2	—
X-rays	169	2.4	—
Prescriptions/materials	145	2.1	—
All other*	369	5.2	—
Inpatient professional services**	287	4.1	4.9
Medical	260	(3.7)	4.6
Surgical	28	(0.4)	0.4
Outpatient total	3,621	51.5	—
Physician	888	12.6	29.2
Medical	794	(11.3)	28.9
Surgical	94	(1.3)	0.3
Laboratory tests	2,086	29.7	107.9
X-rays	151	2.2	2.3
Prescriptions/materials	253	3.6	—
All other†	243	3.4	—

*Includes: Emergency Room services prior to admission, EKGs, blood supplies, respiratory therapy, CT scans, surgery/recovery room charges, anesthesia, ambulance, EEGs, and miscellaneous clinic charges.
**Includes: Hospital visits, hospital surgeries and visits associated with respiratory function testing, EKGs, and EEGs.
†Includes: CT scans, EEGs, EKGs, blood administration, anesthesia, and physical therapy.

nosis to death, at SFGH. Their lifetime costs averaged $27,571,* of which 93.4 percent was for hospital services and 6.6 percent was for inpatient

*It will be noted that the lifetime inpatient expenses of this group are only $4,146 more than the 1984 inpatient expenses of the AIDS patients who died in 1984 (the two groups overlap but are not identical). This is explained by two factors. First, as already noted, this group had a higher percentage of admissions for Kaposi's sarcoma, which are less costly, and a smaller percentage of costly admissions for *Pneumocystis carinii* pneumonia. Second, although the average lifespan of this group was only 224 days, many of these patients had hospital stays 18 to 24 months prior to death, when hospital charges were somewhat lower. Both factors also explain why the average cost per hospital day was $795 for this group, compared with $908 for the decedents who had expenses only in 1984.

Table 21.7
Charges and Number of Services per Patient, by Type of Service, for AIDS Patients
Who Died in 1984 at San Francisco General Hospital
(N = 83)

SERVICE	MEAN CHARGES		MEAN NUMBER
Total	$23,425	100.0%	—
Inpatient total	21,285	90.9	—
Hospital total	19,690	84.1	—
Room	10,291	43.9	25.8
Regular room	7,565	(32.3)	23.8
Intensive care	2,725	(11.6)	2.0
Laboratory tests	5,009	21.4	—
X-rays	864	3.7	—
Prescriptions/materials	722	3.1	—
All other*	2,804	12.0	—
Inpatient professional services**	1,595	6.8	27.1
Medical	1,534	(6.6)	27.1
Surgical	61	(0.2)	† †
Outpatient total	2,140	9.1	—
Physician	403	1.7	12.1
Medical	397	(1.7)	12.0
Surgical	6	(† †)	† †
Laboratory tests	1,078	4.6	51.7
X-rays	154	0.7	2.1
Prescriptions/materials	197	0.8	—
All other†	308	1.3	—

*Includes: Emergency Room services prior to admission, EKGs, blood supplies, respiratory therapy, CT scans, surgery/recovery room charges, anesthesia, ambulance, EEGs, and miscellaneous clinic charges.
**Includes: Hospital visits, hospital surgeries and visits associated with respiratory function testing, EKGs, and EEGs.
† Includes: CT scans, EEGs, EKGs, blood administration, anesthesia, and physical therapy.
† † Less than 0.05.

professional services (Table 21.9). These patients spent an average of 34.7 days in the hospital and had an average of 3.2 hospital admissions over a period of 224 days from diagnosis to death (Table 21.10). The total number of admissions for this group, the total number of hospital and ICU days, and total charges are distributed similarly to those for 1984 admissions shown in Table 21.2, although in this group there was a slightly higher percentage of admissions with Kaposi's sarcoma (18.2 percent compared to 13.3 percent in Table 21.2) and a smaller percentage with *Pneumocystis*

Table 21.8

Charges and Number of Services per Patient, by Type of Service, for
AIDS Patients Diagnosed in 1984 Who Did Not Die in 1984 at
San Francisco General Hospital

(N = 88)

SERVICE	MEAN CHARGES		MEAN NUMBER
Total	$12,040	100.0%	—
Inpatient total	10,190	84.6	—
Hospital total	9,499	78.9	—
Room	5,309	44.1	15.2
Regular room	5,229	(43.4)	15.1
Intensive care	80	(0.7)	0.1
Laboratory tests	2,609	21.7	—
X-rays	318	2.6	—
Prescriptions/materials	484	4.0	—
All other*	780	6.5	—
Inpatient professional services**	691	5.7	12.7
Medical	672	(5.6)	12.7
Surgical	19	(0.2)	† †
Outpatient total	1,850	15.4	—
Physician	376	3.1	11.5
Medical	362	(3.0)	11.4
Surgical	14	(0.1)	0.1
Laboratory tests	980	8.1	44.3
X-rays	143	1.2	2.0
Prescriptions/materials	146	1.2	—
All other†	205	1.7	—

*Includes: Emergency Room services prior to admission, EKGs, blood supplies, respiratory therapy, CT
scans, surgery/recovery room charges, anesthesia, ambulance, EEGs, and miscellaneous clinic charges.
**Includes: Hospital visits, hospital surgeries and visits associated with respiratory function testing,
EKGs, and EEGs.
† Includes: CT scans, EEGs, EKGs, blood administration, anesthesia, and physical therapy.
† † Less than 0.05.

carinii pneumonia (25.9 percent compared with 30.6 percent in Table
21.2). But the distributions of hospital and ICU days and of charges are
very similar for the two groups.

DISCUSSION

Our study found considerably lower costs for treating persons with AIDS
than has been estimated to date. The most frequently cited and best

Table 21.9
Charges and Number of Services per Patient, by Type of Service, from Diagnosis to
Death, for AIDS Patients Who Died in 1984 at San Francisco General Hospital
(N = 85)

SERVICE	MEAN CHARGES		MEAN NUMBER
Total	$27,571	100.0%	—
Hospital total	25,758	93.4	—
Room	13,159	44.7	34.7
Regular room	10,159	(36.8)	32.5
Intensive care	3,000	(10.9)	2.1
Laboratory tests	6,848	24.8	—
X-rays	1,255	4.6	—
Prescriptions/materials	1,018	3.7	—
All other*	3,478	12.6	—
Inpatient professional services**	1,812	6.6	33.2
Medical	1,753	(6.4)	33.1
Surgical	59	(0.2)	†

*Includes: Emergency Room services prior to admission, EKGs, blood supplies, respiratory therapy, CT
scans, surgery/recovery room charges, anesthesia, ambulance, EEGs, and miscellaneous clinic charges.
**Includes: Hospital visits, hospital surgeries and visits associated with respiratory function testing,
EKGs, and EEGs.
†Less than 0.05.

documented estimate, that by Ann Hardy of the Centers for Disease Control (CDC), arrived at a lifetime hospital cost of $147,000 per patient for
the first 10,000 AIDS victims (Hardy 1985; Hardy et al. 1986), as compared
with our estimate of $27,571. Her estimate was based on the assumption
of 167 days of hospital care at a cost of $878 per day, spread over 56 weeks
(or 392 days). Our data show a total of 35 days of hospital care at $795 per
day, over a span of 224 days.

Accounting for the difference in estimated costs

Most of the difference between the two cost figures is due to differences in
the total number of hospital days used by AIDS patients from diagnosis to
death. It is generally agreed that the average length of hospital stay is considerably shorter for AIDS patients in San Francisco than in other cities,
such as New York and Philadelphia. However, a lifetime use of 167 hospital days seems high. Even if we assume that the average length of stay per
admission is 25 days, instead of the 11.7 days shown by our data, and that
AIDS patients who died in 1984 had an average of four hospital admissions from diagnosis to death, this brings the total lifetime use of hospital care to only 100 days—and this is a very liberal estimate.

Table 21.10

Admissions, Hospital Days, and Total Charges, by Diagnosis, for AIDS Patients Who Died in 1984 and Received All Their Inpatient Care, from Diagnosis to Death, at San Francisco General Hospital

(N = 85)

DIAGNOSIS*	ADMISSIONS	HOSPITAL DAYS	INTENSIVE CARE DAYS	TOTAL CHARGES
	(N = 274)	(N = 2,947)	(N = 182)	(N = $2,343,521)
Total	100.0%	100.0%	100.0%	100.0%
Kaposi's sarcoma	18.2	13.6	0.0	12.1
Pneumocystis carinii pneumonia	25.9	46.2	74.7	49.4
Other infectious diseases	17.9	14.4	11.0	14.9
Other neoplasms	0.7	0.2	0.5	0.5
Diseases of blood	11.3	2.4	0.5	2.6
All other	25.9	23.1	13.2	20.5

Average number of admissions per decedent: 3.2
Average number of days from diagnosis to death: 224

*Diagnoses based on ICD-9 codes for discharge diagnosis as follows: Kaposi's sarcoma (173.8); *Pneumocystis carinii* pneumonia (136.3); other infectious diseases (001–139, excluding 136.3); other neoplasms (140–239, excluding 173.8); diseases of the blood (280–289).

Hardy also assumed a higher cost per patient day than our figures indicate: $878 compared with our figure of $795 for patients who died in 1984 and had all their hospital care at SFGH (Table 21.9). Data from New York City show an average daily cost of between $794 and $850 in 1985 (Leicht 1985), which would bring it close to our figure, considering that our cost data are based on charges for patients who died in 1984, some of whom had hospital bills going back to earlier years. Possibly, an average cost per hospital day of $800 for these patients is closer to actual 1984 costs than the $878 assumed by Hardy.

Lowering the bill

If we assume a total of 100 hospital days per AIDS patient from diagnosis to death, at an average cost of $800 per hospital day, this would bring the total lifetime hospital costs of an AIDS patient who died in 1984 to $80,000. This is considerably lower than the $147,000 estimate of Hardy. To arrive at total costs would, of course, require adding charges for outpatient professional services, nursing home, home health and hospice care, and possibly some other services, such as counseling. Our data on the 1984 costs of outpatient care at SFGH suggest that lifetime outpatient professional services may add another $4,000 to $5,000.* We have no firm data on the costs of other medical services, but they are unlikely to add more than another $2,000 to $4,000 per AIDS patient. Thus, total direct medical care costs from diagnosis to death of AIDS patients who died in 1984 may have averaged about $90,000.

Comparing results with a statewide study

A study by the California Department of Health Services (Kizer et al. 1986) has reported on the Medi-Cal (California Medicaid) lifetime costs for AIDS patients in California. Assuming a life expectancy of 18 months, the study's authors estimated the average total Medi-Cal cost for an AIDS patient to be $59,000, which they translated into a "commercial" cost of $91,000. The study contains estimates for the counties of Los Angeles and San Francisco, individually, and for the remainder of the state (Table 21.11).

The estimate, by the California Department of Health Services, of $52,000 for the lifetime cost of treating an AIDS patient in San Francisco

---

*It must be borne in mind, however, that outpatient professional costs may be higher in San Francisco than in other cities because, in San Francisco, outpatient care appears to be substituted for inpatient care to some extent. Thus, the average lifetime outpatient professional charges for an AIDS patient who died in 1984 may have been less nationwide than in San Francisco. The same is true of our very rough estimate of nursing home and home health care costs.

Table 21.11
Estimated Lifetime Costs for AIDS Patients in California

	MEDI-CAL COST	COMMERCIAL COST
Statewide average	$59,000	$ 91,000
Los Angeles County	70,000	109,000
San Francisco County	52,000	74,000
All other counties	65,000	110,000

SOURCE: California Department of Health Services, 1985.

is higher than what our 1984 data for San Francisco General Hospital show, that is, a lifetime cost of $27,571. One reason for this difference is that the Medi-Cal figures include outpatient costs, while our data were limited to inpatient costs. A more important reason, however, is the fact that in our study we counted expenses from the date of a firm diagnosis of AIDS to death while the Medi-Cal study began counting expenses from the date of the first symptoms that *could* indicate AIDS. To quote from the Medi-Cal study:

> The onset date represents the first month that symptoms characteristic of the disorder were noticeable to either the attending physician or the patient. This could mean the month when symptoms such as fever, diarrhea, night sweats, and swollen lymph glands were noted or the onset of an opportunistic infection.

Thus, the "lifetime" of the Medi-Cal AIDS patients was very much longer than that of the AIDS patients in our study, where we adhered to the CDC definition of a diagnosis of AIDS.

A COSTLY DISEASE

Whatever the direct costs of treating AIDS patients, there is no doubt that AIDS is a costly disease. But two points need to be stressed:

Adequate social support services may keep costs down

First, our data show that the costs of treating persons with AIDS appear to be very much lower in San Francisco than in New York, and probably also lower than in Los Angeles and some of the other cities with relatively large numbers of AIDS patients. The reasons for the lower costs in San Francisco are not entirely clear. Part of the explanation may lie in differences in the patient populations. In San Francisco, over 90 percent of AIDS patients are male homosexuals, while in New York, this group accounts for only about 60 percent, with an additional 30 percent being intravenous drug abusers. It is quite likely that the latter patients have few sources of social support and, hence, stay in the hospital longer because there is no alternative place for them to go. In addition, San Francisco has a well-organized gay community which very probably helps patients leave the hospital sooner or stay out of the hospital completely and receive outpatient care. A closer study of the San Francisco social network is clearly indicated. If it is found that the social support services available in San Francisco do indeed keep hospital costs down, other cities may be able to develop similar services, with the result that the costs of treating AIDS patients will decline substantially.

AIDS treatment costs should be kept in perspective

Second, in the public discussions of and concern over the high cost estimates that have been publicized, it is generally forgotten that they are estimates of the *lifetime* direct costs of treating AIDS patients. For example, the $147,000 estimate of Hardy is for the lifetime hospital cost per AIDS patient. This fact tends to be ignored because the lifetime medical costs for AIDS patients are spread over a short time, possibly around six to twelve months on the average, rather than over many years, as in the case of many other diseases. In order to give the estimates some perspective, therefore, it is necessary to compare them not with annual average expenses of other patients but with their lifetime expenses. Unfortunately, there are almost no data on the lifetime direct medical costs of other illnesses. A study by Long et al. (1984) found that terminal cancer patients had average medical expenditures of $21,219 in the last 12 months of life. These data are for 1980, and in 1984 prices these expenditures would be $30,280. Since we have no information about expenses in preceding years, all we can say is that lifetime direct medical costs of cancer patients are probably considerably higher than $30,000.

For patients with end-stage renal disease, there are Medicare data which can be used to make an estimate of lifetime medical expenses for dialysis patients. According to an article by Eggers (1984), Medicare reimbursements per enrollee on dialysis averaged $21,325 in 1979. Translating reimbursements into charges and adjusting this figure to 1984 prices brings average expenses per dialysis patient to $45,873. Eggers's data also show that average Medicare reimbursements per dialysis patient have been very constant over recent years. Eggers, Connerton, and McMullen (1984) indicate that the median life expectancy of dialysis patients is about four years. On the basis of these data, and using a 4 percent discount rate, we have estimated average lifetime medical expenses of renal dialysis patients in 1984 to be about $158,000. That is even higher than the very high estimate of lifetime costs per AIDS patient of Hardy, and considerably higher than our own estimate of about $90,000 for lifetime costs, which we consider a liberal one.

Indirect costs may be very high

This is not to belittle the fact that the medical expenses of AIDS patients are high but merely to put them in perspective. What aggravates the problem is the fact that AIDS patients are concentrated in a few geographic areas, with the result that these communities bear a very heavy burden. Moreover, the direct medical care costs for AIDS patients are only part of the economic costs of this disease. Because the victims are mainly young adults 20 to 40 years old, who are in their most productive period of life, the indirect costs due to morbidity and premature mortality are bound to be very high, probably very much higher than the direct costs and higher than the indirect costs for patients suffering from diseases like end-stage renal disease, over two-thirds of whom were 45 years old and older in 1980 (Eggers 1984).

CONCLUSION

Finally, coping with the challenges of the AIDS epidemic requires that the information and data upon which our health care institutions and communities formulate policy and construct responses be accurate and sound, in order that our decisions be informed ones. During a time of intense attention to and worry about the cost of providing health care in general, overestimating the costs of an already expensive illness places unnecessary pressures on policy-makers and risks faulty decision-making in an atmosphere of panic. Given the scope and complexity of the health care crisis we face, the importance of the careful collection, study, and analysis of costs and other data cannot be underestimated.

APPENDIX

Standard Deviations of Mean Charges

Table 21.1
Mean Inpatient Hospital and Professional Charges per Admission, by Diagnosis, at
San Francisco General Hospital in 1984

	MEAN CHARGE PER ADMISSION	STANDARD DEVIATION	N
All AIDS admissions	$ 9,024	$ 9,483	445
Kaposi's sarcoma	5,695	4,283	59
Pneumocystis carinii pneumonia	14,120	11,006	136
Other infectious diseases	10,682	11,102	73
Other neoplasms	9,665	9,393	9
Diseases of the blood	2,440	2,766	37
All other	6,125	6,540	131

Table 21.5 through 21.8
Mean Inpatient Hospital and Inpatient and Outpatient Professional Charges, for
AIDS Patients Who Received All Their Inpatient and Outpatient Care at
San Francisco General Hospital in 1984

TABLE		MEAN CHARGE PER PATIENT	STANDARD DEVIATION	N
21.5	All AIDS patients	$15,993	$13,833	201
21.6	AIDS patients alive all 12 months	7,026	7,146	30
21.7	AIDS patients who died	23,425	14,523	83
21.8	AIDS patients newly diagnosed who did not die	12,040	11,307	88

Table 21.9
Mean Lifetime Inpatient Hospital and Professional Charges, for AIDS Patients
Who Died in 1984 and Had Received All Their Inpatient Care, from Diagnosis to
Death, at San Francisco General Hospital

	MEAN CHARGE PER PATIENT	STANDARD DEVIATION	N
All AIDS deaths	$27,571	$16,549	85

REFERENCES

California Department of Health Services. 1985. Summary report on California AIDS victims, quantitative analysis. Sacramento Ca., 28 October 1985.

Centers for Disease Control. 1986. Update: Acquired immunodeficiency syndrome—United States. Morbidity and Mortality Weekly Report 35:17-21.

Eggers, P. W. 1984. Trends in Medicare reimbursements for end-stage renal disease: 1974-1979. Health Care Financing Review 6(1): 31-38.

Eggers, P. W., R. Connerton, and M. McMullen. 1984. The Medicare experience with end-stage renal disease: Trends in incidence, prevalence, and survival. Health Care Financing Review 5(3): 69–88.

Groopman, J. E., and A. Detsky. 1983. Epidemic of acquired immunodeficiency syndrome: A need for economic and social planning. Annals of Internal Medicine 99:259-61.

Hardy, A. M. 1985. Statement before the Subcommittee on Health and the Environment, Committee on Energy and Commerce, U. S. House of Representatives. Washington, D.C., 1 November.

Hardy, A. M., K. Rauch, D. Echenberg, W. M. Morgan, and J. W. Curran. 1986. The economic impact of the first 10,000 cases of acquired immunodeficiency syndrome in the United States. Journal of the American Medical Association 255:209-11.

Kizer, K., J. Rodrigues, G. F. McHolland, and W. Weller. 1986. A quantitative analysis of AIDS in California. Sacramento, Calif.: California Department of Health Services, March.

Landesman, S. H., H. M. Ginzburg, and S. H. Weiss. 1985. The AIDS epidemic. New England Journal of Medicine 312:521-25.

Leicht, D. 1985. Statement before the Labor, Health and Human Services, Education and Health Agencies Subcommittee, Appropriations Committee, U. S. Senate. Washington, D.C., 26 September.

Long, S. H., J. O. Gibbs, J. P. Crozier, D. I. Cooper, Jr., J. F. Newman, Jr., and A. M. Larsen. 1984. Medical expenditures of terminal cancer patients during the last year of life. Inquiry 21:315-27.

Moss, A. R., G. McCallum, P. A. Volberding, P. Bacchetti, and S. Dritz. 1984. Mortality associated with mode of presentation in the acquired immune deficiency syndrome. Journal of the National Cancer Institute 73: 1281–84.

Quinn, T. C. 1985. Perspectives on the future of AIDS. Journal of the American Medical Association 253:247-49.

CHAPTER 22

AIDS in New York City: Programs and Costs

JO IVEY BOUFFORD

New York City has the largest number of AIDS patients in the United States—and the number is increasing steadily. As a result, the city of New York and the New York City Health and Hospitals Corporation (HHC) are investing tremendous resources to mount effective programs for the care of persons with AIDS. As Michael Grieco has pointed out (in Chapter 12), it is the demographics of the disease that determine the sorts of programs that are needed, the resources that must be brought to bear, and, inevitably, the health care costs with which we are confronted. This is as true for the community as a whole—and for community-wide health care systems—as it is for any single health care facility facing the problem of AIDS.

In discussing the costs of AIDS in New York City, I want to address three areas of concern:

1. The cost to the city of New York for a variety of AIDS programs mounted by various city agencies.

2. The cost to the New York City Health and Hospitals Corporation as a direct health care services provider.

3. Policy recommendations relating to reimbursement for direct health care services for persons with AIDS.

AIDS PROGRAMS AND COSTS: NEW YORK CITY

Surveillance information on AIDS began to be available in New York City in 1981. Although a number of programs were developed earlier, coordinated planning by the city to cope with the epidemic began in 1984, when we focused on a comprehensive program of services with three characteristics:

1. The improvement of interagency cooperation and the coordination of city agencies with voluntary agencies.

2. The development of service programs that stress case management for individual patients throughout the course of their illness.

221

3. The augmentation, by the municipal sector, of resources for health, education, and social services to promote a service system for persons with AIDS.

In fiscal year 1986, it is estimated that New York City spent approximately $65 million of city tax levy funds on AIDS. Of this amount, $53 million was direct tax levy support for the municipal hospital system's inpatient services for the uninsured and the Medicaid share of services in the municipal system, about $9.5 million was the city's share of Medicaid spent in the voluntary hospital system, and a little under $3 million was for public health education and laboratory support (see Figure 22.1). Furthermore, the cost of municipal hospital outpatient services is in-

Fig. 22.1. Distribution of New York City tax levy expenditures on AIDS for fiscal year 1986 (total = $65 million)

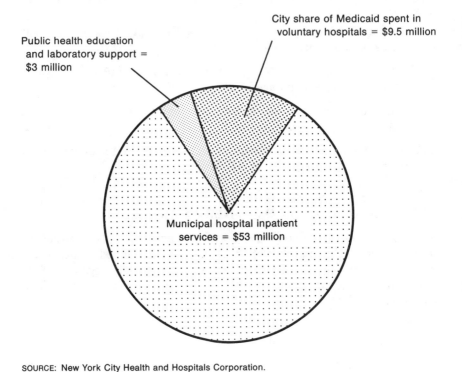

City share of Medicaid spent in
voluntary hospitals = $9.5 million

Public health education
and laboratory support =
$3 million

Municipal hospital inpatient
services = $53 million

SOURCE: New York City Health and Hospitals Corporation.

creasingly significant. State and federal dollars have been more available for housing and community support—through Supplemental Security Income—than for the direct provision of health services.

The array of programs provided by the city of New York includes public health education and surveillance; research and testing; inpatient and ambulatory acute care in the hospital setting; community-based ambulatory care, especially in case finding and dealing with the worried well; home care and community support services; housing and foster care for children with AIDS; and, finally, institutionalized long-term care services.

AIDS PROGRAMS AND COSTS AT HHC

The New York City Health and Hospitals Corporation is the largest municipal hospital system in the United States; its annual operating budget is a little less than $2 billion. HHC's system includes 11 acute care hospitals, five long-term care facilities, and over 40 ambulatory clinics throughout New York City.

HHC's primary mission is to serve *all* patients regardless of their ability to pay. It also has special missions for patients who are in categories that make it harder for them to access services in the private system, especially acute psychiatric patients, drug and alcohol abusers, the homeless, and others. AIDS patients, of course, have become a major focus of attention for HHC in the last few years.

Patients and costs

The population of patients with AIDS-related illnesses has grown steadily in the HHC system, and it is expected to rise further. In March 1985, the average daily census of AIDS patients in the system was 139. By October 1985, that number had increased to 250 patients, where it remained as of the beginning of January 1986. The upward trend is expected to continue, and by 1989 there may be as many as 650 AIDS patients in the HHC system on any given day (see Figure 22.2). Needless to say, this is a burden that is quite dramatic, both in human and economic terms.

Although we do not have the sort of sophisticated cost analysis for HHC that is presented for San Francisco General Hospital by Anne Scitovsky, Mary Cline, and Philip Lee (in Chapter 21), and we are not yet able to track the history of care of a particular patient in the HHC system, HHC does have information on the cost of individual hospital episodes of its AIDS patients. According to the available data, the cost of hospitalization for AIDS patients in the HHC system is about $800 a day, versus an average per diem rate of about $500. In other words, the costs for AIDS patients is about 50 to 60 percent higher than the average medical/surgical per diem rate in the HHC system.

Factors in increased costs at HHC

We think this is attributable to several factors that characterize the acute care requirements of AIDS patients in HHC facilities:

- more intensive nursing care

- increased use of ancillary tests and specialty consultations

- increased use of pharmaceuticals, some of which are experimental and expensive

- increased need for specialized equipment and procedures, such as dialysis

- longer lengths of stay, due in many instances to inadequate post-hospital care arrangements when the patient is ready for discharge

Since HHC treats a disproportionate share of individuals who are substance abusers, as Omar Hendrix has indicated (in Chapter 14), it has a particularly costly mix of AIDS patients. For a sense of the relative numbers, consider that gay and bisexual men who are not intravenous (IV) drug abusers constitute nearly 90 percent of the AIDS population in San Francisco, about 60 percent of the AIDS population in New York City as a whole, and about 16 percent of AIDS patients in HHC facilities. On the other hand, IV drug abusers amount to only about 10 percent of the AIDS population in San Francisco, about 26 percent throughout New York City, and 63 percent of the AIDS patients in HHC hospitals (see Figure 22.3). The service needs of these patients are generally greater than those for non-IV drug abusers; therefore, one would expect HHC data to reflect more costly admissions.

Comparing diagnoses, we find that about 31 percent of the AIDS patients admitted to San Francisco General Hospital in 1984 had *Pneumocystis carinii* pneumonia (see Chapter 21, Table 21.2). Meanwhile, in New York City, about 63 percent of AIDS patients are diagnosed with *Pneumocystis carinii* pneumonia, according to the New York City Department of Health (1985), and about 60 percent of *Pneumocystis carinii* pneumonia patients are IV drug abusers. This may explain some of the more intensive and more costly hospitalizations in HHC facilities.

At HHC, we have taken a more focused look at some of the specific factors in the increased costs of hospitalization—other than the fundamentally poorer health status, to begin with, of many of our patients who are IV drug abusers. An HHC study on nursing care hours, for example, using a patient classification system, indicated that AIDS patients

Fig. 22.2. Average daily census of AIDS patients in New York City Health and Hospitals Corporation facilities

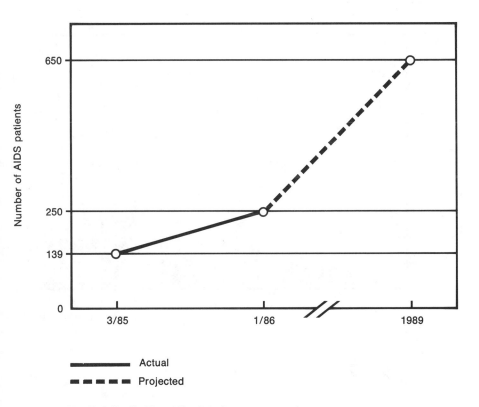

Actual

Projected

SOURCE: New York City Health and Hospitals Corporation..

on the medical/surgical (Med/Surg) units in HHC facilities require about 40 percent more direct nursing care than the average HHC Med/Surg patient, and that pediatric AIDS patients require more than twice the nursing care hours required by the average HHC pediatric patient.

Studies in two of HHC's larger hospitals show that the cost of drug treatment for AIDS patients is twice as high as that for the average patient, that AIDS patients carry about twice as many secondary diagnoses as the average Med/Surg patient, and that the average length of stay (ALOS) for AIDS patients is considerably greater—about 14 days longer—than for the average Med/Surg patient. In early 1986, the ALOS for AIDS patients in

Fig. 22.3. Intravenous drug users in AIDS patient populations in the city of San Francisco, in New York City as a whole, and in New York City Health and Hospitals Corporation facilities

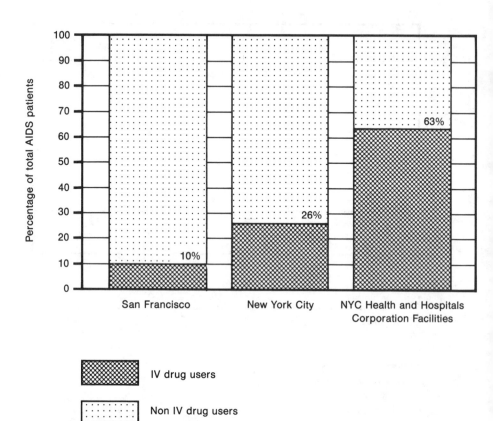

SOURCES: San Francisco Department of Public Health, New York City Department of Health, New York City Health and Hospitals Corporation.

HHC hospitals was 26 days, compared with an 11.7-day ALOS at San Francisco General Hospital (Chapter 21, Table 21.1).

Based on the $800 per day cost of hospitalization for AIDS patients, we estimate that over $90 million will be spent for the direct inpatient costs for AIDS patients in HHC facilities alone in fiscal year 1987, and that about $40 million of this expenditure will be New York City tax levy dollars. I emphasize the municipal share of these expenditures, as well as the municipal hospital role, to dramatize the extraordinary costs of caring for these individuals, especially IV drug abusers, who tend to be concentrated in certain locations. Clearly, this means that certain states and municipalities, in particular those with high substance-abuser populations, will carry a disproportionate share of the costs of the AIDS epidemic. Inevitably, as the epidemic's toll increases, their resources are going to be stressed.

In fact, the resource problem is already compounded by current health insurance methodology—other than private insurance, which in general is less available to the HHC patient population, many of whom are uninsured. A common mode in our system involves "spending down" to Medicaid eligibility. This process incurs considerable cost to individuals, who may lose their jobs, their homes, and other social supports in the community. As a result, their illness leaves them without resources, and the burden for continuing support and care falls directly on the health care provider. As Lambert King has indicated (in Chapter 18), AIDS treatment costs, combined with reimbursment systems that do not take into account the higher costs of caring for AIDS patients, are already imposing additional financial stress on facilities with large populations of these individuals.

The state of New York has recently announced a proposal to designate certain hospitals as Comprehensive AIDS Centers, with preferential reimbursement and, perhaps, an increase in the per diem reimbursement for AIDS patients under Medicaid. Whether this mechanism will be adequate is unclear. Furthermore, it still does not take into account the cost of care for those who are not eligible for Medicaid. Dr. King alludes (in Chapter 18) to the way in which alternate-level-of-care rates and reimbursement rates are calculated on a 1981 base year in New York state, which does not take into account the absence of AIDS patients in 1981 or the presence of AIDS patients today.

REIMBURSEMENT POLICY RECOMMENDATIONS

Looking at the overall data on AIDS patients and at the extent of the epidemic and the problems in its wake, we feel very strongly at the municipal level that the major responsibility for reimbursement for direct health services should be a federal one.

We propose, for example, that AIDS patients be exempted from the two-year waiting period for Medicare eligibility. This has been done for end-stage renal disease patients, and, in view of the fact that between 50 and 70 percent of all AIDS patients die within the 24-month time period between qualification for Supplemental Security Income (SSI) at diagnosis and eligibility for Medicare, SSI eligibility is useless as a health benefit to AIDS patients. In fact, I think the information that Anne Scitovsky, Mary Cline, and Philip Lee present (in Chapter 21) on the total cost of caring for AIDS patients is quite encouraging in relation to the actual financial burden of creating an entitlement program for AIDS patients along the lines of the program for those who suffer with end-stage renal disease. In addition, the availability of an insurance entitlement, such as Medicare, at the beginning of an illness would provide for much more cost-effective case management throughout the range of care in the ambulatory, acute inpatient, and long-term care settings.

We also believe very strongly, at the municipal level, that there should be a diagnosis related group (DRG) developed for AIDS that adequately reflects the costs, lengths of stay, and intensity of illness for these patients. The current DRGs that are used for AIDS, which are largely those of the infectious processes that these patients experience, have weightings of less than one, meaning less than that for the average patient. The ALOS for these diagnoses is between six and eight days, compared with ALOS for most AIDS patients of 11, 23, or 40 days, depending on one's database. While the lack of Medicare entitlement may make the development of a DRG for AIDS seem less important at this point, the fact is that in New York State, at least—and, one might expect, in other states—the DRG-based payment system increasingly will be used as a model for per diem case reimbursement under Medicaid, and perhaps under all-payer systems. The lack of adequate attention to an appropriate DRG for AIDS may thus become more of a problem.

Medicare should also provide access to long-term care services, for which there are tremendous gaps of eligibility. Since Medicare is largely limited to coverage of short-term acute illnesses of the elderly, it does not provide for the chronic in-home care, such as homemaker, personal care, and home health aide services, needed by AIDS patients. Hospice eligibility, too, is unreasonably limited for AIDS patients. Meanwhile, the use of Medicaid home- and community-based service waivers would allow coverage of care for AIDS patients who could be managed at home for less than the cost of providing care in an acute care facility.

With the advent of the new Resource Utilization Groups reimbursement methodology in New York State, and, I expect, in other states, access to long-term care is also going to be a problem for AIDS patients. HHC has had eight AIDS patients in its skilled nursing facilities (SNFs) over the last several months. Their course is a very volatile one: they move very rapidly from what are referred to as "physical A's" in the New York terminology— that is, the least ill patients—to being patients in the most intense category of special care. Four of the eight patients who have been admitted into our SNFs have died within eight weeks of their admission. In view of the reality of AIDS and the need for the provision of a much more comprehesive array of long-term care services, it is clear that some mechanism needs to be developed for a special kind of reimbursement.

CONCLUSION

At the New York City Health and Hospitals Corporation, we believe that AIDS is a catastrophic problem—and a national one. The federal government must step in to take a leadership role and develop some coherent strategy, especially for financing the provision of services, so that local governments and health care providers can be relieved of some of this burden. We in the city of New York, and at the Health and Hospitals Corporation in particular, have in the past and will continue in the future to lobby for appropriate and equitable programs and services for persons with AIDS. Meanwhile, we will continue to bear the cost, as we have in the past, and to meet our obligations to these very important patients.

REFERENCE

New York City Department of Health. 1985. *AIDS—Surveillance update.* 26 December.

CHAPTER 23

A Health Insurer's Perspective on AIDS

LESLIE STRASSBERG

With approximately 10 million subscribers, Empire Blue Cross and Blue Shield is the largest health insurer in the United States. In fact, 80 percent of the population in the New York City area that could potentially be insured by this corporation is, in fact, insured by it. These subscribers represent about $3.6 billion in paid premiums each year to Empire Blue Cross and Blue Shield, and, acting as Medicare intermediary for most of New York State, the corporation pays out an average of $7.5 billion in health insurance benefits annually. That translates into $30 million in benefits each business day. The Empire Blue Cross and Blue Shield benefit is, therefore, an enormous financial injection into the health care economic marketplace in this region of the country.

Since the New York City area has the largest concentration of AIDS and AIDS-related complex cases in the nation, Empire Blue Cross and Blue Shield has a very large interest in the disease and in the course of the epidemic. As a result of that interest, its actuarial department has done some very crude estimates of what Empire Blue Cross and Blue Shield can expect its AIDS claims to be for 1986. Based on 5,000 cases of AIDS in the New York City area, and assuming only $50,000 in expenditures per case for 1986, the estimate is that there will be $250 million in medical costs attributable to AIDS for the year. Empire Blue Cross and Blue Shield estimates that its share of this bill could be between $100 million and $200 million.

Before 1980, there were few AIDS cases to speak of, so on one level this $100 to $200 million in additional benefits represents a brand new infusion of funds into the health care system in this area. The sobering reality we face, however, is that this amount of money is nearly equal to Empire Blue Cross and Blue Shield's entire claim reserve for the protection of its customers. Clearly, the issue of AIDS must have a high priority at Empire Blue Cross and Blue Shield.

230

AIDS STUDIES

Recently, Empire Blue Cross and Blue Shield has embarked on a study of AIDS cases in its enormous patient database. Having 10 million subscribers in the New York City area makes a study of this scope a rather ambitious undertaking. The operating area it encompasses includes 28 counties of New York State: the eastern part of the state, all of New York City, the suburban counties of New York City, and other counties all the way up to Albany, and north to the Canadian border (see Figure 23.1). Based on 10 million subscribers and an average of 85 hospital admissions per 100 eligible subscribers, the study will include nearly 5 million inpatient admissions over the last five years.

The study will attempt to identify all diagnosed AIDS cases in Empire Blue Cross and Blue Shield's database. This is not a very easy task, and the study will take some time to complete. It is hoped that it will be completed by late 1986 and contribute to the ongoing research into the AIDS epidemic in the United States. Then, we hope to make some of the aggregate results available to the public, without compromising the confidentiality of our subscribers.

Empire Blue Cross and Blue Shield is also a sponsor of the Health Services Improvement Fund (HSIF), and through it is supporting a study at the State University of New York at Stony Brook regarding the cost of treatment of AIDS patients in selected hospitals in New York State. In addition, HSIF recently completed a study at St. Luke's-Roosevelt Hospital Center in New York City that focused on resource utilization by AIDS patients in that voluntary acute care hospital.

THE INSURER'S SOCIAL ROLE

Empire Blue Cross and Blue Shield believes that it has more than just a financial role in the AIDS epidemic; we believe it also has a social role. Empire Blue Cross and Blue Shield has always maintained the point of view that it is charged with the responsibility for making coverage available to those in our society who could not purchase coverage on their own, because of health conditions or other reasons. Most insurance companies do very sophisticated underwriting of their applicants. In fulfillment of its social mandate as the Blue Cross and Blue Shield Plan of Eastern New York State, however, Empire Blue Cross and Blue Shield has very liberal underwriting rules. It has open enrollment periods that ensure access to insurance coverage by virtually anyone in the eastern portion of the state.

Fig. 23.1 Empire Blue Cross and Blue Shield operating area,
New York State, by county

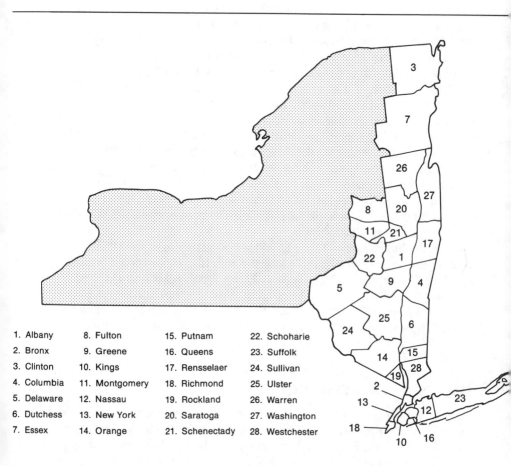

1. Albany	8. Fulton	15. Putnam	22. Schoharie
2. Bronx	9. Greene	16. Queens	23. Suffolk
3. Clinton	10. Kings	17. Rensselaer	24. Sullivan
4. Columbia	11. Montgomery	18. Richmond	25. Ulster
5. Delaware	12. Nassau	19. Rockland	26. Warren
6. Dutchess	13. New York	20. Saratoga	27. Washington
7. Essex	14. Orange	21. Schenectady	28. Westchester

SOURCE: Empire Blue Cross and Blue Shield

As a result of its policies, Empire Blue Cross and Blue Shield has struck a balance between social and economic interests. In doing so, it has a role in the AIDS epidemic both as a financial policy-maker and in helping make health insurance universally available to the general public.

OPPOSITION TO PRESCREENING TESTS

The way Empire Blue Cross and Blue Shield provides health insurance is slightly different from the way most commercial insurance companies operate. Commercial insurers generally are profit-making corporations that compete with one another for lowest claim costs. For example, if one insurer is able to prescreen its applicants better than another insurer, it will likely have lower claim costs than its competitor, thereby earning larger profits. This is fine in a business environment, but it does very little for the social good.

Alarmed by reports of the high costs of treating people with AIDS, many health insurers are now doing sophisticated medical underwriting of persons suspected to be potential AIDS patients, even though they may not have any overt symptoms of infection with the AIDS virus. It is not uncommon to find, for example, that insurers are attempting or have proposals to prescreen applicants by requiring that they submit to ELISA and/or Western blot analysis testing for the presence of antibodies to human T-lymphotropic virus type III/lymphadenopathy-associated virus (HTLV-III/LAV). Although there is no certainty that everybody with HTLV-III/LAV antibodies in their blood will develop AIDS or AIDS-related complex in the future, those whose tests are positive for antibodies are denied insurance coverage by these companies.

Empire Blue Cross and Blue Shield strongly disapproves of these insurers' practices. We believe that it is the social obligation of the entire insurance industry to make coverage available to people at risk for AIDS. Of course, it would be naive for anyone to expect the initiative for restraint in the use of the antibody tests to come from the commercial insurance industry, since the profit-making motive of that segment of the insurance industry would surely mitigate against such policy. The only possible solution to the problem of the unavailability of health insurance coverage likely will be a legislative one. States may have to impose restraints, if they are not voluntarily assumed.

Some solutions of this sort are already in place, as Dennis Altman has indicated (in Chapter 2). Both California and Wisconsin have enacted prohibitions against the use of the HTLV-III/LAV antibody test to prescreen health insurance applicants. In New York, similar legislation has been proposed by Governor Mario Cuomo (Carroll 1986), and James Corcoran, the

Commissioner of Insurance, has stated publicly that he would not permit such tests to be required of insurance applicants (Barron 1985). His policy statement is currently under direct challenge by one of the largest commercial insurers in New York State.

WHAT IS NEEDED

What is urgently needed is some sort of coherent and coordinated local, state, and federal policy regarding AIDS, and I believe that this should be an integration of social and financial policy. Legislation on social policy alone is the equivalent of making empty promises; social policy must be backed by financial policy. For example, we need to have a clear delineation of what an employer's obligations are to employees who have AIDS. It is very easy for an employer to deny having an obligation to someone who was previously employed with the company but who has become disabled by AIDS and is no longer gainfully employed. Such an employee, of course, would no longer be covered by the employer's health insurance benefits. The result is that the employee is then left to the vagaries of public health assistance programs and becomes a burden on the public sector, not to mention the hardships—both medical and social—he or she is likely to undergo. Absent any preventive regulation, the private sector is allowed, therefore, to shift costs that it ordinarily should bear onto the community, which is already confronted with large health care costs.

Empire Blue Cross and Blue Shield makes available to its group customers an insurance conversion policy that provides ongoing individual coverage for premium-paying subscribers. Commercial insurers typically make available a much more modest level of coverage than that provided by Empire Blue Cross and Blue Shield, whose coverage is very comprehensive and includes 120 days of paid-in-full hospitalization, along with basic surgical and medical coverage.

When employers elect not to continue coverage for their employees who have terminated their employment because of disability from AIDS, these people have tended to become wards of the state, with very few having the financial means to pay for their ongoing treatment. What is needed is a uniform policy, so that employers will not be able transfer their financial responsibilities to other employers or to the locality or state, and so that the Blue Cross system is not strained financially to pay for all of these cases that are dumped by other insurers. Empire Blue Cross and Blue Shield certainly wants to pay its fair share of the costs of AIDS, but we also want to see equity in sharing these costs.

CONCLUSION

Empire Blue Cross and Blue Shield also sees a crucial need for public education about AIDS. There is a lot of ignorance, misinformation, and hysteria surrounding AIDS and its effects on people who are in contact with those suffering from AIDS or infected with the AIDS virus. This hysteria has certainly influenced the public's perceptions regarding the treatment of AIDS and its financial costs.

Increased emphasis needs to be placed both on funds for preventive education and on research funding for the prevention and cure of AIDS. In fact, the need for research funding cannot possibly be exaggerated. Substantial research funding probably cannot be expected from the insurance industry, however, even though the insurance industry is left to pay a substantial portion of the bills. By any estimate, the cost of AIDS is going to be great. It must be distributed fairly across not only the local but the national community. In the long run, funding from public and private sources for AIDS prevention and treatment research will accomplish much more than merely paying the bills after people are infected and ill.

REFERENCES

Barron, J. 1985. Insurers study screening for AIDS. *New York Times*, 26 September.

Carroll, M. 1986. Revised bill would limit AIDS test use. *New York Times*, 24 February.

PART EIGHT

Epilogue

AIDS Policy: A Long-Term View
BRUCE C. VLADECK

CHAPTER 24

AIDS Policy: A Long-Term View

BRUCE C. VLADECK

The epidemic of acquired immune deficiency syndrome (AIDS), like other dramatic and highly visible catastrophes, has raised a number of complex and compelling questions for public policy, with implications extending far beyond the more immediate and devastating problems of AIDS victims and the people who care for them. Many of these public policy issues have been explored in the preceding chapters, and there is no need to summarize them here. But at least three issues discussed in this book are so immediately and broadly applicable to other areas of concern that they deserve reiteration.

REBIRTH OF COMMUNITY

The silver lining in the cloud of AIDS, as emphasized by Philip Lee and Peter Arno (in Chapter 1), is the way in which the AIDS crisis has brought forth a remarkable community mobilization in San Francisco and New York City, where volunteers have banded together to care in many ways for victims of AIDS. Dr. Lee's and Dr. Arno's particular emphasis on the way in which this sort of community mobilization appears to run counter to the growing tide of self-interested individualism in much of American life seems to augur hopefully for the reaffirmation of community values in an increasingly atomistic and alienated society. In the same vein, Dr. Arno reports (in Chapter 19) some extraordinary statistics he has collected on the literally thousands of hours of volunteer services provided in both communities.

Yet, David Rothman, discussing the issue of the admission of children with AIDS to the public schools (in Chapter 6), points out that allowing afflicted children into the schools runs counter to the long-standing communitarian tradition of the public health community. The response to children with AIDS is, in fact, more consistent with the civil libertarian approach that individuals be treated as innocent until proven guilty. It is recognition of the legitimate individuality of children with AIDS, not the mores of the broader community, that provides the strongest argument for allowing them to attend school in public classrooms.

The conflict between individualistic and communitarian values is hardly a new one. But it is interesting to note that the particular communities whose spirit has been frequently applauded in these pages—San Francisco and New York's Greenwich Village—are probably not typical of the United States as a whole. Most of us who attended the conference on which this book is based were less sympathetic to proposals in the state of Texas to quarantine AIDS patients, despite the fact that they, too, appeared to have the potential for expressing community solidarity.

There is no real solution to this issue. Individual rights and community solidarity are both values we hold very dear in this society, and the balance between them is always dynamic and tense. But it is useful to be reminded how many issues of central concern to the health of the public also involve this tension. In that regard, the problem of children with AIDS in the public schools is not unrelated to the problems of smoking in public places, of informing workers about potential exposure to toxic substances, or of state laws mandating the use of seat belts in automobiles.

PAYING THE BILL

One example—suggested by a number of contributors to this work—of the decline of the values of social solidarity in contemporary American society is the deterioration of social insurance mechanisms to pay the costs of health care. Increasing emphasis on cost containment and the elimination of cross-subsidization from insurance practices have reduced the willingness of payers, both public and private, to bear the costs associated with caring for anyone but their own.

A discussion of the costs of AIDS, reported here in Chapters 21 through 23, seemed to arrive at the conclusion that, in narrow economic terms, the costs are very substantial in one sense, but not in another. Even if the estimate cited in a study by the Centers for Disease Control (Hardy et al. 1986) was correct—that spending for the care of AIDS patients in hospitals has amounted to about $1.4 billion for the first 10,000 cases (an estimate that is questioned by Anne Scitovsky, Mary Cline, and Philip Lee in Chapter 21)—hospital spending for AIDS would still only account for 0.3 percent of the nation's annual health care bill, or slightly more than one day's total health care expenditures. On the other hand, the costs of caring for AIDS patients have been concentrated in relatively few facilities in a small number of communities. Taxpayers in New York City and San Francisco are bearing a wildly disproportionate share of the costs of the AIDS epidemic, at a time when municipal governments in particular are subject to extraordinary financial stresses. Yet, both the private and public insurance mechanisms by which such costs might in the past have been distributed more widely have weakened considerably in the last four or five years.

Jo Ivey Boufford, President of the New York City Health and Hospitals Corporation, suggests (in Chapter 22) that it would be appropriate, from a public policy standpoint, to treat AIDS as we have treated end-stage renal disease since 1972, by providing immediate Medicare coverage for AIDS patients once the disease is definitively diagnosed. While I think Dr. Boufford's recommendation is eminently sound, I believe it is probably not politically realistic in the current environment of unwillingness on the part of the federal government to maintain existing budgetary commitments, let alone undertake new ones. But that is a comment not on the validity of the proposal but on the political environment, which again speaks directly to prevailing contemporary attitudes about the sharing of social responsibility and social obligations. It is still acceptable, although one wonders for how long, to draw on a national tax base to aid the victims of a local flood or earthquake in this country or elsewhere, but it is not seen as politically realistic to draw on the same national revenue base to assist localities afflicted by the plague of AIDS.

MOVING TOWARD CASE MANAGEMENT

From a personal perspective, as one who has been involved for some time in issues of long-term care for the elderly, I am particularly struck by the extent to which what are being viewed as model programs for the care of AIDS patients are drawing on the lessons we have learned in long-term care over the last decade or so. Indeed, the currently popular terminology in New York State, that of "case management," is drawn directly from the world of geriatric services. The broader lesson is that we are increasingly being forced to recognize how optimal quality of care for people with very serious chronic illness often requires effective utilization of a range of systems (for want of a better term) outside those that have traditionally been narrowly defined as medical. We have become increasingly sensitive to the fact that, in order to provide good care to people with chronic disease, we need to deal effectively with social supports, with problems of housing, with problems of income maintenance, with social services, and so on. This implies an entirely new set of relationships between physicians and other health care and service providers, and it also implies some very different notions about how to pay for services and how to finance them.

As we get technologically more sophisticated about treating patients with acute illness, the care of those with chronic disease will become a larger part of the total activity of the health care system. For most of those with chronic disease—whether they are AIDS patients or elderly arthritics—there are no cures, no magic bullets. We have to learn, and to refine what we have already learned, about entirely new ways of providing services.

NEXT STEPS

Since AIDS is an invariably fatal disease, the more than 30,000 cases diagnosed in this country to date constitute, in and of themselves, a tragedy of enormous dimensions, and current projections for the epidemic's increase are truly staggering in their implications. Dealing with that tragedy, and doing the best we can to care humanely and effectively for those afflicted with the disease, is obviously the primary priority. But other things are at stake in the AIDS epidemic as well. If we are wise and energetic and lucky, science will produce vaccines and a cure before too long. But even if this occurs, some of these other issues will still be with us. They will always be with us. We cannot talk about them, and worry about them, enough.

REFERENCE

Hardy, A. M., K. Rauch, D. Echenberg, W. M. Morgan, and J. W. Curran. 1986. The economic impact of the first 10,000 cases of acquired immunodeficiency syndrome in the United States. *Journal of the American Medical Association* 255:209-11.

Appendices

Acquired Immune Deficiency Syndrome: Case Definition

ACQUIRED IMMUNE DEFICIENCY SYNDROME (AIDS)

Case Definition and Reporting Requirements

A case definition of acquired immune deficiency syndrome (AIDS), for national reporting purposes, was published by the Centers for Disease Control (CDC) in *Morbidity and Mortality Weekly Report* in September 1982. That definition was subsequently published in the *American Journal of Medicine* (Selik, Haverkos, and Curran 1984), as follows:

> Centers for Disease Control Surveillance Definition of AIDS: Diseases must be at least moderately indicative of underlying cellular immunodeficiency and must occur in the absence of known causes of reduced resistance to them. These are listed below in five etiologic categories:
>
> - protozoal and helminthic
> - fungal
> - bacterial
> - viral
> - neoplastic
>
> Within each category, the diseases are listed in alphabetic order. "Disseminated infection" refers to the involvement of liver, bone marrow, or multiple organs, not simply involvement of lungs or multiple lymph nodes. The required diagnostic methods with positive results are shown in parenthesis.

Protozoal and helminthic infections

1. Cryptosporidiosis, intestinal, causing diarrhea for more than one month (on histologic study or stool microscopic study);
2. *Pneumocystis carinii* pneumonia (on histologic study or microscopic study of a "touch" preparation or bronchial washings);
3. Strongyloidosis, causing pneumonia, central nervous system infection or disseminated infection (on histologic study);

4. Toxoplasmosis, causing pneumonia or central nervous system infection (on histologic study or microscopic study of a "touch" preparation).

Fungal infections

1. Candidiasis, causing esophagitis (on histologic study or microscopic study of "wet" preparation from the esophagus or endoscopic findings of white plaques on an erythematous mucosal base);
2. Cryptococcosis, causing central nervous system or disseminated infection (on culture, antigen detection, histologic study or India ink preparation of cerebrospinal fluid).

Bacterial infections

1. "Atypical" mycobacteriosis (species other than tuberculosis or lepra), causing disseminated infection (on culture).

Viral infections

1. Cytomegalovirus, causing pulmonary, gastrointestinal tract or central nervous system infection (on histologic study);
2. Herpes simplex virus, causing chronic mucocutaneous infection with ulcers persisting more than one month, or pulmonary, gastrointestinal tract or disseminated infection (on culture, histologic study or cytologic study);
3. Progressive multifocal leukoencephalopathy (presumed to be caused by a papovavirus) (on histologic study).

Cancer

1. Kaposi's sarcoma in persons less than 60 years of age (on histologic study);
2. Lymphoma limited to the brain (on histologic study).

Case reporting: For the epidemiologic surveillance of AIDS, any patient who has a disease at least moderately indicative of underlying cellular immunodeficiency (as just listed) but who has no known cause of reduced resistance to that disease should be reported by clinicians to their state or local public health department. Those agencies should, in turn, report the case to the AIDS Branch/Division of Viral Diseases, Centers for Disease Control.

Pediatric AIDS

In January 1984, the CDC issued a provisional case definition for AIDS in children, noting that "because children are subject to a variety of congenital immunodeficiencies, confirmation of AIDS diagnoses in children is more complex than in adults. Laboratory testing to exclude congenital conditions is required."

The CDC provisional case definition for pediatric AIDS

For the limited purposes of epidemiologic surveillance, CDC defines a case of pediatric acquired immunodeficiency syndrome (AIDS) in a child who has had:

1. a reliably diagnosed disease at least moderately indicative of underlying cellular immunodeficiency and
2. no known cause of underlying cellular immunodeficiency or any other reduced resistance reported to be associated with that disease.

The diseases accepted as sufficiently indicative of underlying cellular immunodeficiency are the same as those used in defining AIDS in adults, with the exclusion of congenital infections, e.g., toxoplasmosis or herpes simplex virus infection in the first month after birth or cytomegalovirus infection in the first 6 months after birth.

Specific conditions that must be excluded in a child are:

1. Primary immunodeficiency diseases—severe combined immunodeficiency, DiGeorge syndrome, Wiskott-Aldrich syndrome, ataxia-telangiectasia, graft versus host disease, neutropenia, neutrophil function abnormality, agammaglobulinemia, or hypogammaglobulinemia with raised IgM.
2. Secondary immunodeficiency associated with immunosuppressive therapy, lymphorecticular malignancy, or starvation.

Revised Case Definition of AIDS

In June 1985, following the annual meeting of the Conference of State and Territorial Epidemiologists (held on June 2-5 in Madison, Wisconsin), the CDC issued a revised surveillance definition of AIDS for national reporting. The refinements in case definition that follow reflect the discovery and isolation of human T-lymphotropic virus type III/lymphadenopathy-associated virus (HTLV-III/LAV) as the apparent infective agent that causes AIDS:

A. In the absence of the opportunistic diseases required by the current case definition, any of the following diseases will be considered indicative of AIDS if the patient has a positive serologic or virologic test for HTLV-III/LAV:

(1) disseminated histoplasmosis (not confined to lungs or lymph nodes), diagnosed by culture, histology, or antigen detection;
(2) isosporiasis, causing chronic diarrhea (over 1 month), diagnosed by histology or stool microscopy;
(3) bronchial or pulmonary candidiasis, diagnosed by microscopy or by presence of characteristic white plaques grossly on the bronchial mucosa (not by culture alone);
(4) non-Hodgkin's lymphoma of high-grade pathologic type (diffuse, undifferentiated) and of B-cell or unknown immunological phenotype, diagnosed by biopsy;
(5) histologically confirmed Kaposi's sarcoma in patients who are 60 years old or older when diagnosed.

B. In the absence of the opportunistic diseases required by the current case definition, a histologically confirmed diagnosis of chronic lymphoid interstitial pneumonitis in a child (under 13 years of age) will be considered indicative of AIDS unless test(s) for HTLV-III/LAV are negative.

C. Patients who have a lymphorecticular malignancy diagnosed more than 3 months after the diagnosis of an opportunistic disease used as a marker for AIDS will no longer be excluded as AIDS cases.

D. To increase the specificity of the case definition, patients will be excluded as AIDS cases if they have a negative result on testing for serum antibody to HTLV-III/LAV, have no other type of HTLV-III/LAV test with a positive result, and do not have a low number of T-helper lymphocytes or a low ratio of T-helper to T-suppressor lymphocytes. In the absence of test results, patients satisfying all other criteria in the definition will continue to be included.

AIDS Infections and Malignancies

Clinical manifestations of AIDS, according to the CDC surveillance definition and classification system for HTLV-III/LAV infections (1986), include the following secondary infectious diseases:

- *Pneumocystis carinii* pneumonia (PCP)
- chronic cryptosporidiosis
- toxoplasmosis
- extra-intestinal strongyloidiasis
- isosporiasis
- candidiasis (esophageal, bronchial, or pulmonary)
- cryptococcosis
- histoplasmosis
- mycobacterial infection with *Mycobacterium avium* complex or *M. kansasii*
- cytomegalovirus infection
- chronic mucocutaneous or disseminated herpes simplex virus infection
- progressive multifocal leukoencephalopathy
- oral hairy leukoplakia
- multidermatomal herpes zoster
- recurrent *Salmonella* bacteremia
- nocardiosis
- tuberculosis
- oral candidiasis (thrush)

Malignancies associated with HTLV-III/LAV infection:

- Kaposi's sarcoma
- non-Hodgkin's lymphoma (small, noncleaved lymphoma or immunoblastic sarcoma)
- primary lymphoma of the brain

AIDS-RELATED COMPLEX (ARC)

Although the CDC has issued no definition of ARC, and ARC is not reportable to the CDC (but may be reportable to some state and local health departments), clinicians have used the term since 1983 to describe an AIDS-related syndrome that carries at least a likelihood (the degree of which is as yet undetermined) of progression to full-scale AIDS. A diagnosis of ARC requires the presence of two or more symptoms of AIDS, plus two or more laboratory findings that are indicative of otherwise unexplained immunodeficiency or are consistent with CDC-defined AIDS.

According to Lawrence Mass, M.D. (1985), "More recent and less widely used terms that have been used to characterize ARC conditions include a syndrome of 'wasting' [weight loss] and that of progressive generalized lymphadenopathy (PGL). The former meets ARC criteria and is believed by some observers to be characteristically prodromal; that is, irreversible and progressive to full-blown AIDS in the majority of patients, and in a relatively short period of time. PGL and lymphadenopathy syndrome (LAS) also meet ARC criteria but are thought to have far less likelihood of progression to full-blown AIDS."

CLASSIFICATION SYSTEM FOR HTLV-III/LAV INFECTIONS

The extent of HTLV-III/LAV infection and related disease in the United States is constantly being reassessed and the CDC's definition of AIDS/ARC itself is subject to change as more is learned about the manifestations of infection. In recognition of the complexity of the situation and in order "to provide a means of grouping patients infected with HTLV-III/LAV according to the clinical expression of the disease," the CDC has devised and published a classification system for HTLV-III/LAV-related illnesses. The complete system is detailed in the CDC's *Morbidity and Mortality Weekly Report*, issue of 23 May 1986; it is summarized here.

The system, which applies only to persons already diagnosed as having HTLV-III/LAV infection, classifies the manifestations of infection into four mutually exclusive groups. According to the CDC, "classification in a particular group is not explicitly intended to have prognostic significance, nor to designate severity of illness."

- Group I (Acute infection) includes patients with transient signs and symptoms that appear at the time of or shortly after initial infection with the AIDS virus, as identified by laboratory studies. Patients in Group I are to be reclassified in another group following resolution of this acute syndrome.

- Group II (Asymptomatic infection) includes patients who have no signs or symptoms of AIDS virus infection. Patients in this category may be subclassified based on hematologic and/or immunologic laboratory studies and their results.

- Group III (Persistent generalized lymphadenopathy) includes patients with persistent generalized lymphadenopathy but without findings that would lead to classification in Group IV. Patients in this category may also be subclassified on the basis of laboratory studies and results.

- Group IV (Other disease) includes patients with clinical symptoms and signs of HTLV-III/LAV infection other than or in addition to lymphadenopathy. These patients are assigned to one or more subgroups based on clinical findings. The subgroups are: A. constitutional disease; B. neurologic disease; C. secondary infectious diseases; D. secondary cancers; E. other conditions resulting from AIDS virus infection. These subgroups are not mutually exclusive and do not represent any a priori hierarchy of severity of illness.

According to the CDC, "this classification system does not imply any change in the definition of AIDS used by CDC since 1981 for national reporting. Patients whose clinical presentations fulfill the surveillance definition of AIDS are classified in Group IV. However, not every case in Group IV will meet the surveillance definition."

CONCLUSION

Early in 1986, health officials, researchers, and epidemiologists were estimating that from 5 to 50 percent of persons infected with HTLV-III/LAV will ultimately develop CDC-defined AIDS over a period of months to years (Boffey 1986). The incubation period preceding symptomatic disease has been estimated to be from 2.5 to 7.5 years, and recent data indicate that it can be longer. According to a report from the National Academy of Sciences in October 1986, studies suggest "at least 25 to 50 percent of infected persons will progress to AIDS within five to ten years after infection," and "the possibility that the percentage is higher cannot be ruled out" (Russell 1986).

REFERENCES

Boffey, P. 1986. AIDS in the future: Experts say deaths will climb sharply. New York Times, 14 January.

Centers for Disease Control. 1982. Update on acquired immune deficiency syndrome (AIDS)—United States. Morbidity and Mortality Weekly Report 31:507–14.

———. 1984. Update: Acquired immunodeficiency syndrome (AIDS)—United States. Morbidity and Mortality Weekly Report 32:688–91.

_____. 1985. Revision of the case definition of acquired immunodeficiency syndrome for national reporting—United States. *Morbidity and Mortality Weekly Report* 34:373–75.

_____. 1986. Classification system for human T-lymphotropic virus type III/lymphadenopathy-associated virus infections. *Morbidity and Mortality Weekly Report* 35:334–39.

Mass, L. 1985. *Medical answers about AIDS*. 2nd ed. New York: Gay Men's Health Crisis.

Russell, C. 1986. Experts say AIDS fight must be stepped up. *Washington Post*, 30 October.

Selik, R. M., H. W. Haverkos, and J. W. Curran. 1984. Acquired immune deficiency syndrome (AIDS) trends in the United States, 1978-1982. *American Journal of Medicine* 76:493–500.

AIDS Statistical Update, Surveys, and Projections

In January 1986, when the United Hospital Fund and the Institute for Health Policy Studies held their public policy conference on acquired immune deficiency syndrome (AIDS), the cumulative number of AIDS cases that had been reported in the United States was 16,458 (Centers for Disease Control 1986a). Nine months later, as of 29 September 1986, the number of AIDS cases reported to the Centers for Disease Control had climbed to 25,650—an increase of 9,192 cases (56 percent)—and the number of known deaths had climbed to 14,345 (56 percent) (Centers for Disease Control 1986b).

While the conference on which the articles in this volume are based focused largely upon the effects of and responses to the AIDS epidemic in the United States, AIDS is an international health problem. As of 4 October 1986, according to the World Health Organization, the number of AIDS cases recorded worldwide since the disease was first diagnosed five years ago stood at 31,646 (Netter 1986). Thus, in addition to the tables in this appendix that update data shown in related tables in the text, additional data on local, national, and international aspects of the disease have been provided in order to enhance the statistical picture.

This appendix is divided into five parts:

I. United States Statistical Update
II. AIDS in Europe
III. AIDS in Africa
IV. AIDS in the Americas and the Far East
V. Projections for the Future.

I. UNITED STATES STATISTICAL UPDATE

The updated tables that follow provide the means to compare the demographics and other aspects of the epidemic as they stood at the time

253

of the conference and at the approximate time when these edited proceedings went to press. Where practical and feasible, these tables correspond directly to tables in the text, as follows:

- Table B.1 compares the distribution of AIDS cases by major metropolitan area in the United States for December 1985 and September 1986, and relates to Table 1.1 (in Chapter 1).

- Table B.2 compares the demographics of AIDS in the United States by patient group for January and September 1986, and relates to Table 1.2 (in Chapter 1).

- Table B.3, categorizing U.S. AIDS cases by race/ethnic group, relates to Table 8.1 (in Chapter 8).

Where it would have been unwieldly or impractical to reproduce the exact format of a table in the text, data are presented somewhat differently. For example, while Table B.4 relates to Table 12.2 (in Chapter 12), it contains updated and comparative data for New York City only, instead of for New York City and the United States (the latter already updated, as mentioned, in Table B.2). Similarly, the data presented in the text in Table 12.3 (comparing aspects of the epidemic in New York City and San Francisco) have been updated in Table B.5 for AIDS cases in New York City, in Table B.6 for AIDS cases in San Francisco, and in Table B.7, where data for each city through September 1986 are compared.

Although efforts have been made to achieve data consistency, it should be noted that statistics for apparently identical data segments may be seen to vary a bit from table to table. In part, this derives from the fact that different data sources may have been used for different tables, and the apparent discrepancies—largely minor ones—reflect differences in the methods of data collection and/or in the reporting periods and dates among the various sources. The data in these tables have been obtained from three sources:

- the Centers for Disease Control (CDC), in Atlanta

- The New York City Department of Health, AIDS Surveillance Office

- the San Francisco Department of Public Health, Bureau of Communicable Disease Control

The figures for cumulative AIDS cases for a particular location reported by the CDC on a given day may be different from the total obtained from the local health department for the same or a proximate date. There are two factors involved in this discrepancy: one is that there is often a lag in the reporting of AIDS cases to the CDC by the local surveillance offices; the other involves the way in which the CDC assigns

Table B.1
Cumulative Reported AIDS Cases,
by Selected Standard Metropolitan Statistical Areas,
December 1985 and September 1986

METROPOLITAN AREA	DECEMBER* 1985	SEPTEMBER** 1986	INCREASE NUMBER	PERCENT
New York City	4,923	7,608	2,685	54.5
San Francisco	1,730	2,657	927	53.6
Los Angeles	1,306	2,172	866	66.3
District of Columbia	483	739	256	53.0
Miami	475	729	254	53.5
Houston	402	724	322	80.1
Newark	373	632	259	69.4
Chicago	323	566	243	75.2
Philadelphia	284	483	199	70.1
Dallas	236	417	181	76.7
Atlanta	223	384	161	72.2
Boston	221	386	165	74.7
Jersey City	179	300	121	67.6
Nassau County (N.Y.)	159	286	127	79.9
Ft. Lauderdale	153	269	116	75.8
San Diego	147	276	129	87.8
Seattle	141	236	95	67.4
New Orleans	125	214	89	71.2
West Palm Beach	122	173	51	41.8
Anaheim	114	180	66	57.9
Baltimore	114	182	68	59.6

*Data as of 20 December 1985.
**Data as of 29 September 1986.
SOURCE: Centers for Disease Control, provisional data.

cases to a particular locality. For CDC reporting purposes, an AIDS case belongs to the city where the patient first noticed symptoms of the illness and not necessarily to the city where it was diagnosed. For example, although a person may be diagnosed with AIDS in San Francisco, if he or she first noticed symptoms while a resident of New York, the case will be assigned to New York City in CDC statistical reports, but the New York City Department of Health statistics may not include that case in its local tally. As a result, the respective reports of the CDC and the New York City Department of Health, for approximately the same dates, may show different totals for AIDS cases in New York.

Table B.2
Cumulative AIDS Cases by Patient Group,
United States, January and September 1986

	JANUARY*		SEPTEMBER**	
PATIENT GROUP	NUMBER	PERCENT	NUMBER	PERCENT
Adult				
Homosexual/bisexual men not IV drug users	10,600	65.3	16,590	65.6
Homosexual/bisexual men and IV drug users	1,310	8.1	1,997	7.9
IV drug users	2,766	17.0	4,322	17.1
Hemophilia patients	124	0.8	215	0.8
Heterosexual contacts	182	1.1	425	1.7
Transfusion recipients	261	1.6	436	1.7
None of the above/other				
No identified risks †	586	3.6	777	3.1
Born outside U.S. † †	398	2.5	534	2.1
SUBTOTAL	16,227	100.0	25,296	100.0
Pediatric				
Parent with AIDS or at increased risk for AIDS	175	75.8	283	79.9
Hemophilia patients	11	4.8	15	4.2
Transfusion recipients	33	14.3	46	13.0
None of the above/other	12	5.2	10‡	2.8
SUBTOTAL	231	100.0	354	100.0
TOTAL	16,458		25,650	

Note: Percents may not total due to rounding.
*Data as of 13 January 1986.
**Data as of 29 September 1986.
† Includes persons who died before risk group could be determined.
† † Includes persons without other identified risks who were born in countries in which heterosexual transmission is believed to play a major role, although precise means of transmission have not yet been fully defined.
‡ Since January, two pediatric cases in this category have been reclassified.
SOURCE: Centers for Disease Control, provisional data.

An additional element of variance derives from the constant refinement of data and reclassification of cases that the data collection and reporting agencies do as a normal part of updating their research and surveillance. The number of AIDS cases reported for 31 December 1985 in a particular locale in early January may be revised upward or downward in a

Table B.3
Cumulative Reported AIDS Cases by Race/Ethnic Group,
United States, January and September 1986

RACE/ETHNIC GROUP	JANUARY*		SEPTEMBER**		PEDIATRIC**	
	CASES	PERCENT	CASES	PERCENT	CASES	PERCENT
White	9,611	59.6	15,272	60.4	67	18.9
Black	4,041	25.0	6,192	24.5	206	58.2
Hispanic	2,287	14.2	3,554	14.0	78	22.0
Other/Unknown	199	1.2	278	1.1	3	0.8
TOTAL	16,138	100.0	25,296	100.0	354	100.0

Note: Percents may not total due to rounding.
*Data as of 6 January 1986.
**Data as of 29 September 1986.
SOURCE: Centers for Disease Control, provisional data.

later report issued in March, as additional cases diagnosed in December but reported later are added, or some of the reported December cases are reclassified and dropped in the interim. For these reasons, data are almost always reported as "provisional."

Finally, numbers may differ because areas designated in different reports may have the same name but may not be the same geographically. When the CDC refers to San Francisco, it is referring to the Standard Metropolitan Statistical Area (SMSA) known as San Francisco; however, when the San Francisco Department of Health reports data for San Francisco, it is referring to the city and county of San Francisco only, an area smaller and less populous than the SMSA of the same name and, naturally, having fewer AIDS cases than the SMSA. These differences can be detected, for example, if the cumulative number reported by the CDC for the San Francisco SMSA as of 29 September 1986, in Table B.1, is compared with the number reported by the San Francisco Department of Public Health as of 30 September 1986, in Table B.6.

II. AIDS IN EUROPE

At the first meeting on AIDS convened by the World Health Organization (WHO) Regional Office for Europe, in Aarhus, Denmark, in October 1983, ten European nations reported a cumulative total of 215 cases of AIDS.

Table B.4
Cumulative AIDS Cases by Patient Group,
New York City, December 1985 and September 1986

PATIENT GROUP	DECEMBER 1985*		SEPTEMBER 1986**	
	NUMBER	PERCENT	NUMBER	PERCENT
Adult				
Homosexual/bisexual men not IV drug users†	3,027	58.1	4,399	57.2
Homosexual/bisexual men and IV drug users	305	5.9	406	5.3
IV drug users	1,462	28.1	2,271	29.5
Hemophilia patients	8	0.1	13	0.2
Heterosexual contacts	80	1.5	156	2.0
Transfusion recipients	38	0.7	57	0.7
None of the above/other				
Other	109	2.1	163	2.1
No identified risks	51	1.0	53	0.7
Born outside U.S.††	130	2.5	178	2.3
SUBTOTAL	5,210	100.0	7,696	100.0
Pediatric				
Parent with AIDS or at increased risk for AIDS	87	84.4	124	87.9
Hemophilia patients	—	—	1	0.7
Tranfusion recipients	8	7.8	8	5.7
None of the above/other	8	7.8	8	5.7
SUBTOTAL	103	100.0	141	100.0
TOTAL	5,313		7,837	

Note: Percents may not total due to rounding.
*Data as of 20 December 1985.
**Data as of 15 September 1986.
† Includes homosexual/bisexual cases whose IV drug use status is unknown.
†† Includes persons born in countries in which most AIDS cases have not been associated with known risk factors.
SOURCE: New York City Department of Health, preliminary data.

These countries were: Denmark, France, the Federal Republic of Germany, Greece, Italy, the Netherlands, Spain, Sweden, Switzerland, and the United Kingdom. Nine months later, in July 1984, these same nations reported a total of 421 cases of AIDS (Centers for Disease Control 1984). The number of AIDS cases has continued to rise in Europe and, according to WHO, the cumulative total stood at 3,127 as of 3 October 1986 (Netter

Table B.5
Cumulative AIDS Cases by Selected Characteristics,
New York City, December 1985 and September 1986

	DECEMBER 1985*		SEPTEMBER 1986**		INCREASE	
	NUMBER	PERCENT	NUMBER	PERCENT	NUMBER	PERCENT
Total Cases†	5,313		7,837		2,524	47.5
By race/ethnic group						
White	2,474	46.6	3,537	45.1	1,063	43.0
Black	1,636	30.8	2,441	31.1	805	49.2
Hispanic	1,165	21.9	1,805	23.0	640	54.9
Other/unknown	38	0.7	54	0.7	16	42.1
Cases by patient group						
Homosexual/bisexual	3,332	62.7	4,805	61.3	1,473	44.2
IV drug user	1,462	27.5	2,271	29.0	809	55.3
Transfusion w/blood						
or blood products	46	0.9	65	0.8	19	41.3
Hemophilia/Coagulation						
disorder	8	0.2	14	0.2	6	75.0
Heterosexual contact	80	1.5	156	2.0	76	95.0
Child of parent with or						
at risk for AIDS	87	1.6	124	1.6	37	42.5
Unknown/other	298	5.6	402	5.1	104	34.9
Cases male	4,779	89.9	7,014	89.5	2,235	46.8
Cases female	534	10.1	823	10.5	289	54.1
Adult cases	5,210	98.1	7,696	98.2	2,486	47.7
Pediatric cases††	103	1.9	141	1.8	38	36.9
Cases/100,000 pop.‡	74		109		35	47.3

*Data as of 20 December 1985.
**Data as of 15 September 1986.
†Figures include both adult and pediatric cases unless otherwise indicated.
††Pediatric cases refer to patients under 13 years of age at diagnosis.
‡Based on 1984 population figures.
SOURCE: New York City Department of Health, Office of Epidemiologic Surveillance and Statistics, preliminary data.

1986). Cumulative European AIDS cases and their distribution by country as of 30 June 1986 (the most recent date for which comprehensive data is available), based on data published by WHO and the U. S. Centers for Disease Control, are summarized in Tables B.8 and B.9.

AIDS was recognized in Europe at about the same time as in the United States, and systematic surveillance for the disease began in WHO's Eu-

Table B.6
Cumulative AIDS Cases by Selected Characteristics,
San Francisco, December 1985 and September 1986

	DECEMBER 1985*		SEPTEMBER 1986**		INCREASE	
	NUMBER	PERCENT	NUMBER	PERCENT	NUMBER	PERCENT
Total Cases†	1,631		2,428		797	48.9
By race/ethnic group						
White	1,431	87.7	2,112	87.0	681	47.6
Black	82	5.0	139	5.7	57	69.5
Hispanic	93	5.7	145	6.0	52	55.9
Other/unknown	25	1.5	32	1.3	7	28.0
Cases by patient group						
Homosexual/bisexual	1,591	97.5	2,352	96.9	761	47.8
IV drug user	12	0.7	28	1.2	16	133.3
Transfusions w/blood or						
blood products	12	0.7	20	0.8	8	66.7
Hemophilia/Coagulation						
disorder	2	0.1	2	0.1	—	—
Heterosexual contact	3	0.2	8	0.3	5	166.7
Child of parent with or						
at risk for AIDS	3	0.2	3	0.1	—	—
Unknown/other	8	0.5	15	0.6	7	87.5
Cases male	1,618	99.2	2,403	99.0	785	48.5
Cases female	13	0.8	25	1.0	12	92.3
Adult cases	1,628	99.8	2,423	99.8	795	48.8
Pediatric cases††	3	0.2	5	0.2	2	66.7
Cases/100,000 pop.‡	229		341		112	48.9

*Data as of 31 December 1985.
**Data as of 30 September 1986.
†Figures include both adult and pediatric cases unless otherwise indicated.
††Pediatric cases refer to patients under 13 years of age at diagnosis.
‡Based on 1984 population figures.
SOURCE: San Francisco Department of Public Health, Bureau of Communicable Disease Control, provisional data.

ropean Region nations in 1982. AIDS data for Europe are collected by the WHO European Collaborating Centre on AIDS, located in Paris, to which 27 countries were reporting in mid-1986. By 30 June 1986, an average of 38 new AIDS cases per week were being reported in Europe (while the U. S. rate at that time was 236 new cases per week). Four countries—the Federal Republic of Germany, France, Italy, and the United Kingdom—accounted

Table B.7
Cumulative AIDS Cases by Selected Characteristics,
New York City and San Francisco, September 1986

	NEW YORK CITY*		SAN FRANCISCO**	
	NUMBER	PERCENT	NUMBER	PERCENT
Total Cases †	7,837	100.0	2,428	100.0
By race/ethnic group				
White	3,537	45.1	2,112	87.0
Black	2,441	31.1	139	5.7
Hispanic	1,805	23.0	145	6.0
Other/unknown	54	0.7	32	1.3
Cases by patient group				
Homosexual/bisexual	4,805	61.3	2,352	96.9
IV drug user	2,271	29.0	28	1.2
Transfusion w/blood or blood products	65	0.8	20	0.8
Hemophilia/Coagulation disorder	14	0.2	2	0.1
Heterosexual contact	156	2.0	8	0.3
Child of parent with or at risk for AIDS	124	1.6	3	0.1
Unknown/other	402	5.1	15	0.6
Cases male	7,014	89.5	2,403	99.0
Cases female	823	10.5	25	1.0
Adult cases	7,696	98.2	2,423	99.8
Pediatric cases † †	141	1.8	5	0.2
Cases/100,000 pop. ‡	109		341	

*Data as of 15 September 1986.
**Data as of 30 September 1986.
 † Figures include both adult and pediatric cases unless otherwise indicated.
† † Pediatric cases refer to patients under 13 years of age at diagnosis.
 ‡ Based on 1984 population figures.
SOURCE: New York City Department of Health, Office of Epidemiologic Surveillance and Statistics; San Francisco Department of Public Health, Bureau of Communicable Disease Control; preliminary data.

for 2,086 cases, 69 percent of the 3,041 total cases (World Health Organization 1986a). The demographic profile of the AIDS cases in Europe reported to the WHO center as of 30 June 1986 is summarized in Table B.10.

The European nations with the highest rates of AIDS per million population, as of 30 June 1986, were Switzerland (21.1 cases per million), Den-

Table B.8
Cumulative AIDS Cases Reported in 27 Countries of the
World Health Organization European Region,
1 October 1984 through 30 June, 1986

COUNTRY	OCTOBER 1984	MARCH 1985	JUNE 1985	SEPTEMBER 1985	DECEMBER 1985	MARCH 1986	JUNE 1986
Austria	—	13	18	23	28	34	36
Belgium	—	81	99	118	139	160	171
Czechoslovakia	—	—	—	—	—	4	4
Demark	31	41	48	57	68	80	93
Federal Repub. of Germany	110	162	220	295	377	459	538
Finland	4	5	6	10	10	11	11
France	221	307	392	466	573	707	859
German Dem. Republic	—	—	—	—	—	—	—
Greece	2	7	9	10	13	14	22
Hungary	—	—	—	—	—	—	—
Iceland	—	—	—	—	—	2	2
Ireland	—	—	—	—	8	9	10
Israel	—	—	—	—	—	23	24
Italy	10	22	52	92	140	219	300
Luxembourg	—	—	1	3	3	3	3
Malta	—	—	—	—	—	—	5
Netherlands	26	52	66	83	98	120	146
Norway	4	8	11	14	17	21	24
Poland	—	—	—	—	—	—	—
Portugal	—	—	—	—	18	24	28
Romania	—	—	—	—	—	1	1
Spain	18	29	38	63	83	145	177
Sweden	12	22	27	36	42	50	57
Switzerland	33	51	63	77	100	113	138
United Kingdom	88	140	176	225	287	340	389
U. S. S. R.	—	—	—	—	—	—	—
Yugoslavia	—	—	—	1	2	3	3
TOTAL	559	940	1,226	1,573	2,006	2,542	3,041

—Data not available.
SOURCES: World Health Organization, European Collaborating Centre on AIDS; U. S. Public Health Service, Centers for Disease Control.

Table B.9
Cumulative AIDS Cases Reported in
World Health Organization European Region
Countries, October 1983 to October 1986

PERIOD ENDING	CUMULATIVE CASES	INCREASE	
		NUMBER	PERCENT
October 1983	215		
July 1984	421	206	95.8*
October 1984	559	138	32.8
December 1984	762	203	36.3
March 1985	940	178	23.4
June 1985	1,226	286	30.4
October 1985	1,573	347	28.3
December 1985	2,006	433	27.5
March 1986	2,542	536	26.7
June 1986	3,041	499	19.6
October 1986†	3,127	86	2.8

*The reporting period between October 1983 and July 1984 is approximately nine months, resulting in an apparently larger percentage increase compared to the other reporting periods.
†Preliminary and incomplete data, reported as of 3 October 1986, should not be construed to indicate a decrease in the incidence of AIDS in Europe.
SOURCES: World Health Organization, European Collaborating Centre on AIDS; U. S. Public Health Service, Centers for Disease Control.

mark (18.3), Belgium (17.3), and France (15.7). However, these rates were low compared with the United States, where the rate was then about 93 cases per million population (these rates are based on 1985 population estimates). Furthermore, a significant proportion of AIDS cases in Belgium—over two-thirds as of 31 December 1985—have been diagnosed in persons of non-European origin, mostly Zairians (World Health Organization 1986b).

Homosexual/bisexual males account for between 60 and 95 percent of total AIDS cases in 10 of the 17 European countries with more than five cases. In Austria, Greece, Ireland, and Israel, that risk group accounts for 40–56 percent of the total cases; in Belgium, Italy, and Spain, homosexual/bisexual men comprise less than 30 percent of total cases.

Although heterosexual intravenous (IV) drug users account for only 12 percent of AIDS cases overall in Europe, in Italy and Spain they account for 51 percent and 46 percent respectively (together equaling 73 percent of all European AIDS cases linked to IV drug use). Nineteen percent of Aus-

Table B.10
Demographics of Cumulative AIDS Cases
Reported in World Health Organization European Region
Countries, 30 June 1986

PATIENT GROUPS	NUMBER	PERCENT
Adult Europeans	2,615	88.7
Adult Non-Europeans	333	11.3
TOTAL	2,948	100.0
Non-Europeans by place of origin		
Africa	186	55.9
Americas	131	39.3
Other/Unknown	16	4.8
TOTAL	333	100.0
Europeans		
Assessed by risk group		
Homosexual/bisexual	1,877	71.8
Heterosexual IV drug users	317	12.1
Homosexual/bisexual IV		
drug users	64	2.4
Hemophiliacs	112	4.3
Transfusion recipients	54	2.1
No known risk factor	148	5.7
Not assessed by risk group	43	1.6
TOTAL	2,615	100.0
Non-Europeans		
Associated with known risk group	106	31.8
Not associated with known		
risk group	204	61.3
Not assessed by risk group	23	6.9
TOTAL	333	100.0
Adults	2,948	96.9
Children	93	3.1
TOTAL	3,041	100.0
Children by risk group		
Parent with or at risk for AIDS	62	66.7
Transfusion/hemophilia-related	27	29.0
Risk factor unknown	4	4.3
TOTAL	93	100.0

SOURCE: World Health Organization, *Weekly Epidemiological Record* 61:305–06.

trian AIDS cases, 9 percent of those in Switzerland, 6 percent in the Federal Republic of Germany, and 4 percent in Norway also belong in this category. Meanwhile, in France, the Netherlands, and the United Kingdom, heterosexual IV drug users are about 3 percent of the individual national totals (World Health Organization 1986a).

Although homosexual/bisexual males accounted for more than two-thirds of European AIDS cases in mid-1986, their percentage of the total over time has gradually diminished from a higher share to a level comparable to that in the United States. Concurrently, there has been a steady increase in the percentage of AIDS cases among heterosexual IV drug users in Europe, who accounted for about 4 percent of total cases there in June 1985 (see Table B.11), but for nearly 11 percent of the total by June 1986 (see Table B.12). While heterosexual IV drug users account for a much higher percentage (over 17 percent) of AIDS cases in the United States (Table B.12), both the United States and Europe have experienced similar increases in the percentage of cases related to IV drug use over the history of the epidemic. The rapid spread of AIDS among IV drug users in Europe has been demonstrated by studies conducted in various countries in 1985 that showed a high and growing frequency—20 to 50 percent—of serologic markers for HTLV-III/LAV infection in this segment of the risk population (World Health Organization 1986c). This trend is significant because epidemiologists believe that heterosexual IV drug users play an important role in the spread of AIDS from the established risk groups into the general population.

Heterosexual contact has been thought to be the predominant mode of virus transmission in European AIDS cases that fall into patient categories with unknown risk or no risk factor (Centers for Disease Control 1986c). Of the 310 non-Europeans with AIDS who were assessed for risk group membership as of 30 June 1986, 66 percent were not associated with any known risk group (Table B.10). Many came from regions, such as Africa and the Carribean, where most AIDS patients are heterosexuals who do not fit into any of the known risk categories. Of the 175 persons of non-European origin who had been diagnosed with AIDS by 31 December 1985, the majority lived in Europe before developing AIDS symptoms, but about one-third of them had come to Europe after becoming ill (World Health Organization 1986b).

As of 31 December 1985, 12 European countries—Austria, Denmark, France, the Federal Republic of Germany, Greece, Ireland, Italy, Norway, Portugal, Spain, Sweden, and the United Kingdom—had reported cases of AIDS in hemophilia patients, and 7 countries—Belgium, Denmark, France, the Federal Republic of Germany, Italy, the Netherlands, and the United Kingdom—had reported AIDS in blood tranfusion recipients (World Health Organization 1986b). Screening of blood donors for an-

Table B.11
Distribution of Cumulative AIDS Cases in Europe
by Patient Group and Percentage of Total,
July 1984 through September 1985

	PERIOD ENDING					
PATIENT GROUP	07/84	10/84	12/84	03/85	06/85	09/85
Homosexual or bisexual males	318	432	537	661	853	1,085
	(75.5%)	(77.3%)	(70.5%)	(70.3%)	(69.6%)	(69.0%)
Heterosexual IV drug users	5	7	11	25	48	90
	(1.2)	(1.3)	(1.4)	(2.7)	(3.9)	(5.7)
Hemophilia patients	12	17	20	28	39	53
	(2.9)	(3.0)	(2.6)	(3.0)	(3.2)	(3.4)
Transfusion recipients	2	3	8	16	25	35
	(0.5)	(0.5)	(1.0)	(1.7)	(2.0)	(2.2)
Homosexual/bisexual IV drug users	3	5	11	12	18	24
	(0.7)	(0.9)	(1.4)	(1.3)	(1.5)	(1.5)
No risk factor:						
Males	56	63	112	122	149	167
	(13.3)	(11.3)	(14.7)	(13.0)	(12.2)	(10.6)
Females	25	31	48	57	70	84
	(5.9)	(5.5)	(6.3)	(6.1)	(5.7)	(5.3)
Unknown	—	1	15	19	24	35
	—	(0.2)	(2.0)	(2.0)	(2.0)	(2.2)
TOTAL	421	559	762	940	1,226	1,573
	(100.0)	(100.0)	(100.0)	(100.0)	(100.0)	(100.0)

Note: Percents may not total due to rounding.
SOURCE: Centers for Disease Control, *Morbidity and Mortality Weekly Report* 33:609, 34:29, 34:149, 34:474, 34:585, 35:43.

tibodies to the AIDS virus has been implemented in most European countries and measures to exclude blood donors who are members of AIDS risk groups have been undertaken. It is thought that the prevention of AIDS transmission by blood transfusion is now effective in most of the European countries where AIDS has been reported (Centers for Disease Control 1986c).

Table B.12
Distribution of Cumulative Adult AIDS Cases by Patient Group,
United States and Europe, 30 June 1986

PATIENT GROUP	UNITED STATES		EUROPE	
	NUMBER	PERCENT	NUMBER	PERCENT
Homosexual/bisexual males	14,298	65.3	1,877	63.7
Homosexual/bisexual				
IV drug users	1,746	8.0	64	2.2
Heterosexual IV drug users	3,755	17.2	319	10.8
Hemophilia patients	175	0.8	112	3.8
Transfusion recipients	361	1.6	54	1.8
Heterosexual contacts	359	1.6	—	—*
Risk group not reported**	—	—	104	3.5
No identified risk	1,169†	5.3	352	11.9
Unknown	—	—*	66	2.2
TOTAL	21,893	100.0	2,948	100.0

Note: Percents may not total due to rounding.
*Data for this category included in no-identified-risk group.
**Cases in non-Europeans who are members of undesignated individual risk groups.
†Includes persons born in countries in which most AIDS cases have not been associated with known risk factors but where heterosexual transmission is believed to play a major role.
SOURCES: Centers for Disease Control, provisional data; World Health Organization, *Weekly Epidemiological Record* 61:305-06.

The distribution of AIDS cases by age and sex have remained roughly similar for the United States and Europe. In the United States, as of 30 June 1986, 68 percent of persons with AIDS were 20–39 years old, and 89 percent were males (Centers for Disease Control 1986b). In Europe, data for 30 June 1986 show that 63 percent of AIDS patients were in the 20–39 age range, and 90 percent were males (World Health Organization 1986a). Case-fatality rates for AIDS patients over time are also about equal for Europe and the United States—in the 52–56 percent range.

Although the total number of AIDS cases reported in Europe by October 1986—3,127 cases—was only a fraction of the 25,650 cases that had been reported in the United States as of approximately the same date, it seems clear that AIDS is going to be a significant health problem in Europe, too. Just how significant is difficult to predict, but according to Dr. Jean-Baptiste Brunet, director of WHO's European Collaborating Centre on AIDS (Zinman 1986a), present trends suggest that there may be more than 20,000 cases of AIDS in Europe by June 1988. While total numbers may never reach the level of the United States, over the long term AIDS in the European health care community will probably require a similarly substantial commitment of resources for AIDS preventive education, research, and treatment.

III. AIDS IN AFRICA

As serious as the AIDS epidemic is in the United States, and as serious as it is becoming in Europe, the scope of the problem appears to be even greater in Africa, where surveys of HTLV-III/LAV antibody seropositivity suggest that as many as two million people—estimates range from 5 percent to more than 15 percent of the population—are infected with the virus. According to Dr. Fakhri Assaad, director of the Division of Communicable Diseases of the World Health Organization (WHO) in Geneva, as many as 50,000 people, most of them in central and equatorial Africa, already have AIDS (Chase 1986). In addition, studies indicate that in Africa, unlike the demographics of the disease elsewhere, AIDS patients and those infected with HTLV-III/LAV are almost exclusively heterosexual people (Clumeck, Van de Perre, et al. 1985), and males and females are affected in about equal proportion (Mann et al. 1986).

Because of difficulties in collecting health data in many African countries, information about AIDS and its incidence in Africa is still somewhat limited, and comprehensive statistics are not yet available. AIDS data collection in Africa is further complicated both by the lack of diagnostic laboratories for testing, and by the fact that some national governments in Africa have been slow—and even reluctant—to collect and report data on AIDS. Because some researchers have reported evidence suggesting that AIDS may have originated in Africa and may have been transmitted to humans from the African green monkey, one of several species of monkeys and apes which harbor simian retroviruses similar to HTLV-III/LAV, some African governments feel that Africans are being wrongly blamed—by implication—for the disease. Thus, to admit that AIDS exists in Africa amounts to complicity in what is regarded as a public health slander. This has resulted, in Africa, in cases of official indifference to AIDS and in an unwillingness in some instances to recognize, report, or even discuss the disease. In Zambia and Kenya, for example, officials respectively have referred to reports of the Africa-AIDS connection as "propaganda," and "a new form of hate campaign" (Altman 1985a). These attitudes are gradually changing, however, as the seriousness of the situation and the threat to public health become undeniable. Furthermore, the opinion that AIDS originated in Africa is by no means universal among AIDS researchers.

What is known is that Kaposi's sarcoma (KS), a cancer seen in AIDS patients in the United States and Europe, has long been endemic to equatorial Africa and that KS there seems to have increased and become more virulent in recent years (Altman 1985b). It was, in fact, the KS-AIDS relationship seen in the United States and Europe and cases of AIDS diagnosed in patients of African origin in Europe that drew the attention of health officials and researchers to Africa. Of additional significance was a new wasting syndrome known in Africa as "slim disease," first reported in Uganda but spreading to other countries, and apparently linked to the AIDS virus. As of 31 December 1985, AIDS had been diagnosed in Europe in 175 natives of 23 African countries (see Table B.13), and several studies in Africa had definitely established the presence and spread of both AIDS virus and AIDS itself.

Table B.13
Distribution and Percent of AIDS Cases Among Africans
Diagnosed in Europe, by Country of Origin, 31 December 1985
(N = 175)

COUNTRY	NUMBER	PERCENT
Algeria	2	1.1
Angola	1	0.6
Burundi	5	2.9
Cameroon	3	1.7
Cape Verde	1	0.6
Central African Republic	3	1.7
Chad	3	1.7
Congo	15	8.5
Egypt	1	0.6
Gabon	4	2.3
Ghana	2	1.1
Kenya	1	0.6
Madagascar	1	0.6
Mali	3	1.7
Morocco	1	0.6
Namibia	1	0.6
Rwanda	5	2.9
Senegal	2	1.1
Togo	1	0.6
Tunisia	1	0.6
Uganda	1	0.6
Zaire	115	65.7
Zambia	3	1.7

SOURCE: World Health Organization, *Weekly Epidemiological Record* 61:126.

The profile of African AIDS patients has been found to be remarkably different in one significant aspect from what physicians and researchers have been accustomed to seeing in Europe and North America, but there are also some significant similarities. None of a group of 23 African AIDS patients included in a 1979–1981 study in Belgium, for example, had a history of homosexuality, bisexuality, or drug addiction, or had received blood transfusions in the five years before onset of symptoms (Clumeck, Sonnet, et al. 1984). Several of the patients in the study had come to Belgium from Zaire, seeking treatment for unexplained weight loss and chronic diarrhea; others had lived in Belgium for 4 to 48 months, but had returned frequently to Africa for visits. Subsequent information collected about some of these patients and others diagnosed in Kigali, Rwanda revealed a high correlation between seropositivity for HTLV-III/LAV antibody and sexual promiscuity (that is, heterosexual promiscuity, including, among male patients, frequent contact with female prostitutes), and that 24 percent of a group of female patients with AIDS or AIDS-related complex were, in fact, professional prostitutes, none of whom had a history of drug addiction. This and other studies suggest that parenteral drug use has not been involved to any great extent in the spread of AIDS among heterosexuals in Africa (Clumeck, Van de Perre, et al. 1985), unlike the situations in the United States and Europe.

In Rwanda, a study by Clumeck, Robert-Guroff, et al. (1985) found that 67 (80 percent) of a group of 84 Rwandese prostitutes attending a sexually transmitted diseases clinic in Butare between January 1983 and July 1984 were seropositive for antibodies to the AIDS virus. The researchers concluded that "prostitutes could be an important human reservoir of the AIDS agent among the heterosexual population in Central Africa," a hypothesis that seems to be buttressed by the high prevalance of seropositivity they detected among male clients of prostitutes in Rwanda. The same study also found that 12.5 percent of a control group of healthy Africans and 15.5 percent of randomly assessed Rwandese blood donors—who were also asymptomatic—had antibodies to HTLV-III/LAV and were apparently healthy carriers of the disease. Limited data from screening programs at blood banks in the United States where AIDS risk group members have been discouraged from donating blood indicate that antibody seroprevalence nationally is less than 0.04 percent (Schorr, et al. 1985).

Whereas transfusions of blood and blood products account for only 1.8 percent of AIDS cases in the United States, the importance of this means of transmission in the African epidemic is still unknown, but it is being investigated. Among a cohort of AIDS patients studied in Zaire, blood transfusion in the three year period before onset of AIDS was found to be a risk factor in 9 percent of the cases (Mann et al. 1986). The reuse of poorly or improperly sterilized hypodermic needles in medical procedures, and traditional practices such as scarification and tattooing, as well as visits to practitioners of folk medicine, have also been identified as possible means of infection in Africa.

Researchers cannot say with certainty how long AIDS has been present in Africa. Exploring the Africa-AIDS connection in a series of articles in the *New York Times*, Lawrence K. Altman (1985a) reported, however, that studies and comparisons of stored blood collected in Africa as long ago as 1963 have indicated the presence of the AIDS virus or one closely resembling it in at least four countries—Kenya, Uganda, Zaire, and Burkina Faso. These and other findings suggest that the disease has been slowly spreading in central and East Africa for perhaps two decades. Dr. Luc Montagnier, of the Pasteur Institute in Paris, has reported that, whereas examinations of stored blood indicated infection with AIDS virus in about one percent of the population in some areas of Zaire in the mid-1970's, more recent tests show 10 percent of the people infected. Rates of infection shown in a number of studies of stored blood collected at different times from different areas of the African continent since the mid-1960's have varied widely (Altman 1985a). Researchers and scientists have disagreed over whether these findings confirm an African origin for AIDS.

Among American experts who support the African-origin hypothesis are Dr. Robert Gallo, of the National Cancer Institute, and Dr. William A. Haseltine of Harvard Medical School and the Dana-Farber Cancer Institute in Boston. Research into the suspected connection between the African green monkey and AIDS is being conducted by Dr. Max Essex of the Harvard School of Public Health, and others. On the other hand, in the fall of 1985, Dr. Peter Piot, a microbiologist and AIDS researcher at the Institute of Tropical Medicine in Antwerp, Belgium, maintained that the origin of AIDS was uncertain and that it would be difficult to prove Africa as the site (Altman 1985a). Although some officials have suggested that determining the geographical origin of AIDS is a low priority endeavor, a number of researchers believe that tracing the disease to its roots may provide data helpful in treating it and developing a vaccine.

Whatever its origin, recent studies of AIDS and the rate of AIDS virus infection in Africa point to a serious and increasing public health problem. Moreover, some researchers assert that AIDS has been occurring in epidemic form in central Africa since the late 1970s (Kreiss et al. 1986). When WHO convened its first workshop on AIDS in Africa, in the Central African Republic in October 1985, participants came from nine African nations: Burundi, Cameroon, Central African Republic, People's Republic of the Congo, Gabon, Rwanda, Uganda, United Republic of Tanzania, and Zaire. International experts in clinical medicine, microbiology, epidemiology, and public health took part in the conference, initiating a process of information exchange on AIDS in central Africa and collaboration between WHO and the nations of the region in efforts to confront and deal with the disease. For reporting purposes in Africa, WHO employs a case definition of AIDS (known in Africa as SIDA, the acronym for the French syndrome d'immunodéficit acquis) that is similar to the definition established for the United States by the Centers for Disease Control (see Appendix A).

Although only 911 confirmed cases of AIDS were reported from Africa at the time of the Second International Conference on AIDS, in Paris in June 1986, researchers and WHO officials have arrived at much higher estimates of illness—50,000 people with AIDS, 2 million infected—by extrapolating from confirmed cases and apparent rates of AIDS virus infection among various population subgroups (Holland 1986). It is thought that for every known case of AIDS there are between 50 and 100 infected carriers of the AIDS virus. WHO officials report, for example, that blood tests indicate that six to eight percent of childbearing women in Kinshasa, the capital of Zaire, are infected with HTLV-III/LAV (Zinman 1986b).

The male-female ratio of the AIDS patients in the Kinshasa study of Mann et al. was 1:1.1, while in the United States the male-female ratio has been in the 13:1 range. The distributions by age range of the adult Kinshasa patients and adult AIDS patients in the United States are roughly comparable: in Kinshasa, 75 percent of patients were between 20 and 39 years of age and 91 percent were 20–49 years old; in the United States, 68 percent of AIDS patients are in the 20–39 age range, and 89 percent are in the 20–49 group (Centers for Disease Control 1986d). According to Mann et al., men with AIDS in Kinshasa tended to be older than women (mean ages 37.4 and 30.0 respectively), and the case rate for Kinshasa women 20 to 29 years old was found to be 269 percent higher than that for men.

Given the apparent rate of AIDS infection among the adult population, including childbearing women, children in Africa are also likely to be affected by AIDS in significant numbers, but the full extent of the disease in the lowest age groups is unknown. According to Clumeck, Robert-Guroff, et al. (1985), studies conducted in Zaire and Uganda have indicated seropositivity in 35 to 67 percent of children in areas of those countries. However, diagnosis of pediatric AIDS in Africa is problematic because of a high incidence of illnesses with similar manifestations, such as diarrhea and weight loss, that are prevalent in general among African children. Until better and more comprehensive diagnostic procedures and facilities are available and in use, surveillance of pediatric AIDS in Africa will continue to be inadequate.

Meanwhile, Dr. Bela M. Kapita, a Kinshasa physician, has reported that some 1,000 people have contracted AIDS in that city since 1983 (Holland 1986), that AIDS is common among female prostitutes there, and that 60 percent of prostitutes tested in Nairobi, Kenya and nearly 90 percent of those in Rwanda carry the AIDS virus (Chase 1986). Dr. Kapita's figures correlate closely with those cited by others, including Mann et al., Kreiss et al., and Clumeck, Robert-Guroff et al.

The study of AIDS infection in Nairobi prostitutes by Kreiss et al. (1986) suggests how AIDS has spread—and may continue spreading—in Africa. It involved two groups of prostitutes, 64 of lower socioeconomic status (LSS) and 26 of higher socioeconomic status (HSS), along with 40 male clients of a sexually transmitted disease (STD) clinic, and a control group of 42 medical personnel. Sixty-six percent of the LSS group were seropositive for antibody to HTLV-III/LAV; varying high percentages of the group were also positive for other STDs, including 55 percent for syphilis. In the HSS group, 31 percent were seropositive; although 31 percent also had serum reactive for syphilis, in general their rates of other STDs were significantly lower than those of the LSS group. Of the STD clinic patients, eight percent were seropositive for AIDS virus antibody, as was one member (two percent) of the control group. Although the seropositive subjects were found generally to have immunologic abnormalities associated with AIDS virus infection, none had opportunistic infections, Kaposi's sarcoma, weight loss, fever, diarrhea, or fatigue typical of AIDS. Still, over half of the seropositive group did have generalized lymphadenopathy. None of the study subjects used intravenous drugs, but most of the prostitutes had a history of intramuscular injections for medical treatment. This was also true of nearly all of the STD clients, whose rate of seropositivity for AIDS virus antibody was considerably lower than that of the prostitutes.

Kreiss et al. reported that studies of stored serum samples indicated that the AIDS virus had been introduced into the subject population since 1980, and that data suggested its spread from central Africa. They also noted that seropositivity among the prostitutes was associated with sexual contact with males from Rwanda, Uganda, and Burundi. The sexual contacts of the LSS group, with the highest rate of infection, were exclusively African. According to the researchers, however, they "found no association between HTLV-III antibody and nationality." Citing the possibility that heterosexual males might continue to spread the AIDS virus among urban prostitutes across the continent, Kreiss et al. observed that an urgent need exists in Africa for public health programs to modify sexual behavior and limit sexual contact with persons in high-risk groups.

Although the studies cited in this appendix section suggest that AIDS virus infection is already widespread and spreading in central and equatorial Africa, reports to the World Health Organization indicate that the incidence of the disease appears to vary across the continent. As of 17 December 1985, Kenya had recorded 10 AIDS cases, four of which affected persons from other African countries. Eight of the patients had died (World Health Organization 1985). In Accra, Ghana, 310 persons belonging to groups at risk of acquiring AIDS were tested for antibody to HTLV-III/LAV at the University of Ghana's Noguchi Memorial Institute for Medical Research. All were negative. No cases had been reported by Ethiopia, as of 6 January 1986, but AIDS education and epidemiological research were beginning to be undertaken there (World Health Organization 1986d). A report from Zimbabwe on surveillance of blood donors in that country between February and October 1985 indicated that 3.2 percent of donors showed seropositivity for antibody to HTLV-III/LAV, and that 11.8 percent of 69 Kaposi's sarcoma patients tested positive for the AIDS virus. However, no AIDS cases were confirmed in Zimbabwe (World Health Organization 1986e).

Representatives of the World Health Organization African Region nations met in Brazzaville in March 1986 to discuss recommendations and adopt a comprehensive plan of action to control AIDS in Africa. A status report as of 6 March 1986 indicated that AIDS cases had been reported in seven countries (not identified). Twenty-one of the member countries had a range of AIDS-related activities underway, including information and education programs, formal AIDS surveillance programs, antibody-testing, and the development of National AIDS Committees, as urged by WHO (World Health Organization 1986f). The government of Zaire, for example, had already authorized Project SIDA, an AIDS research program, in October 1983, and had begun systematic surveillance for AIDS in Kinshasa in June 1984. Results from this surveillance were reported in the 20 June 1986 issue of the *Journal of the American Medical Association* (Mann et al. 1986), and have been discussed earlier in this appendix.

Perhaps the most striking aspect of AIDS in Africa is that it appears to be spread to a great extent through heterosexual—predominantly vaginal—intercourse, but other methods of transmission—involving blood or blood product transfusions, contaminated hypodermics or medical instruments, folk medicine practices, ritual scarification, and transmission from infected mother to infant—are certainly involved. Although homosexuality and bisexuality are not seen to be common in Africa, neither type of sexual behavior can be ruled out for possible involvement at some level in the AIDS epidemic there. While AIDS surveillance in Africa has not been underway long enough to result in comprehensive statistics on mortality, there is no evidence that the case fatality rate in Africa is any lower than it is elsewhere.

The reports and studies of AIDS and AIDS virus infection in Africa add up to what appears to be an already critical public health situation. One thing is certain, the game of denial in which some African govern-ments have been involved cannot continue for very much longer; reality must be faced. To delay preparing for the burden AIDS imposes on health care systems, to fail to implement programs of education and prevention, and to continue to ignore the mounting evidence of the epidemic's pre-sence and spread will leave those nations and their populations vulnerable to a mammoth public health catastrophe. Indeed, if it is true, as some researchers believe, that at least 20 to 30 percent of AIDS-infected people will develop AIDS within 10 years (Eckholm 1986), and if the estimates by WHO officials that some two million Africans are infected with HTLV-III/ LAV are also correct, then there may be over 600,000 cases of AIDS in Af-rica alone by the middle of the next decade. The potential also exists for many more than that number.

IV. AIDS IN THE AMERICAS AND THE FAR EAST

The Americas

Discussions of AIDS tend to focus on the United States, Europe, and Af-rica, where most of the cases have been diagnosed, but the incidence of the disease is also increasing in other parts of the world. Table B.14 lists cumulative AIDS cases and total deaths over the 1982–1986 period in those nations of the Americas which had a total of 10 or more cases as of 30 June 1986.

According to data published by the World Health Organization (1986g) on 26 September 1986, there were a total of 24,752 confirmed cases of AIDS and 13,345 deaths from AIDS in the Americas as of 30 June 1986. These figures include the confirmed AIDS cases and deaths in the countries that were not included in Table B.14 because they had fewer than 10 cases.

Australia

The World Health Organization (1986h) has reported a cumulative total of 203 AIDS cases in Australia as of 29 April 1986. Males accounted for 195 (96.1 percent) of the cases; 8 patients (3.9 percent) were females. The case fatality rate for AIDS patients in Australia at the time of the report was 48.8 percent. The demographics of the Australian cases in that report are summarized in Table B.15.

Table B.14
AIDS Cases and Deaths in Selected Countries of the Americas, Cumulative Totals,
1982 through 30 June 1986

COUNTRY	CUMULATIVE AIDS CASES					DEATHS
	1982	1983	1984	1985	1986	
Argentina	—	6	11	42	58	29
Bahamas	—	—	—	38	68	21
Bermuda	—	—	5	27	42	26
Brazil	5	50	188	540	754	365
Canada	25	81	217	513	638*	321
Chile	—	—	4	8	12	6
Costa Rica	—	2	6	9	12	10
Dominican Repub.	—	4	8	39	62	30
French Guiana	—	3	6	31	31†	15
Guadeloupe	2	4	11	16	16†	14
Haiti	—	232	340	377	501	111
Mexico	—	8	18	33	161	67
Saint Lucia	—	—	1	10	10†	2
Trinidad/Tobago	—	9	16	71	108	71
United States	1,147	4,069	9,553	18,561	22,162	12,181
Venezuela	—	—	9	32	40	22
TOTAL	1,179	4,468	10,393	20,347	24,675	13,291

*Data through 14 July 1986.
† 1986 data not received.
—No reported cases or data not available.
SOURCE: World Health Organization, Weekly Epidemiological Record 60:153; 61:88, 301.

Japan

The World Health Organization (1986i) has reported that 11 cases of AIDS had been confirmed in Japan as of 31 October 1985. All patients were males; six were categorized as homosexuals, and five were hemophiliacs. The first AIDS case diagnosed in Japan was confirmed in March 1985. Of the remaining patients, five were confirmed in May, two in July and three in October. Six of the 11 patients—two homosexuals and four hemophiliacs from the groups diagnosed in May, July, and October—had died by the reporting date.

V. PROJECTIONS FOR THE FUTURE

By the beginning of 1987, the rate of AIDS incidence in the United States was 126 cases per million population (1980 census; Centers for Disease

Table B.15
Cumulative AIDS Cases and Deaths in Australia,
by Patient Group, 29 April 1986

PATIENT GROUP	NUMBER	PERCENT	DEATHS	PERCENT
Homosexual/bisexual male	176	86.7	79	79.8
Homosexual/bisexual IV				
drug user	2	1.0	2	2.0
IV drug user	—	—	—	—
Transfusion recipient	19	9.4	14	14.1
Hemophiliac	3	1.5	3	3.0
Heterosexual partner of person				
with or at risk for AIDS	2	1.0	1	1.0
Other/unknown	1	0.5	—	—
TOTAL	203	100.0*	99	100.0

*Percents may not total due to rounding.
SOURCE: World Health Organization, *Weekly Epidemiological Record* 61:168.

Control 1986e). At the time of the Second International Conference on AIDS in Paris, in late June 1986, predictions for the growth and spread of the epidemic were ominous. Researchers at the conference reported estimates of up to 100,000 current AIDS cases worldwide and the director general of the World Health Organization asserted that somewhere between 5 and 10 million people are infected with the AIDS virus (Holland 1986).

In the United States at about the same time, officials of the U. S. Public Health Service (USPHS) issued a report indicating their belief that, based on current trends, there will be a cumulative total of 270,000 AIDS cases in the country by 1991—a more than tenfold increase in only five years—and that the death toll will climb to 179,000 (66 percent) by then. All but 25 percent of the new AIDS cases included in those figures are expected to be among persons already infected as of 1986. For 1991 alone, federal officials are predicting 74,000 new cases and 54,000 deaths, compared to estimates of about 16,000 new cases and 9,000 deaths for 1986 (Eckholm 1986). These figures are based on federal estimates of 1.5 million currently infected individuals, 20–30 percent of whom are expected to develop AIDS within the next decade. In addition, an undetermined but substantial percentage of others who are infected but do not develop full-scale AIDS may suffer a variety of AIDS-related illnesses that may require long-term medical attention.

The population subgroups affected by AIDS are not expected to change in any major way in the United States. If official projections are correct, about 65–70 percent of AIDS cases will continue to be among men in the homosexual/bisexual risk group, and about 25 percent will be intravenous drug users (8 percent of AIDS cases are both homosexual/ bisexual and drug users). The proportion of cases linked to heterosexual intercourse is expected to rise from the 1986 level of about 4 percent to around 9 percent—about 7,000 cases annually—by 1991. Hemophiliacs and those infected as a result of blood transfusions may continue to account for small percentages of AIDS cases, but those proportions will diminish over time as the effect of antibody testing of donated blood reduces AIDS virus transmission by that route. Meanwhile, the cumulative total of pediatric AIDS cases by 1991 is expected to exceed 3,000.

As grim as these official predictions for the epidemic's increase seem, there are some scientists who believe that the AIDS epidemic will be even worse. Dr. William A. Haseltine, an AIDS researcher at the Dana-Farber Cancer Institute in Boston has remarked, for example, that "We expect upward of one million people to die of [AIDS] in the next ten years," and that it could be "considerably worse" or "moderately worse" than that (Colen 1986).

With uncertainty about the absolute numbers of people who will be suffering from AIDS or AIDS-related illnesses in the years ahead, not to mention the inability to predict the course of medical research and treatments that may or may not be developed, it is difficult to estimate what the long-range financial costs of treating AIDS patients will be in the United States. In their June 1986 report, estimating that within five years some 145,000 people annually will need medical treatment because of AIDS, USPHS officials predicted annual national health care costs for AIDS of between $8 and $16 billion, or about 2.5 percent of total U. S. spending on health care. These estimates were based on a projected average annual cost of $46,000 for care per patient. However, the report cautioned that costs may turn out to be 10 to 50 percent higher because of a number of variables and nonmedical costs that may be involved in AIDS but are difficult to estimate (Russell 1986).

Through 1986, the costs of providing treatment and care for people with AIDS have been concentrated in a few urban areas, where most of the AIDS cases have occurred. As of 29 September 1986, the eight metropolitan areas reporting more than 500 AIDS cases accounted for 62 percent of total U. S. cases but for only 16 percent of the U. S. population (see Table B.16), and three cities—New York, San Francisco, and Los Angeles— with only 8.7 percent of the U. S. population, accounted for nearly 50 percent of all AIDS cases that had been reported to the Centers for Disease Control. New York and San Francisco together have reported 40 percent of the cases, but officials predict that their share of AIDS patients will shrink to less than 20 percent of the total by 1991, as the incidence of the disease

Table B.16
Distribution of AIDS Cases
and Population Among Selected United States
Standard Metropolitan Statistical Areas (SMSAs),
29 September 1986

| SMSAs | AIDS CASES* | | POPULATION† | | |
	NUMBER	PERCENT	MILLIONS	PERCENT	CASES/MILLION
New York City	7,620	29.7	9.12	4.0	835.5
San Francisco	2,657	10.4	3.25	1.4	817.5
Los Angeles	2,175	8.5	7.48	3.3	290.8
Washington, D.C.	741	2.9	3.06	1.3	242.2
Miami	729	2.8	1.63	0.7	447.2
Houston	722	2.8	2.91	1.3	248.1
Newark	632	2.5	1.97	0.9	320.8
Chicago	565	2.2	7.10	3.1	79.6
SUBTOTAL	15,841	61.8	36.52	16.0	433.8
Remainder of U.S.	9,809	38.2	191.11	84.0	51.3
TOTAL	25,650	100.0	227.63	100.0	112.7

*Data as of 29 September 1986.
†Population data reported in 1980 census.
SOURCE: Centers for Disease Control, provisional data.

becomes more geographically generalized (Pear 1986). As a result, more and more localities can expect to find AIDS an increasingly challenging and expensive public health problem in the years ahead.

REFERENCES

Altman, L. K. 1985a. Linking AIDS to Africa provokes bitter dispute. *New York Times,* 21 November.

_____. 1985b. Rare cancer tied to AIDS takes new form in Africa. *New York Times,* 09 December.

Centers for Disease Control. 1984. Update: Acquired immunodeficiency syndrome—Europe. *Morbidity and Mortality Weekly Report* 33:607–09.

_____. 1985. Update: Acquired immunodeficiency syndrome—United States. *Morbidity and Mortality Weekly Report* 34:245–48.

_____. 1986a. Update: Acquired immunodeficiency syndrome—United States. *Morbidity and Mortality Weekly Report* 35:17–21.

_____. 1986b. *Acquired Immunodeficiency Syndrome (AIDS) Weekly Surveillance Report,* provisional data, 29 September.

_____. 1986c. Update: Acquired immunodeficiency syndrome—Europe. *Morbidity and Mortality Weekly Report* 35:35–46.

_____. 1986d. *Acquired Immunodeficiency Syndrome (AIDS) Weekly Surveillance Report*, provisional data, 18 August.

_____. 1986e. *Acquired Immunodeficiency Syndrome (AIDS) Weekly Surveillance Report*, provisional data, 29 December.

Chase, M. 1986. AIDS has spread 'almost everywhere' in Africa, Zaire doctor tells parley. *Wall Street Journal*, 24 June.

Clumeck, N., J. Sonnet, H. Taelman, F. Mascart-Lemone, M. De Bruyere, P. Vandeperre, J. Dasnoy, L. Marcelis, M. Lamy, C. Jonas, L. Eyckmans, H. Noel, M. Vanhaeverbeek, J. Butzler. 1984. Acquired immunodeficiency syndrome in African patients. *New England Journal of Medicine* 310:492–97.

Clumeck, N., M. Robert-Guroff, P. Van de Perre, A. Jennings, J. Sibomana, P. Demol, S. Cran, R. C. Gallo. 1985. Seroepidemiological studies of HTLV-III antibody prevalence among selected groups of heterosexual Africans. *Journal of the American Medical Association* 254:2599–602.

Clumeck, N., P. Van de Perre, M. Carael, D. Rouvroy, and D. Nzaramba. 1985. Heterosexual promiscuity among African patients with AIDS. *New England Journal of Medicine* 313:182.

Colen, B. D. 1986. AIDS: How fast, far will it spread? *Newsday*, 10 June.

Eckholm, E. 1986. Broad alert over AIDS: Social battle is shifting. *New York Times*, 17 June.

Holland, S. 1986. World AIDS cases may total 100,000, doctors estimate. *Washington Post*, 24 June.

Kreiss, J. K., D. Koech, F. A. Plummer, K. K. Holmes, M. Lightfoote, P. Piot, A. R. Ronald, J. O. Ndinya-Achola, L. J. D'Costa, P. Roberts, E. N. Ngugi, and T. C. Quinn. 1986. AIDS virus infection in Nairobi prostitutes: Spread of the epidemic to East Africa. *New England Journal of Medicine* 314:414–18.

Mann, J. M., H. Francis, T. Quinn, P. K. Asila, N. Bosenge, N. Nzilambi, K. Bila, M. Tamfum, K. Ruti, P. Piot, J. McCormick, and J. W. Curran. 1986. Surveillance for AIDS in a central African city. *Journal of the American Medical Association* 255:3255–59.

Netter, T. W. 1986. AIDS cases are said to rise sharply worldwide. *New York Times*, 5 October.

Pear, R. 1986. Tenfold increase in AIDS death toll is expected by '91. *New York Times*, 13 June.

Russell, C. 1986. AIDS could join America's top 10 killers in five years. *Washington Post*, 13 June.

Schorr, J. B., A. Berkowitz, P. D. Cumming, A. J. Katz, and S. G. Sandler. 1985. Prevalence of HTLV-III antibody in American blood donors. *New England Journal of Medicine* 313:384–85.

World Health Organization. 1985. Acquired immune deficiency syndrome: Kenya. *Weekly Epidemiological Record* 60:394.

_____. 1986a. Acquired immunodeficiency syndrome (AIDS): Situation in the WHO European region as of 30 June 1986. *Weekly Epidemiological Record* 61:305–06.

_____. 1986b. Acquired immunodeficiency syndrome (AIDS): Situation in Europe as of 31 December 1985. *Weekly Epidemiological Record* 61:125–28.

_____. 1986c. *Guidelines on AIDS in Europe*. Copenhagen: World Health Organization, Regional Office for Europe, 28.

_____. 1986d. Acquired immune deficiency syndrome: Ethiopia; Ghana. *Weekly Epidemiological Record* 61:26–27.

_____. 1986e. Acquired immune deficiency syndrome: Zimbabwe. *Weekly Epidemiological Record* 61:18.

_____. 1986f. Acquired immunodeficiency syndrome (AIDS): Plan of action for control in the African Region. *Weekly Epidemiological Record* 61:93.

_____. 1986g. Acquired immunodeficiency syndrome (AIDS) in the Americas—Update. *Weekly Epidemiological Record* 61:301.

_____. 1986h. Acquired immune deficiency syndrome: Australia. *Weekly Epidemiological Record* 61:168.

_____. 1986i. Acquired immune deficiency syndrome: Japan. *Weekly Epidemiological Record* 61:27.

Zinman, D. 1986a. Steep AIDS rise expected in Europe. *Newsday,* 23 June.

_____. 1986b. Health chief sees world AIDS peril. *Newsday,* 24 June.

AIDS Resources and Organizations

The following list of AIDS resources and organizations with AIDS-related programs is separated into two categories: national and local. National organizations are listed alphabetically by name. Local organizations are listed alphabetically by state and city. These lists are by no means complete or definitive. New organizations offering AIDS-related services are constantly forming, and existing health- and social service-related organizations are constantly becoming involved in AIDS activities as the impact of the epidemic spreads. At the same time, organizations also go out of existence or sometimes merge their activities with other groups.

Consulting some of the AIDS-related national organizations may be useful in locating additional resources in a particular locality. The AIDS Action Council, the National AIDS Network, and the U. S. Conference of Mayors, for example, all publish continually updated directories of service organizations.

Note: The inclusion of any organization or group on this list constitutes neither endorsement nor recommendation of its services or materials by either the United Hospital Fund of New York or the Institute for Health Policy Studies. Similarly, the omission of any organizations or groups from the list should not be construed to reflect negatively upon any of those organizations or groups. One caveat: Addresses and telephone numbers are subject to change; consulting local telephone directory information services is recommended if organizations cannot be reached at numbers listed.

NATIONAL ORGANIZATIONS

AIDS Action Council
729 8th Street, S.E., Suite 200
Washington, DC 20003
202/547-3101

AIDS Information
U. S. Public Health Services
Room 721-H, HHH Building
200 Independence Avenue S.W.
Washington, DC 20201
202/245-6867

283

AIDS Information Exchange
U. S. Conference of Mayors
1620 Eye Street, N.W.
Washington, DC 20006
202/293-7330

American Association of Physicians
for Human Rights
1050 W. Pacific Coast Highway
Harbor City, CA 90710
213/548-0491

American Cancer Society
777 Third Avenue
New York, NY 10017
212/371-2900

American College Health Association
15879 Crabbs Branch Way
Rockville, MD 20855
301/963-1100

American Foundation for AIDS Re-
search (AmFAR)
East: 40 West 57th Street
         New York, NY 10019-4001
         212/333-3118
West: 9601 Wilshire Boulevard
         Los Angeles, CA 90210-5294
         213/273-5547

American Health Foundation
Ford Foundation Building
320 East 42nd Street
New York, NY 10017
212/953-1900

American Hospital Association
AIDS Activities
840 North Lake Shore Drive
Chicago, IL 60611
312/280-6130

American Management Association
135 West 50th Street
New York, NY 10020
212/586-8100

American Medical Association
535 N. Dearborn
Chicago, IL 60610
312/645-5000

American Psychological Association
1200 17th Street, N.W.
Washington, DC 20036
202/955-7600

American Public Health Association
1015 Fifteenth Street, N.W.
Washington, DC 20005
202/789-5600

American Red Cross
17th & D Streets, N.W.
Washington, DC 20006
202/737-8300

Association of State and Territorial
Health Officials
1311A Dolly Madison Boulevard
McClean, VA 22101
703/556-9222

Centers for Disease Control
AIDS Task Force
1600 Clifton Road
Atlanta, GA 30333
404/329-2891
    AIDS Hotline
    800/447-2437

Coalition Clearinghouse
1615 H Street, N.W.
Washington, DC 20062
202/463-5970

The Documentation of AIDS Issues
and Research Foundation, Inc.
(DAIR)
2336 Market Street, Suite 33
San Francisco, CA 94114
415/928-0292

Gay Rights National Lobby
P. O. Box 1892
Washington, DC 20013
202/546-1801

Lambda Legal Defense and
Education Fund
132 West 43rd Street
New York, NY 10036
212/944-9488

National AIDS Network
729 8th Street, S.E.
Washington, DC 20003
202/546-2424

National Coalition of Gay Sexually
   Transmitted Disease Services
P. O. Box 239
Milwaukee, WI 53201
414/277-7671

National Gay Task Force
1517 U Street, N.W.
Washington, DC 20009
202/332-6483

National Hemophilia Foundation
Soho Building
110 Greene Street, Room 406
New York, NY 10012
212/219-8180

National Institute of Allergy
   and Infectious Diseases
AIDS Bibliography
9000 Rockville Pike
Building 5, Room 135
Bethesda, MD 20205

National Institute on Drug Abuse
Parklawn Building
5600 Fishers Lane
Rockville, MD 20857
202/443-6500

National Lesbian and Gay Health
   Foundation
P. O. Box 65472
Washington, DC 20035
202/797-3708

United States Conference of
   Local Health Officers
1620 Eye Street, N.W.
Washington, DC 20006
202/293-7330

United States Conference of Mayors
Attn: Health Program
1620 Eye Street, N.W.
Washington, DC 20006
202/293-7330

STATE AND LOCAL ORGANIZATIONS

Persons who find no organizations or resources in their vicinity among
those listed below should get in touch with their local public health agencies. The public health departments of most states and many cities already
have established AIDS programs, or at the very least may be sources of additional information and referral.

ALABAMA

Birmingham AIDS Outreach
P. O. Box 73062
Birmingham, AL 35253
205/930-0440

Mobile AIDS Support Group
2451 Fillingim Street
Mobile, AL 36617
205/690-8158

West Alabama AIDS Network
2810 8th Street
Tuscaloosa, AL 35401
205/354-0067

ALASKA

Alaska AIDS Project
P. O. Box 200070
Anchorage, AK 99520
907/276-3920

ARIZONA

Mobilization Against AIDS
351 E. Thomas Rd. #508
Phoenix, AZ 85102

Arizona AIDS Fund Trust
5150 North 7th Street
Phoenix, AZ 85014
602/277-1929

Tucson AIDS Project
80 West Cushing Street
Tucson, AZ 85701
602/792-3772

ARKANSAS

Arkansas AIDS Foundation
P. O. Box 1033
Camden, AR 71701
501/370-1149

AIDS Support Group
409 Walnut Street
Little Rock, AR 72205
501/663-6455

CALIFORNIA

Berkeley Gay Men's Clinic
2339 Durant Avenue
Berkeley, CA 94704-1670
415/548-2570 or 848-9220

Pacific Center AIDS Project
P. O. Box 908
Berkeley, CA 94701
415/548-8283

AIDS Response Program
Gay & Lesbian Community Services
    Center
12832 Garden Grove Boulevard
Garden Grove, CA 92643
714/534-0862

Long Beach AIDS Service Group
2025 East 10th Street
Long Beach, CA 90804
213/439-3948

Aid for AIDS
8235 Santa Monica Boulevard
West Hollywood, CA 90069
213/656-1107

AIDS Project/Los Angeles (APLA)
3670 Wilshire Blvd. #300
Los Angeles, CA 90010
213/738-8200

Gay and Lesbian Community Services
    Center
1213 N. Highland Avenue
Hollywood, CA 90038
213/464-7276

South California Mobilization
    Against AIDS
1428 N. McCadden Pl.
Los Angeles, CA 90028
213/463-3928

Minority AIDS Council
5882 West Pico Boulevard
Los Angeles, CA 90019
213/936-4949

California Department of Health
    Services—AIDS Activities
P. O. Box 160146
Sacramento, CA 95816-0146
916/445-0553

Sacramento AIDS/KS Foundation
900 K Street, #103
Sacramento, CA 98514
916/488-2437

Hemophilia Council of CA, AIDS
    Project
4304 Third Avenue
San Diego, CA 92103
619/543-1355

Owen Clinic
University of CA Medical Center
255 Dickinson Street
San Diego, CA 92103
619/294-3995

San Diego AIDS Project
4304 3rd Avenue
P. O. Box 81082
San Diego, CA 92138
619/294-2437
  Hotline: 619/260-1304

AIDS Health Project
333 Valencia Street, 4th Floor
San Francisco, CA 94103
415/626-6637

AIDS InterFaith Network
890 Hayes Street
San Francisco, CA 94117
415/558-9644

Hospice of San Francisco
225 30th Street
San Francisco, CA 94141
415/285-5622

Lesbian & Gay Health Services
  Coordinating Committee
San Francisco Dept. of Public Health
101 Grove Street
San Francisco, CA 94102
415/558-2541

People with AIDS/SF
1040 Ashbury, #5
San Francisco, CA 94117
415/665-3787

San Francisco AIDS Foundation
333 Valencia Street, 4th Floor
San Francisco, CA 94103
415/864-4376
  Hotline: 415/863-2437

Shanti Project
890 Hayes Street
San Francisco, CA 94117
415/558-9688

Westside Community Mental Health
  Center
1153 Oak Street
San Francisco, CA 94117
414/431-9000

AIDS Foundation of Santa Clara
  County
715 North First Street
San Jose, CA 95112
408/298-2437

Tri-County AIDS Task Force
300 San Antonio Road
Santa Barbara, CA 93110
805/967-2311

COLORADO

Colorado AIDS Project
P. O. Box 18529
Denver, CO 80218
303/837-0166

CONNECTICUT

AIDS Coordinator
Connecticut State Department
  of Health Services
150 Washington Street
Hartford, CT 06106
203/566-5058

Hartford Gay Health Collective
P. O. Box 6723
Hartford, CT 06105
203/723-5194

AIDS Project/New Haven
P. O. Box 636
New Haven, CT 06503
203/624-2437

DELAWARE

Delaware Lesbian and Gay Health
  Advocates (DLGHA)
214 North Market St.
Wilmington, DE 19801
302/652-3310

DISTRICT OF COLUMBIA

AIDS Action Project
Whitman-Walker Clinic
2335 18th Street, N.W.
Washington, D.C. 20009
202/332-5295

St. Francis Center
3800 Macomb Street, N.W.
Washington, D.C. 20016
202/234-5613

FLORIDA

AID Center One
604 S. W. 12th Avenue
Ft. Lauderdale, FL 33312
305/764-3123

Gainesville AIDS Community
  Network
P. O. Box 8488
Gainesville, FL 32605
904/371-1428

AIDS Education Project
901 Doval Street
Key West, FL 33040
305/294-8302

Health Crisis Network
P. O. Box 52-1546
Miami, FL 33152
305/326-8833

Tampa AIDS Network
2903 S. Concordia
Tampa, FL 33629
813/839-5939

GEORGIA

AID Atlanta (AIDA)
811 Cypress Street, N.W.
Atlanta, GA 30308
404/872-0600

HAWAII

Life Foundation
320 Ward Avenue, Suite 104
Honolulu, HI 96814
808/942-2437

IDAHO

Idaho AIDS Foundation
Boise, ID
208/345-2277

ILLINOIS

Gay Community AIDS Project
P. O. Box 713
Champaign, IL 61820
217/351-2437

AIDS Action Project
Howard Brown Memorial Clinic
2676 N. Halsted Street
Chicago, IL 60614
312/871-5777

INDIANA

Indiana AIDS Task Force
7026 North Temple Avenue
Indianapolis, IN 46220
317/929-3466

IOWA

Central Iowa AIDS Project
2116 Grand Avenue
Des Moines, IA 50312
515/243-4235

KANSAS

Kansas AIDS Network
P. O. Box 2655
Topeka, KN 66601
913/357-7499

KENTUCKY

AIDS Crisis Task Force
P. O. Box 11442
Lexington, KY 40575
606/233-0444

LOUISIANA

Baton Rouge MCC AIDS Project
Box 64996
Baton Rouge, LA 70896
504/928-3726

NO/AIDS Task Force
P. O. Box 2616
New Orleans, LA 70176
504/529-3009

Foundation for Health Education
P. O. Box 51537
New Orleans, LA 71051
504/928-2270

MAINE

The AIDS Project
P. O. Box 10723
Portland, ME 04104
207/775-1267

Central Maine Health Foundation
P. O. Box 3113
Lewiston, ME 04240
207/782-6113

MARYLAND

Health Education Resource Center
101 W. Read Street, Suite 819
Baltimore, MD 21201
301/985-1180

Gay Community Center of Baltimore
   Health Clinic
241 West Chase Street
Baltimore, MD 21201
301/837-2050

MASSACHUSETTS

AIDS Action Committee
661 Boylston Street, Suite 4
Boston, MA 02116
617/437-6200

Haitian Committee on AIDS
   in Massachusetts
117 Harvard Street
Dorchester, MA 02124

MICHIGAN

United Community Services
   of Metropolitan Detroit
51 West Warren Avenue
Detroit, MI 48201
313/833-0622

Wellness Networks, Inc.
P. O. Box 1046
Royal Oaks, MI 48068
313/876-3582

MINNESOTA

Minnesota AIDS Project
2025 Nicollet Avenue, #200
Minneapolis, MN 55404
612/870-7773

MISSISSIPPI

Mississippi Gay Alliance
P. O. Box 8342
Jackson, MS 39204
601/353-7611

MISSOURI

Good Samaritan Project
P. O. Box 10087
Kansas City, MO 64111
816/452-2255

AIDS Project/Springfield
718 North Kansas Expressway
Springfield, MO 65802
417/864-8373

St. Louis Task Force on AIDS
P. O. Box 2905
St. Louis, MO 63103
314/367-1140

MONTANA

Billings AIDS Support Network
P. O. Box 1748
Billings, MT 59103
406/252-1212

NEBRASKA

Nebraska AIDS Project
P. O. Box 3512
Omaha, NE 68103
402/342-4233

NEVADA

Southern Nevada Social Services
P. O. Box 71014
Las Vegas, NV 89109
702/733-9990

NEW HAMPSHIRE

Citizen Alliance Gay/Lesbian Rights
P. O. Box 756
Concord, NH 03301
603/223-2355

NEW JERSEY

South Jersey Against AIDS
1616 Pacific Avenue, Suite 201
Atlantic City, NJ 08401
609/347-8799

NJ Lesbian & Gay AIDS Awareness
St. Michael's Medical Center
268 High Street
Newark, NJ 01702
201/596-0767

AIDS Office
Division of Communicable Diseases
New Jersey Department of Health
Health & Agriculture Building
Trenton, NJ 08625
609/292-7300

NEW MEXICO

New Mexico Service Office
124 Quincy, N.E.
Albuquerque, NM 87108
505/266-0911

New Mexico Physicians for
  Human Rights
P. O. Box 1361
Espanola, NM 87532
505/753-2779

New Mexico AIDS Services
209A McKenzie Street
Santa Fe, NM 87501
505/984-0911

NEW YORK

AIDS Institute
New York State Health Department
Empire State Plaza
Corning Tower—Room 1931
Albany, NY 12237
    Hotline: 800/462-1884

Haitian Coalition on AIDS
255 Eastern Parkway
Brooklyn, NY 11238
718/735-3568
    Hotline: 718/855-0972

Western NY AIDS Program
Buffalo AIDS Task Force, Inc.
P. O. Box 38, Bidwell Station
Buffalo, NY 14222
716/847-2441

AIDS Institute
10 East 40th Street
New York, NY 10016
212/340-3388

AIDS Resource Center (ARC)
P. O. Box 792, Chelsea Station
New York, NY 10011
212/206-1414

Beth Israel Medical Center
Department of Public Affairs
First Avenue at 16th Street
New York, NY 10003
212/420-2069

Gay Men's Health Crisis (GMHC)
Box 274
132 West 24th Street
New York, NY 10011
212/807-6655

People with AIDS (PWA) Coalition
P. O. Box 197
Murray Hill Station
New York, NY 10156

New York City Department of Health
Bureau of Public Health Education
125 Worth Street, Box 46
New York, NY 10013
212/485-8111

AIDS Task Force of Central NY
P. O. Box 1911
Syracuse, NY 13201
315/475-2430

Mid-Hudson Valley AIDS Task Force
(MHVATF)
P. O. Box 1640
White Plains, NY 10602-1640
914/997-5149
    AIDSLINE 914/997-1614

NORTH CAROLINA

Metrolina AIDS Project
P. O. Box 32662
Charlotte, NC 28232
704/333-2437

Lesbian & Gay Health Project
P. O. Box 3203
Durham, NC 27705
919/683-2182

OHIO

Health Issues Task Force
P. O. Box 14925
Public Square Station
Cleveland, OH 44114
216/651-1448

Dayton AIDS Task Force
665 Salem Avenue
Dayton, OH 45406
513/455-1889

AIDS Volunteers of Cincinnati
P. O. Box 19009
Cincinnati, OH 45219
513/421-7585

Columbus AIDS Task Force
65 S. 4th Street
Columbus, OH 43201
614/224-0411

OKLAHOMA

Tulsa AIDS Task Force
1711 S. Jackson, Unit FF
Tulsa, OK 74107
918/584-4093

Gay & Lesbian Community Center
2135 N. W. 39th Street
Oklahoma City, OK 73112
405/524-2437

OREGON

Cascade AIDS Project
408 S. W. Second Avenue
Portland, OR 97204
503/223-5907

Willamette AIDS Council
P. O. Box 5388
Eugene, OR 97405
503/687-4013

PENNSYLVANIA

AIDS Service Center
P. O. Box 1656
Allentown, PA 18105

Philadelphia AIDS Task Force
P. O. Box 7259
Philadelphia, PA 19101
215/545-6686 or 732-2437

Pittsburgh AIDS Task Force
P. O. Box 2763
Pittsburgh, PA 15230

Lehigh Valley AIDS Service Center
A-22 Springridge
Whitehall, PA 18052
215/433-3320

PUERTO RICO

AIDS Foundation of Puerto Rico
Box 3847, Fernandez/Juncos Sta.
Santurce, PR 00910
809/728-6169

RHODE ISLAND

Rhode Island AIDS Project
22 Hayes Street
Providence, RI 02905
401/277-6545

SOUTH DAKOTA

Public Health Center
1320 S. Minnesota Avenue
Sioux Falls, SD 57105
605/335-5020

TENNESSEE

AIDS Response Knoxville
P. O. Box 2343
Knoxville, TN 27901
615/521-6546

Nashville CARES
P. O. Box 25107
Nashville, TN 37202
615/321-0118

TEXAS

Austin AIDS Project
P. O. Box 4874
Austin, TX 78765
512/452-9550

Dallas Gay Alliance AIDS Task Force
P. O. Box 190712
Dallas, TX 75219
214/528-4233

KS/AIDS Foundation of Houston, Inc.
P. O. Box 66973
Houston, TX 77006
713/524-2437

San Antonio AIDS Foundation
P. O. Box 120113
San Antonio, TX 78212
512/733-3429

UTAH

AIDS Project Utah
P. O. Box 8485
Salt Lake City, UT 84108
801/486-2437

VERMONT

CARES
203 Elmwood Avenue
Burlington, VT 05401
802/862-5917

VIRGINIA

Richmond AIDS Information
  Network
1721 Hanover Avenue
Richmond, VA 23219
804/355-4428

WASHINGTON

Northwest AIDS Foundation
P. O. Box 3449
Seattle, WA 98114
206/326-4166

Shanti
P. O. Box 20698
Seattle, WA 98102
206/322-0279

WEST VIRGINIA

Mountain State AIDS Network
Box 57
Morganstown, WV 26505
304/292-5789

WISCONSIN

Madison AIDS Support Group
P. O. Box 731
Madison, WI 53701
608/255-1711

Brady East STD Clinic
1240 East Brady Street
Milwaukee, WI 53202
414/273-2437

Milwaukee AIDS Project
P. O. Box 92505
Milwaukee, WI 50302
414/273-2437

Index

About the Authors

DENNIS ALTMAN, M.A., is a professor of political science at La Trobe University, Bundoora, V.I.C., Australia. At the time of the conference, he was a policy fellow at the Institute for Health Policy Studies, School of Medicine, University of California, San Francisco.

PETER S. ARNO, PH.D., is an assistant professor in the Department of Health Care Administration, Baruch College/Mount Sinai School of Medicine of The City University of New York. At the time of the conference, he was a Pew postdoctoral fellow at the Institute for Health Policy Studies, School of Medicine, University of California, San Francisco.

RONALD BAYER, PH.D., is an associate for policy studies at The Hastings Center, Hastings-on-Hudson, New York.

JO IVEY BOUFFORD, M.D., is president of the New York City Health and Hospitals Corporation. Dr. Boufford is a pediatrician.

JOSEPH A. CIMINO, M.D., is a professor and chairman of the Department of Community and Preventive Medicine, New York Medical College, Valhalla, New York.

MARY W. CLINE is a research assistant at the Palo Alto Medical Research Foundation, Palo Alto, California.

RICHARD DUNNE is executive director of Gay Men's Health Crisis, New York City.

EMILY FRIEDMAN, a writer, lecturer, researcher, and health policy analyst, is a contributing editor for *Healthcare Forum and Hospitals*, a contributing writer to *Medical World News*, and a consultant to The Robert Wood Johnson Foundation Community Programs for Affordable Health Care.

MICHAEL H. GRIECO, M.D., J.D., is chief of the divisions of Allergy, Clinical Immunology, and Infectious Diseases at St. Luke's-Roosevelt Hospital Center, New York City.

OMAR L. HENDRIX, M.P.A., is senior director of the Office of Planning, New York City Health and Hospitals Corporation.

NANCY R. HOLLAND is executive director of the American Blood Commission.

RALPH C. JOHNSTON, JR., PH.D., is coordinator of the AIDS Education Project at the State University of New York (SUNY), Stony Brook.

LAMBERT N. KING, M.D., PH.D., is medical director and vice president for professional affairs at St. Vincent's Hospital and Medical Center, New York City.

MATHILDE KRIM, PH.D., is co-chair of the American Foundation for AIDS Research (AmFAR) and an associate research scientist at St. Luke's-Roosevelt Hospital Center and at the College of Physicians and Surgeons, Columbia University, New York City.

PHILIP RANDOLPH LEE, M.D., is a professor of social medicine and director of the Institute for Health Policy Studies at the School of Medicine, University of California, San Francisco.

PETER W. A. MANSELL, M.D., is medical director of the Institute for Immunological Disorders and deputy department chairman and professor of clinical cancer prevention at the Department of Cancer Prevention, The University of Texas System Cancer Center, M. D. Anderson Hospital and Tumor Institute, Houston.

JOHANNA PINDYCK, M.D., is senior vice president of The New York Blood Center and director of The Greater New York Blood Program, New York City.

DAVID J. ROTHMAN, PH.D., is Bernard Schoenberg professor of social medicine and the director of the Center for the Study of Society and Medicine at the College of Physicians and Surgeons, Columbia University, New York City.

HARVEY M. SAPOLSKY, PH.D., a professor of public policy and organization at the Massachusetts Institute of Technology, Cambridge, has written on various aspects of health policy and defense policy and is coauthor of *The American Blood Supply*.

ANNE A. SCITOVSKY, M.A., is chief of the health economics department at the Research Institute of the Palo Alto Medical Foundation, Palo Alto, California, and lecturer at the Institute for Health Policy Studies, School of Medicine, University of California, San Francisco.

MERVYN F. SILVERMAN, M.D., M.P.H., formerly the director of the San Francisco Department of Public Health, is president of the American Foundation for AIDS Research (AmFAR) and director of The Robert Wood Johnson Foundation AIDS Health Services Program.

LESLIE STRASSBERG is assistant vice president for actuarial services at Empire Blue Cross and Blue Shield, New York City.

ROBERT G. SULLIVAN, J.D., is a partner in the law firm of Lipsig, Sullivan and Liapakis, New York City.

BRUCE C. VLADECK, PH.D., is president of the United Hospital Fund.

PAUL A. VOLBERDING, M.D., is chief of the divisions of AIDS Activities and Medical Oncology at San Francisco General Hospital and an associate professor at the School of Medicine, University of California, San Francisco.

TIMOTHY WESTMORELAND, J.D., is assistant counsel for the Subcommittee on Health and the Environment, House of Representatives, United States Congress, Washington, D.C.

ACKNOWLEDGMENTS

For their assistance in compiling and/or updating statistics, appreciation is expressed to the following organizations and their respective staffs: the New York City Department of Health, AIDS Epidemiology and Surveillance Unit; the San Francisco Department of Public Health, Bureau of Communicable Disease Control; the United States Public Health Service, Centers for Disease Control; the World Health Organization, United Nations Headquarters, New York City. Appreciation is also expressed to Janis Hoagland, for proofreading with an editor's eye, and, likewise, to Carol Ewig, Toni Heisler, and Noreen Nash.

Current Publications

HEALTH POLICY

AIDS Public Policy Dimensions

Based on the proceedings of a major national conference, cosponsored by the United Hospital Fund and the Institute for Health Policy Studies of the University of California, San Francisco, this book examines health policy and related socio-medical issues, including acute care, community services, and financial implications, raised by the epidemic of acquired immune deficiency syndrome.
345 pp. $30.00   ISBN: 0-934459-35-5

Medicare and Extended Care: Issues, Problems, and Prospects

This 17-chapter book, based on a national conference, presents a comprehensive examination of extended care and its place in the health care system. It identifies patients who would benefit from extended care, describes model extended care programs, and includes financial perspectives on providing such care as it was originally conceived.
April 1987 $34.00 plus postage & handling
Available from Rynd Communications, 99 Painters Mill Road, Owings Mills, Md. 21117, or call 1-800-446-2221.

Hospitals and the Uninsured Poor: Measuring and Paying for Uncompensated Care

The proceedings of a national conference addressing the issues of financing health care for the uninsured poor. It explores the dimensions of the problem and describes federal and state initiatives in the waiver states of Maryland, Massachusetts, New Jersey, and New York, as well as in the non-waiver states of California, Florida, and Pennsylvania. National policy and research perspectives are provided.
192 pp. 1985 $30.00
ISBN: 0-934459-00-2

Health Care of Homeless People

Based on the proceedings of a national conference, this state-of-the-art guide identifies and discusses health and public policy issues in caring for the homeless, and provides specific information on medical treatment, psychiatric intervention, and program planning. Barriers to successful model programs are described.
349 pp. 1985 $29.95 plus postage & handling
Available from Springer Publishing Company, 536 Broadway, New York, N.Y. 10012.

ANNUAL INFORMATION SERVICES

Health and Health Care in New York City: Local, State, and National Perspectives
1987 Edition

An annual publication providing a graphic overview of health and health care in New York City, New York State, and the nation. Designed to provide a framework for decision making and planning, the chart book depicts the most recent trends in population, health status, availability and use of health facilities, and health care manpower and finances. Data are preceded by a narrative overview.
132 pp. 1987 $30.00
ISBN: 0-934459-46-0

Health Facilities in Southern New York: A Guide to Inpatient, Outpatient, and Long-Term Care
1987 Edition

A directory of health care facilities in New York City, Long Island, and the Northern Metropolitan area containing information on location, ownership, and certified beds of all facilities as well as detailed information on the capacity and utilization of hospital inpatient, outpatient, and long-term care services. Hospital statistics reflect 1985 operation. Hospital addresses, phone numbers, and chief executive officers are listed.
70 pp. 1987 $20.00
ISBN: 0-934459-38-X
Previous editions are available at a cost of $15.00 each

SPECIAL STUDIES

Health Expenditures in New York City, 1983
Paper Series 1

A United Hospital Fund paper providing an overview of health care spending patterns in New York City in 1983, by object of expenditure and source of funds. Selected trend analyses and national comparisons are included.
32 pp. 1985 $5.00
ISBN: 0-934459-09-6
1984 and 1985 updates are included free of charge.

The Financial Condition of New York City Voluntary Hospitals: The First Year of NYPHRM
Paper Series 2

A multi-dimensional approach is utilized in this important publication to describe the changes in the financial status of voluntary hospitals in New York State, including the first-year effects of the New York Prospective Hospital Reimbursement Methodology (NYPHRM). The hospitals' 1983 annual operating results, cash position, capital structure, and age of plant are examined and then compared to hospitals in the rest of New York State, the Northeast region, and the nation.
24 pp. 1985 $5.00
ISBN: 0-934459-10-X
A 1984 update is included free of charge.

Is Counting the Dead Enough? Strategies for Monitoring Health Care Needs and Health Status in New York City
Paper Series 3

The measurement of the health status and consequent health care needs of New Yorkers has traditionally relied on such indicators as mortality and gross morbidity. However, in an era of sophisticated survey and research tools, more accurate and sensitive measures are possible. In this paper, several promising approaches to measurement, surveying, and information analysis are examined, and measures that detect problems earlier in the course of illness are called for.
36 pp. 1986 $5.00
ISBN: 0-934459-34-7

New York's Role as a Center for Health Care: An Analysis of Nonresident Patients Served by New York City Hospitals
Paper Series 4

The role of New York City hospitals in caring for patients residing outside the city is examined in this paper. It includes a review and assessment of the flow of patients and analyzes the impact of out-of-city patients on New York City's hospital industry. In addition, a detailed comparison of case mix and length of stay for resident and nonresident patients in 1982 is presented.
40 pp. 1986 $5.00
ISBN: 0-934459-29-0

New Directions in Health Care: Consequences for the Elderly
Paper Series 5

Recent changes in the financing of health care for the nation's elderly promise to have a profound effect on this large and particularly vulnerable group in our society. This paper explores the

complex and interrelated changes in demography and health status, financing, organization and delivery of services, and regulation of care, and their impact on the elderly. It describes a research design that would measure, primarily with quantitative data, the direction and magnitude of these changes.
36 pp. 1986 $5.00
ISBN: 0-934459-30-4

Home Care in New York City: Providers, Payers, and Clients
Paper Series 6

Because the development of home care services has been fragmented and incremental, data essential to informed public policy decisions are neither readily available nor fully adequate. To fill the gap, this paper provides a summary overview of home care in New York City, including descriptions of services, providers, beneficiaries, and costs, integrates existing data, and critically examines the important policy issues in the field.
44 pp. 1987 $5.00
ISBN: 0-934459-11-8

Getting Care: Poor Children and New York City Hospitals
Paper Series 7

This paper explores the use of New York City's hospital outpatient departments and emergency rooms by children. It highlights the importance of age, geographic access, and insurance coverage in the use of ambulatory care facilities. Analyses are presented using the United Hospital Fund's 1984 Patient Origin Information System (POIS) for such factors as the type of hospital visited and the medical reason for the visit, and the implications of these findings for ambulatory health care policy are discussed.
March 1987 $5.00
ISBN: 0-934459-39-8

PATIENT ORIGIN AND COMMUNITY REPORTS

New York City Community Health Atlas

This comprehensive atlas presents and integrates data from the Patient Origin Information System (POIS), the 1980 Census, and other sources to provide a picture of health needs and service patterns in each of the communities within New York City. Maps depict demographic and health service patterns in New York City and delineate variations in population characteristics and health service use among the city's zip code areas. The health care atlas is designed to meet the needs of researchers and analysts investigating citywide patterns of community health care and of planners and facility managers interested in better understanding specific neighborhoods.
216 pp. 1985 $40.00
ISBN: 0-934459-15-0

POIS Report Series
Inpatient Hospital Use in New York City 1985

A component of the Patient Origin Information System (POIS) providing comprehensive information on the residence, insurance coverage, and clinical service of all inpatients in New York City hospitals in 1985, and similar information on city residents who received hospital care elsewhere in the state. Volume I depicts overall patterns of hospital use by residents of each borough and by nonresident patients. Volumes II and III provide detailed community profiles showing the specific hospitals at which residents of each zip code area received care, the clinical service used, and the patients' insurance coverage.
1987 Complete 3-volume set, $125.00
ISBN: 0-934459-42-8
Volume I (Overview) only, $30.00
ISBN: 0-934459-43-6
Three-volume sets of 1980 and 1982 data are available for trend analysis and com-

parative study. The costs are $80.00 and $100.00, respectively.

POIS Report Series
Ambulatory Care in
New York City 1984

The ambulatory care component of the Patient Origin Information System (POIS) providing comprehensive information on who uses New York City hospitals, which services they use, and how they pay for their care. All outpatient department and emergency room visits in New York City hospitals during the second quarter of 1984 are included. Volume I depicts overall patterns of hospital use and community dependence on individual facilities. Volumes II and III provide detailed community profiles on outpatient department and emergency room visits, respectively.
1985 Complete 3-volume set, $60.00
ISBN: 0-934459-16-9
Volume I (Overview) only, $25.00
ISBN: 0-934459-17-7
A 3-volume set of 1983 data is also available for trend analysis and comparative study. The cost is $100.00.

VOLUNTARY PROGRAMS

The State of New York City's
Municipal Hospital System, Fiscal
Years 1985 and 1986

Based on the findings of the United Hospital Fund's City Hospital Visiting Committee, a century-old citizens' group, this annual publication reports on conditions affecting patient care in New York City's public hospitals. It provides an overview of the management, financial condition, staffing, and individual facilities, and suggests needed improvements. The publication is based on meetings with the management of the New York City Health and Hospitals Corporation and site visits to each of the municipal hospitals, neighborhood family care centers, and satellite facilities.
38 pp. 1986 $5.00
ISBN: 0-934459-37-1

Public Concerns, Community
Initiatives: The Successful
Management of Nursing Home
Consumer Information Programs

Based on a national conference, this is a comprehensive resource for the step-by-step organization of nursing home consumer information programs. The book advocates community involvement in nursing homes as a proven means of improving the quality of life of nursing home residents and as a way of strengthening public policy in long-term care. It describes in detail the role of the consumer and legal issues in nursing home advocacy programs, and provides specific information on setting up a program and working with volunteers.
268 pp. 1985 $25.00
ISBN: 0-934459-27-4

POLICY DISCUSSION PAPERS

The **President's Letter** is comprised of bimonthly papers that highlight important health policy issues. Available free of charge, the **President's Letter** series provides balanced, informed discussion and fresh perspectives on significant and complex problems.
N/C

Order Form

Publications (specify title)	Code	Quantity	Price	Total
	LEAVE BLANK			

10% discount for orders of 5 or more publications

Mailing and handling $2.50

TOTAL

Enclosed is a check for $ _____

Name _____

Title _____

Organization _____

Address _____

City/State/Zip _____

Telephone (_____) _____

☐ Please send complete *Current Publications* catalog.
☐ Please send additional information about the United Hospital Fund.

Mail to: Publications Program, United Hospital Fund, 55 Fifth Avenue, New York, NY 10003 Attn: Sally J. Rogers.

For office use only.

AD				
SC	FC	OC	P.O. #	CHECK #	DATE	$ AMOUNT

2451